CONTRIBUTOR LIST

AUTHORS AND CONTRIBUTORS

Authors

Rebecca Hill, PhD(c), DNP, MSN, FNP-C, CNE
Assistant Professor
MGH Institute of Health Professions
Boston, Massachusetts

Emily J. Karwacki Sheff, MS, RN, FNP-BC
Assistant Professor
Partnership Liaison, Project REEP
Rivier University
Nashua, New Hampshire

Contributors

Amy Bruno, PhD, ANP-BC
Assistant Professor
MGH Institute of Health Professions
Boston, Massachusetts

Tammi Magazzu, MSN, WHNP-BC, APRN
Instructor in Nursing
MGH Institute of Health Professions
Boston, Massachusetts

Vicki Moran, PhD, RN, MPH, CNE, CDE, PHNA-BC, TNS
Assistant Professor
Saint Louis University
St. Louis, Missouri

Kaveri M. Roy, DNP, RN
Assistant Professor
MGH Institute of Health Professions
Boston, Massachusetts

Cindy Stern, MSN, RN, CCRP
Senior Administrator
Penn Center Cancer Network
Penn Medicine
Philadelphia, Pennsylvania

Linda Turchin, RN, MSN, CNE
Professor Emeritus
Fairmont State University
Fairmont, West Virginia

Bradley Patrick White, MSN, RN
Instructor in Nursing
MGH Institute of Health Professions
Boston, Massachusetts

REVIEWERS

Cynthia Arceneaux, MSN, RN, FNP-BC
Instructor
Lamar State College–Port Arthur
Port Arthur, Texas

Mary B. Beerman, MN, RN, CCRN-K
Instructor
Georgia Gwinnett College
Lawrenceville, Georgia

Linda K. Bennington, PhD, RN
Senior Lecturer
Old Dominion University
Virginia Beach, Virginia

Kysha Cerisier, DNP, AGACNP-BC, FNP-BC
Instructor
Azure College
Fort Lauderdale, Florida

Rebecca Cox-Davenport, PhD, RN
Assistant Professor
Lander University
Fountain Inn, South Carolina

Felicia Crump, PhD, MS, MSN, RN
Assistant Program Director/Instructor
Northeast Mississippi Community
    College
Booneville, Mississippi

Heraldine Flores, MSN, RN, CPN
Lead Pediatric Nursing Faculty
Baker College of Clinton Township
Clinton Township, Michigan

Kathleen Fraley, MSN, RN
Professor
St. Clair County Community College
Port Huron, Michigan

Denise L. Garee, PhD, MSN, RN, CEN
Adjunct Faculty
Indian River State College
Fort Pierce, Florida
President
4N6 Nurse Consulting, LLC
Vero Beach, Florida

Selena Gilles, DNP, ANP-BC, CNEcl, CCRN
Clinical Assistant Professor
New York University
New York, New York

Kimberly A. Guard, MSN, RN
Associate Professor
Global Studies Advisor
Ivy Tech Community College
Richmond, Indiana

Katherine M. Hagerott, MSN, BA, RN
Assistant Professor
Mount Saint Mary's University
Los Angeles, California

Amanda Huber, DNP, APRN, FNP-C
Assistant Professor
Galen College of Nursing
Louisville, Kentucky

Cindy Johnson, PhD, RN
Clinical Assistant Professor
Berry College
Mount Berry, Georgia

Katie Morales, PhD, RN, CNE
Assistant Professor
Berry College
Mount Berry, Georgia

Vicki Moran, PhD, RN, MPH, CNE, CDE, PHNA-BC, TNS
Assistant Professor
Saint Louis University
St. Louis, Missouri

Bobbie J. Perdue, PhD
Professor Emerita
Syracuse University
Syracuse, New York
Adjunct Faculty
Jersey College School of Nursing
    City
Tampa, Florida

Barbara Rome, MS, RN, CNE, PhD Candidate
Associate Professor
Queensborough Community
    College
Bayside, New York

Shelley Sadler, RN, MSN, APRN, WHNP-BC
Instructor
Morehead State University
Morehead, Kentucky

E'Loria Simon-Campbell, PhD, RN
Assistant Professor Tenure Track,
    SHSU-ACUE Fellow
Sam Houston State University
Woodlands, Texas

Leigh A. Snead, MSN, RN
Assistant Professor
University of Arkansas at Little
    Rock
Little Rock, Arkansas

Linda Turchin, RN, MSN, CNE
Professor Emeritus
Fairmont State University
Fairmont, West Virginia

Tamie Verbance, MSNEd, BSN, RN
Clinical Coordinator/Instructor
Treasure Valley Community
    College
Ontario, Oregon

Patti Wentz, MSN, RN, CNE
Director of Nursing, RN Program
ECPI University
Greenville, South Carolina

Jennifer Wilson-Hicks, MSN-Ed, RN
Nursing Faculty
Pittsburgh Technical College
Oakdale, Pennsylvania

Lippincott®
Pharmacology Review for NCLEX-RN®

Rebecca Hill, PhD(c), DNP, MSN, FNP-C, CNE

Emily J. Karwacki Sheff, MS, RN, FNP-BC

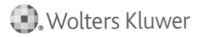
. Wolters Kluwer

Philadelphia • Baltimore • New York • London
Buenos Aires • Hong Kong • Sydney • Tokyo

Executive Product Manager & Editor: Renee A. Gagliardi
Content Strategist: Bernadette Enneg and Michael Marino
Editorial Coordinator: Julie Kostelnik
Production Project Manager: Sadie Buckallew
Design Coordinator: Elaine Kasmer
Art Director: Jennifer Clements
Manufacturing Coordinator: Karin Duffield
Marketing Manager: Sarah Schuessler
Prepress Vendor: SPi Global

Copyright © 2020 Wolters Kluwer

This book is protected by copyright. No part of this book may be reproduced or transmitted in any form or by any means, including as photocopies or scanned-in or other electronic copies, or utilized by any information storage and retrieval system without written permission from the copyright owner, except for brief quotations embodied in critical articles and reviews. Materials appearing in this book prepared by individuals as part of their official duties as U.S. government employees are not covered by the above-mentioned copyright. To request permission, please contact Wolters Kluwer at Two Commerce Square, 2001 Market Street, Philadelphia, PA 19103, via email at permissions@lww.com, or via our website at shop.lww.com (products and services).

9 8 7 6 5 4 3 2

Printed in China

Library of Congress Cataloging-in-Publication Data
Names: Hill, Rebecca (Rebecca Russo), author. | Karwacki Sheff, Emily J., author.
Title: Lippincott pharmacology review for NCLEX-RN / Rebecca Hill, Emily J. Karwacki Sheff.
Other titles: Pharmacology review for NCLEX-RN
Description: 1st edition. | Philadelphia : Wolters Kluwer, [2020] | Includes bibliographical references and index.
Identifiers: LCCN 2019017473 | ISBN 9781975109837 (paperback)
Subjects: | MESH: Pharmacological Phenomena | Drug Therapy—methods | Study Guide | Nurses Instruction
Classification: LCC RM301.28 | NLM QV 18.2 | DDC 615.1—dc23 LC record available at https://lccn.loc.gov/2019017473

This work is provided "as is," and the publisher disclaims any and all warranties, express or implied, including any warranties as to accuracy, comprehensiveness, or currency of the content of this work.

This work is no substitute for individual patient assessment based upon healthcare professionals' examination of each patient and consideration of, among other things, age, weight, gender, current or prior medical conditions, medication history, laboratory data and other factors unique to the patient. The publisher does not provide medical advice or guidance and this work is merely a reference tool. Healthcare professionals, and not the publisher, are solely responsible for the use of this work including all medical judgments and for any resulting diagnosis and treatments.

Given continuous, rapid advances in medical science and health information, independent professional verification of medical diagnoses, indications, appropriate pharmaceutical selections and dosages, and treatment options should be made and healthcare professionals should consult a variety of sources. When prescribing medication, healthcare professionals are advised to consult the product information sheet (the manufacturer's package insert) accompanying each drug to verify, among other things, conditions of use, warnings and side effects and identify any changes in dosage schedule or contraindications, particularly if the medication to be administered is new, infrequently used or has a narrow therapeutic range. To the maximum extent permitted under applicable law, no responsibility is assumed by the publisher for any injury and/or damage to persons or property, as a matter of products liability, negligence law or otherwise, or from any reference to or use by any person of this work.

shop.lww.com

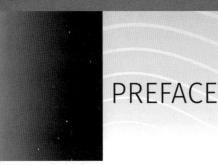

PREFACE

Bringing Pharmacology to Life!

The NCLEX-RN has steadily increased the percentage of questions pertaining to pharmacologic and parenteral therapies. Nurses, the last line of defense for clients in avoiding medication errors, are required to understand the application of medications to provide safe and effective care. Pharmacology, however, does not exist in isolation. It is critical to apply knowledge of pharmacology in relation to medical diagnoses, health assessment findings, and diagnostics to treat clients holistically.

This first edition pharmacology review text for the NCLEX-RN seeks to provide the most critically important information about medications in conjunction with a brief synopsis of the medical conditions, assessment findings, and diagnostic indicators associated with those medications. The authors strived to present this information in a succinct and logical way to enhance retention of information and strengthen pharmacology knowledge when preparing to take the NCLEX-RN examination.

How to Use this Book

Each chapter of this text will include a brief overview of the disorders the medications are used to treat. Next, each disorder will be broken down to include clinical pearls of assessment, signs and symptoms, diagnostics, and pertinent lab values. Following this, the medications will be provided to include a brief synopsis (class of medication, prototype medication, mechanism of action, side effects, critical information about the medication, and indications). Call out boxes pertaining to Safety Alerts, Black Box Warnings, or Lifetime Considerations will be highlighted as applicable in each chapter. At the end of each chapter, there will be NCLEX-style practice questions, with accompanying rationales. These practice questions, written by the authors and contributors, have all been assessed for their rigor via Lippincott® NCLEX-RN PassPoint. These questions should be used to apply the information you have learned throughout your nursing education and reviewed within this text to help prepare you for the pharmacology content on the NCLEX-RN® examination.

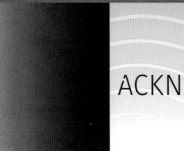

ACKNOWLEDGMENTS

I would like to thank my students for the constant push and request for pharmacology resources, from which this idea was created. Thank you also to our contributors, the experts that made this book a reality. Emily, you have been a fantastic coauthor to work with on this journey! To my husband, Jon, you are my biggest cheerleader. I am so grateful for your confidence in me and for your support with every project I take on. Mom, your unending love, support, and countless hours of childcare mean more to me than you will ever know. To my children, Avery, Jonathan, and Theodore: you are my inspiration and the force that keeps me striving to do and be more. I love you.

Rebecca Hill, PhD(c), DNP, MSN, FNP-C, CNE
Assistant Professor
MGH Institute of Health Professions
Boston, Massachusetts

I would like to thank my nursing mentors who have encouraged and supported my journey in nursing education and publication—my mother-in-law, Barbara Sheff; my first nursing director on White 10 at MGH, Marita Prater; and Professor Janice Bell Meisenhelder. Thank you to each of you—I have no doubt I would not be where I am today in my career without each of your support. I would also like to thank our chapter contributors. Without your hard work and expertise, this book would not be here! Lastly, I would like to thank my amazing husband, Eric, and three wonderful children, Jacob, Ryan, and Zachary. Eric, your encouragement and support are the world to me. Thank you for giving me the space to thrive and grow in my career, without your help I could never make it all happen! And boys, the amount of times I have sat next to you writing while you did your homework or in the car during your football or soccer practices are countless. I do everything I do for the three of you. All my love, mom.

Emily J. Karwacki Sheff, MS, RN, FNP-BC
Assistant Professor
Partnership Liaison, Project REEP
Rivier University
Nashua, New Hampshire

ABOUT THE AUTHORS

Dr. Rebecca Hill, PhD(c), DNP, MSN, FNP-C, CNE earned a DNP, MSN, and post-master's certificate in nursing education from Duke University; a BSN from the University of Rhode Island and is a current PhD candidate at Boston College Connell School of Nursing. She is a certified nurse educator with 11 years of teaching experience in traditional baccalaureate and direct-entry nursing programs. Dr. Hill is an assistant professor of nursing at the MGH Institute of Health Professions in Boston, Massachusetts. Her research interests span both education and clinical topics, with her current focus on the study of problematic feeding in infants. She has a special interest and dedication to the understanding of predictors of student success in pre-licensure courses and on the NCLEX-RN® exam, has worked as a

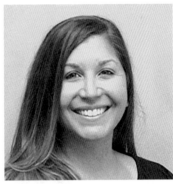

Permission by MGH Institute of Health Professions

subject matter expert for several pharmacology textbooks and online adaptive quiz programs, and is an item writer for pharmacology and adult-health reference materials. Dr. Hill maintains clinical practice as a family nurse practitioner in family medicine and urgent care. She has served as faculty representative at the National Student Nurses' Association annual convention and as president of two chapters of Sigma Theta Tau International. Dr. Hill was recently awarded the M. Louise Fitzpatrick Scholarship Award for her professional and scholastic accomplishments in nursing.

Emily Karwacki Sheff, MS, RN, FNP-BC is currently a PhD candidate in nursing education at Villanova University. She earned her master's degree in nursing from Boston College and a bachelor's of science from Northeastern University in behavioral neuroscience. She has 14 years of teaching experience in both accelerated and traditional nursing programs, teaching at both the baccalaureate and master's level. She has taught pharmacology for the past 11 years and is currently an assistant professor of nursing and the Partnership Liaison for HRSA grant, Project REEP at Rivier University in Nashua, New Hampshire. Her research interests includes nursing workforce development, and work engagement and has been published and invited to

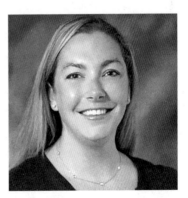

Courtesy of John Gauvin, Studio

present at regional, national and international conferences. In addition, Ms. Sheff has contributed as a content expert to several textbooks and study guides and has extensive experience in developing online learning course. Besides teaching, Ms. Sheff has practiced in urgent care as a family nurse practitioner and volunteers as an abstract/grant peer reviewer for Sigma Theta Tau International. She has recently been named as one of New Hampshire Union Leaders 40 Under Forty for 2019.

CONTENTS

1 BASIC PRINCIPLES OF PHARMACOLOGY

PHARMACOLOGY BASICS

- ◆ The benefits and risks must be considered when using any medication to diagnose, treat, or prevent disease.
- ◆ There are several considerations when using medications, as there is always a risk of side and/or adverse effects associated with the introduction of a medication into the body. Most importantly, the medication should be as effective, safe, and selective as possible.
- ◆ Other considerations include cost, ease of administration, and drug interactions. Unfortunately, no drug is perfect, and this can lead to medication nonadherence.

NURSING CONSIDERATIONS IN PHARMACOLOGY

- ◆ Before administering medication, the nurse should collect the client's vital signs, perform a focused physical assessment, and identify drug-specific knowledge. This information will allow the nurse to evaluate medication effectiveness, identify the presence of side and/or adverse effects, and provide essential client education based on the level of readiness to learn.
- ◆ All medication orders should be checked carefully and compared with the client's current medical issues and known allergies. Therefore, the nurse must have adequate knowledge of pharmacology.
- ◆ Client identity must be verified using two identifiers (e.g., name and date of birth).
- ◆ The nurse should hold a medication and consult the prescriber if any component of the medication order is unclear or the nurse is uncertain of the rationale for administering the medication.
- ◆ Client education is a major component of medication administration by the nurse. Clients should be taught the basics surrounding any medication prescribed, including
  - Generic and brand name of the medication
  - Prescribed dose
  - Duration, timing, and routine (e.g., in the morning, with or without food)
  - Administration route (e.g., oral, injection, etc.)
  - When and how to notify the prescriber for side effects (e.g., drowsiness, nausea, dizziness, etc.)
  - When and how to notify the prescriber about adverse effects (e.g., angioedema, bronchospasm, allergic reactions, etc.)
  - Expected response to the medication
  - When the client should expect to notice the effect of the medication
  - Special considerations for storage, refills
  - Any contraindications with other medications, foods, or beverages
  - Ways to improve medication effectiveness (e.g., taking vitamin C with iron supplements)
- ◆ Nurses have several resources for obtaining medication information, including pharmacists, the prescriber, drug reference guides, and reliable Internet sources.

The Nursing Process and Pharmacology

◆ Figure 1-1 illustrates the five steps in the nursing process: assessment, diagnosis, planning, implementation, and evaluation. It is helpful to begin with assessment as the first step when approaching clinical situations. Infrequently, and usually only in emergency situations, the nurse will bypass the assessment phase of the process to institute lifesaving measures.

◆ NCLEX tip: When questions ask the nurse to prioritize client care in a clinical scenario, refer back to the nursing process. Most often, assessment of a client will be the priority nursing action.

◆ Assessment: The nurse should obtain baseline information prior to the administration of any medication so that the medication effectiveness can be properly evaluated. This assessment will also help alert the nurse to the development of side and/or adverse effects.

◆ Diagnosis: This phase allows the nurse to identify potential and actual problems related to medication administration. This may include the potential for side and/or adverse effects, and the ability of the client to adhere to the medication regimen.

◆ Planning: The nurse will develop goals, priorities, and interventions specific to the medication(s) administered. The overall goal of medication administration is to achieve maximum benefit with minimal harm to the client. Prioritization with medication administration should be focused on life-threatening situations that require immediate intervention.

◆ Implementation: Similar to the planning phase, the implementation phase allows the nurse to complete the action of medication administration and follow through with the interventions designed during the planning phase. Interventions focus on methods to increase the effectiveness of medications and include the use of nonpharmacologic adjuncts in nursing care, proper drug administration using the six rights of medication administration, and providing appropriate client education and consideration of client safety measures.

◆ Evaluation: The nurse should conduct evaluation following medication administration, specifically identifying the effectiveness of the regimen, the presence of side and/or adverse effects, and client compliance and satisfaction with the prescribed medication(s).

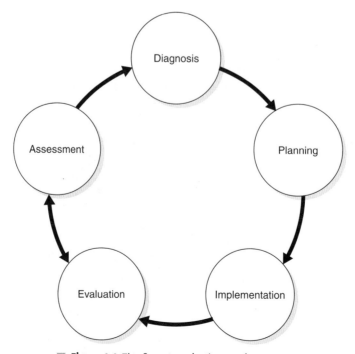

Figure 1-1 The five steps in the nursing process.

Medication Names

◆ There are names medications can be classified by: chemical, generic, and trade (brand).
  ● Chemical names are the chemical nomenclature. This is not used in nursing practice but is required during drug development.
  ● Each medication has only one generic name. This is the name nurses are required to know and is assigned by the United States Adopted Names Council.
  ● Trade or brand name is the name given to medication by the pharmaceutical marketer. One generic medication can have several brand names, making it confusing for a client. In most cases, the trade and generic versions of medication are equivalent, and the generic form is usually less expensive.

Pharmacokinetics and Pharmacodynamics

◆ **Pharmacokinetics** describes what the human body does to a medication as it passes through the human body. Many factors can affect pharmacokinetics, such as water solubility, fat solubility, the degree of dissociation, and molecular weight of the medication. There are four components of pharmacokinetics: absorption, distribution, metabolism, and excretion. Most medications are metabolized by the liver and excreted by the kidneys. For this reason, baseline assessments of liver and kidney function should be a consideration by the nurse prior to starting any new medication. Dysfunction of the liver and/or kidneys may warrant a reduction of medication dosage by the prescriber.
  ● **Absorption** is the way a medication enters the bloodstream after it is administered. This is dependent on the route of administration. Medications that are given intravenously are absorbed immediately and completely into the bloodstream. In contrast, oral medications must dissolve and cross gastrointestinal cell membranes prior to entering the bloodstream. For this reason, the route of administration is a major consideration when deciding how quickly a medication's effect is needed. For example, in emergency situations, a quicker rate of absorption is needed so that the medication's effect is rapid. Except for the intravenous route, all other routes of administration have obstacles that impede absorption and will have interpatient variability regarding when the medication will take effect. This variability depends on factors such as blood flow, surface area at the site of administration, perfusion and circulation, gastric pH, and the presence or absence of food in the stomach (for oral administration).
  ● The many routes of administration include:
    ▶ Oral
    ▶ Intravenous
    ▶ Intramuscular
    ▶ Subcutaneous
    ▶ Topical
    ▶ Inhaled
    ▶ Suppositories (rectal or vaginal)
    ▶ Direct injection to a certain area (e.g., intrathecal injection)
  ● **Distribution** is the process by which a medication exits the bloodstream and enters cells to exert its effect(s). Blood flow and a medication's ability to enter cells affect the degree and rate of distribution. The body's protective features, such as the blood–brain barrier, also impact how well a medication can exit the bloodstream and enter cells. The extent to which a medication binds to protein, such as albumin, will impact the time it takes the medication to exert its pharmacologic effect(s).

NURSING ADMINISTRATION If a medication needs to be taken on an empty stomach to enhance absorption, it should be administered 1 hour before or 2 hours after a meal, unless otherwise specified.

SAFETY ALERT! When a medication is highly bound to protein, there is only a small amount of free drug available to exert an effect. When administering two or more medications that compete for protein-binding sites, the nurse must monitor for potential medication toxicity if one or more of the medications is removed from the protein binding sites and more free drug is available for use.

- **Metabolism** is the breakdown of a medication, commonly by the liver, usually to an inactive form. This is also known as biotransformation. The liver can also metabolize medications to produce other outcomes, such as activation of a medication, or promotion of toxicity due to metabolites, or decreasing toxicity by drug inactivation. Most commonly, metabolism allows for inactivation, followed by excretion of a medication by the kidneys. Metabolism of a medication varies from client to client and is dependent on several factors. Pediatric clients less than 3 years of age have underdeveloped livers, which leads to decreased ability to metabolize medications. Older adults have decreased ability to metabolize medications as liver function declines. Some medications are inactivated by the liver following oral administration. This is known as the **first-pass effect**. Medications that are largely metabolized when first entering the liver may not be available to use and may need to be administered by an alternate route that bypasses the liver or at a higher oral dose. The effectiveness of metabolism will also alter a medication's **half-life**, which is the time it takes for 50% of a medication to be removed from circulation. With a fully functioning liver, it takes several half-lives for a medication to be eliminated.
- **Excretion** is the mechanism through which a medication is removed from the body. Excretion is dependent on renal function and perfusion. Like metabolism, young children and older adults are at risk of impaired excretion due to less-than-optional renal function. Medications can also be excreted in other ways, such as through the sweat, via exhalation, or through feces or bile.
- ◆ **Pharmacodynamics** describes what a medication does to the body. Most commonly, medications bind to receptors within the body to either enhance or suppress actions that the body would, under perfect conditions, do on its own. A medication will not create a new or novel effect beyond what a human body would be capable of doing.
  - Medications that enhance/activate an endogenous action are known as **agonists**.
  - Medications that block/deactivate an endogenous action are known as **antagonists**.
  - A third class, known as **partial agonists**, enhance an endogenous action, but with lesser intensity than agonists.
- ◆ There are some medications that do not bind to receptors and exert an action through a chemical reaction. An example is an antacid.
- ◆ What any one medication does to the body is highly dependent on the individual client. Every client is different; a dose that works for one client may be too high or too low of a dose for another person. For this reason, a standard dose for every medication has been created, known as the **average effective dose** (ED_{50}). This standard dose has been determined to be effective in 50% of clients, meaning medication titration will be necessary for the other 50% of clients receiving the medication. Therefore, it is imperative that nurses know how to evaluate for effectiveness, sub- and supratherapeutic signs and symptoms of medications they administer.

◆ In addition to the standard dose, medication also has a known **therapeutic index**. This is the ratio between the lethal dose and the ED_{50} of a medication. As a general rule, medications with a wider or larger therapeutic index are safer, as it allows for more of a dosage adjustment before becoming lethal or subtherapeutic.

SAFETY ALERT! Medications with a narrow or small therapeutic index have a higher potential for toxicity. These medications frequently require serum drug level testing periodically to be sure toxicity is not developing.

Medication Errors and Their Prevention

◆ Medication errors can occur for many reasons. Most commonly, confusion between two drug names, human error, and miscommunication lead to medication errors.
◆ Nurses are the last line of defense between the client and a medication error.
◆ To decrease the frequency of medication errors, nurses should be aware of their resources for learning about medications and know whom to contact to verify any medication orders that are unclear or confusing.
◆ To prevent errors:
  ● Medication orders should not be handwritten.
  ● Computerized medication administration systems should be used whenever possible.
  ● Medication reconciliation should occur at admission, at the time of transfer between hospital units, and prior to discharge.
  ● Orders should include only those abbreviations approved by the Joint Commission, American Medical Association, and Institute for Safe Medication Practices.
  ● Medications should be verified three times prior to administration, following the six rights:
    ▶ Right medication
    ▶ Right client
    ▶ Right dose
    ▶ Right route
    ▶ Right time
    ▶ Right documentation

Adverse Effects of Drugs

Drug Abuse
◆ Some drugs, such as morphine and other narcotics, lead to dependence in some clients.
◆ Using a medication beyond medical necessity may constitute drug abuse.
  ● Physical and/or psychological dependence can result from drug abuse.
  ● When the medication is stopped, the client can undergo a withdrawal syndrome. Some aspects of withdrawal can be fatal if left untreated.
◆ It is important to remember that substance abuse disorders are treatable.
◆ The Comprehensive Drug Abuse Prevention and Control Act, passed in 1970, devised regulations for the prescription of medications that have a high risk of abuse. Here, five categories (I–V) are assigned to medications with abuse potential. These controlled substances require special licensing of prescribers to be eligible to prescribe the medications and require monitoring and special handling. Schedule I represents the medications with the highest potential for abuse that lack any acceptable medical use, such as heroin.

Toxicology: Poisoning/Overdose

◆ Many medications can be classified as poisons, especially when taken at lethal doses.
  ● Identification of the poison is the first critical step.
  ● Contacting the National Poison Control Center Hotline (1-800-222-1222) should occur once the poison is identified.
◆ Most commonly, poisonings occur in children due to accessibility of medications that have not been properly secured away from children.
◆ Nursing management focuses on supportive care, emphasizing airway, breathing, and circulation, in conjunction with implementation of methods to remove the poison from the body.
◆ Poison removal can be done with medications or other methods.
◆ Many medications have antidotes that can counteract the poison ingested.
◆ Poisons ingested orally less than 1 hour ago can be treated with medications or other methods to decrease the gastric absorption:
  ● Activated charcoal absorbs the poison. It is most effective when given within 30 minutes of poison ingestion but may be beneficial for up to 4 hours after poison ingestion.
  ● Gastric lavage flushes/irrigates the stomach, and then the fluid is suctioned from the stomach. Lavage can be used for poison ingested within 1 hour of treatment initiation.
  ● Cathartics are laxatives that accelerate the elimination of the harmful substance through the gastrointestinal tract.
  ● For poisons ingested more than 1 hour ago and already in the bloodstream, hemodialysis may be used to remove the poison.

SAFETY ALERT! Activated charcoal, lavage, and/or cathartics should not be administered to clients with gastric perforations or bowel obstructions or those at risk for gastric perforation.

Special Considerations

◆ Medication dosing and therapy should be catered to each client because individuals react to medication differently. Assessment of how a medication affects a client allows for adjustments to be made to increase the benefit of the medication and decrease the risk for harm. Some of the most common reasons for variation in how a medication affects a client include age, renal and liver function, and body size. More specifically, certain populations require vigilance in dosing such as clients with certain genetic predispositions, women who are pregnant and/or breast-feeding, clients that are very young, and the elderly population.
◆ **Pharmacogenomics** is the study of how medications differ in effect related to genetic composition. Most commonly, drug metabolism (biotransformation) is altered due to genetic factors. Medications are currently created in a "one size fits all" manner, despite the knowledge that not all individuals react to medications in the same way. One medication that may adequately control a client's blood pressure, for example, may not have any impact on another client's blood pressure whatsoever. The study of pharmacogenomics is very new, with clinical trials under way to help tailor the treatment of medical conditions with genetics as a key component in the treatment regimen.
◆ Variability in clients' genetic makeup can alter the way medications are metabolized. Some client's can be known as "poor metabolizers," while others may be "ultra-rapid metabolizers." These metabolic differences will impact the rate of metabolism, specifically within

the cytochrome P-450 system. For example, a client who is a poor metabolizer of CYP450 2C9 will metabolize warfarin at a much slower rate. Clinically, this will mean the client will need a much lower dose of warfarin to prevent excessive anticoagulation secondary to slow breakdown of the medication.

◆ Ethnic origin should also be considered, as the genetic makeup varies by ethnicity. For example, Asian clients metabolize medications in the CYP450 2D6 system (e.g., SSRIs) more slowly, necessitating lower dosages to prevent toxicity.

◆ Figure 1-2 provides a graphic representation explaining the genetic differences that may lead to alterations in medication action.

◆ Pediatric organ systems are not fully developed, placing pediatric clients at a higher risk of medication sensitivity and toxicity. Similar to pregnancy and lactation, very few medications have been tested for safety in children. All phases of pharmacokinetics are altered in pediatric clients. Absorption of oral medications is increased because the gastric emptying time is slower. The thin skin of young children leads to faster absorption of medications delivered through the skin. Distribution is altered because the amount of protein circulating in the bloodstream is lower than that of an adult. This leads to higher levels of free circulating medication available to exert an effect. The blood–brain barrier is also not completely developed, which can result in heightened effects on the central nervous system. The liver is not completely developed until close to 3 years of age, slowing metabolism of medications,

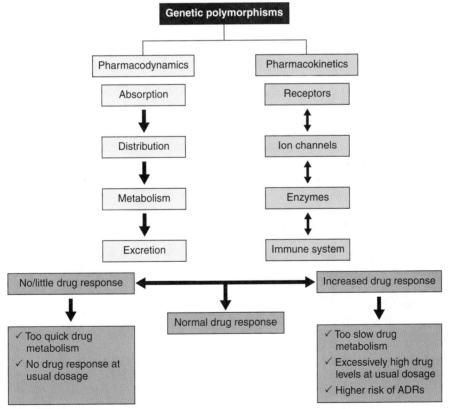

■ **Figure 1-2** Genetic variations in medication action (From: Ahmed, S., Zhou, Z., Zhou, J., & Chen, S-Q. (2016). Pharmacogenomics of drug metabolizing enzymes and transporters: Relevance to precision medicine. *Genomics, Proteomics & Bioinformatics, 16*(2), 152–153. doi: 10.1016/j.gpb.2016.03.008. Under a creative common license: https://creativecommons.org/licenses/by/4.0/legalcode.)

which can lead to toxic levels. The kidneys are also not fully developed until 1 year of age, leading to limitations in drug elimination. Because of the pharmacokinetic alterations in young children, dosing is either weight based or calculated based on body surface area.

◆ The geriatric population of adults are more sensitive to medications due to altered pharmacokinetic properties. **Polypharmacy**, the use of multiple medications at the same time to treat acute and chronic illnesses, places geriatric clients at higher risk for drug–drug interactions. Reduced blood flow to the gastric mucosa can alter absorption. Distribution of medications throughout the body differs in older adults due to the decreased amount of total protein, lower amounts of body water and lean mass, and higher amounts of body fat. With age, liver function and hepatic blood flow decline, slowing drug metabolism. Renal function also declines with age and is the most common reason for drug toxicity in older adults. For this reason, creatinine clearance is the gold standard of renal function evaluation in the older population. These alterations in pharmacokinetics frequently require decreases in dosing of medications to avoid adverse effects and toxicity. Serum drug levels are frequently monitored for medications with narrow therapeutic ranges.

◆ During pregnancy, medications have the potential to affect the fetus when the medication passes through the placenta. With breastfeeding, some medications may be present in breast milk, which may affect neonates, infants, and/or children that are breastfed. Most medications have not been tested for safety in pregnancy, and therefore, the risk–benefit ratio is always a major consideration prior to prescribing medications for women of childbearing age. Birth defects caused by medication is known as **teratogenesis**. The Federal Drug Administration created drug categories that define the risk of all medications to the fetus. These five categories are set to be phased out by 2020 and are therefore not included in this chapter. Similar to pregnancy, few studies have been conducted on medication safety during breastfeeding. Usually, the amount of medication in breast milk is low enough that it will not cause harm to a child. However, all medications taken by a breastfeeding woman should be considered carefully, with special attention to dosing, scheduling, and timing of breastfeeding in association with the dosing schedule.

Practice Questions

1. The nurse is preparing to administer a newly prescribed antibiotic to a 72-year-old client. Which assessment data would require the nurse to hold the medication and notify the prescriber?

    1. White blood cell count (WBC) 16,000/μL (16 × 10⁹/L)
    2. Serum creatinine 0.6 mg/dL (53.04 μmol/L)
    3. Alanine aminotransferase (ALT) 120 U/L (2 μkat/L)
    4. Serum albumin 4.2 g/dL (42 g/L)

2. The nurse is preparing to administer morning medications to four clients. Which client has the **greatest** risk of medication toxicity?

    1. A 38-year-old client with a serum albumin level of 6.2 g/dL (62 g/L)
    2. A 52-year-old client with renal failure on hemodialysis
    3. A 67-year-old client receiving three medications that are highly protein bound
    4. A 74-year-old client prescribed four medications for hypertension

3. A client is receiving a medication with a narrow therapeutic index. What is the **priority** action by the nurse?

    1. Review the client's most recent renal and liver function tests.
    2. Request an order for a serum medication level immediately.
    3. Discuss decreasing the dose of the medication with the prescriber.
    4. Assess the client for signs and symptoms of medication toxicity.

4. A pediatric client is prescribed amoxicillin 25 mg/kg/day divided in two daily doses. The medication is available as 125 mg/5 mL. The client weighs 18 pounds. What is the total daily dose for the client? Round answer to the nearest tenth.

    _____ mg

5. A client with terminal cancer has been taking morphine 15 mg PO every 4 hours for the past several weeks. Upon assessment, the client reports to the nurse that the pain has been increasing steadily over the last 2 days without much relief from the prescribed morphine. What is the **priority** action by the nurse?

    1. Contact the prescriber to request a more frequent dosing schedule.
    2. Review the client's vital signs to evaluate for the presence of toxicity.
    3. Assess the client for signs or symptoms of physical dependence.
    4. Suggest nonpharmacologic techniques to enhance effectiveness of the medication.

6. A client has been prescribed diphenhydramine 500 mg for the treatment of a mild allergic reaction. After reviewing a drug reference manual, the nurse identifies that the dose is incorrect. What is the **priority** action by the nurse at this time?

    1. Hold the medication and notify the prescriber.
    2. Administer the recommended dose as listed in the drug reference manual.
    3. Contact the pharmacist to double-check the dose parameters.
    4. Assess the client for signs of anaphylaxis.

7. A nursing student is explaining the process of pharmacokinetics to her nurse preceptor. What statement, if made by the student, would require the preceptor to intervene?

　　1. "When you take a medication orally, there are several factors within your gastrointestinal tract that can alter how well a medication will work for you."

　　2. "The amount of protein in your bloodstream will directly affect how well you metabolize medications."

　　3. "Frequently, dosing adjustments are needed because everyone reacts to medications differently."

　　4. "If a medication is destroyed by the liver when ingested, you may need to use an injectable form."

8. A nurse is administering a one-time dose of a medication at 0800 that has a half-life of 6 hours. The client wants to know when the effects of the medication will wear off. Which is the appropriate response by the nurse?

　　1. "I will ask the prescriber to come speak with you about this."

　　2. "Since this is a one-time dose, you will likely not notice any effects of the medication."

　　3. "It will take approximately 24 hours for the effects to wear off."

　　4. "You will notice a slow decline of effects within 6 hours."

9. A client calls the nurse to inquire about medication administration. The directions provided state to take the medication on an empty stomach. The client reports taking the medication with breakfast this morning. Which response by the nurse is correct?

　　1. "Please take another dose of the medication now to increase its effectiveness."

　　2. "You may notice more side effects by taking the medication with food today."

　　3. "Please come to the clinic so that we can examine you for medication toxicity."

　　4. "The medication may be less effective when taken with food. Take it 1 hour before breakfast tomorrow."

10. A client presents to the emergency department following accidental overdose of a medication 3 hours ago. What is the **priority** action by the nurse?

　　1. Prepare the client for hemodialysis.

　　2. Assess the client's vital signs.

　　3. Insert a nasogastric tube.

　　4. Obtain bloodwork for analysis of liver function.

11. The nurse has administered the prescribed dose of an analgesic medication to a client. When considering the nursing process, what is the nurse's **next** responsibility to the client?

　　1. Planning nonmedication interventions

　　2. Evaluating effectiveness of therapy

　　3. Updating the plan of care as needed

　　4. Assessing vital signs

12. Which statement made by a client suggests the need for further education regarding a newly prescribed medication?
    1. "I'm paying for this prescription, so I'd like it written for the generic form."
    2. "There seems to be several brand names for this medication; it's confusing."
    3. "I prefer a trade named version of the medication since they are generally more effective."
    4. "I'm glad I don't have to use the medication's chemical name when refilling the prescription."

13. In order to evaluate the effectiveness of an antibiotic medication, which nursing intervention will the nurse implement?
    1. Assess for nausea and vomiting.
    2. Monitor and compare vital signs.
    3. Identify existence of relevant allergies.
    4. Determine risk for adverse drug interactions.

14. What would be the significance of bright red streaked stool reported by a client prescribed heparin?
    1. The client may be allergic to the medication.
    2. The next dose of the medication should be increased.
    3. The dosage will need to be evaluated for possible reduction.
    4. The client should avoid eating beets, cranberries, and red gelatin.

15. A client with a brain tumor must be monitored for problems related to what aspect of medication pharmacokinetics?
    1. Absorption
    2. Distribution
    3. Metabolism
    4. Excretion

16. A client with which medical condition is presented with the greatest challenge to the effective function of a nicotine patch?
    1. Second-degree burns
    2. Atherosclerosis
    3. Crohn disease
    4. Peptic ulcer

17. A client has been newly prescribed a nightly sedative. Which nursing action would the nurse engage in during the implementation phase of the nursing process to assure effective, relevant nursing care? Select all that apply.
    1. Encouraging the client to use the call bell for assistance during the night
    2. Educating the client to the possibility of morning grogginess
    3. Inquiring the next morning as to how the client slept
    4. Closing the door to minimize noise from the hallway
    5. Offering the client an extra blanket for warmth

18. Which client report suggests that the client is at high risk for nonadherence for a newly prescribed medication? Select all that apply.
    1. "I really, really hate giving myself injections."
    2. "I don't think my insurance will cover this prescription."
    3. "I was told I'd have to take this medication for the rest of my life."
    4. "It's so unfair that I got sick and now have to take this medication."
    5. "This medication makes me really nauseous and too sleepy to drive."

19. The nurse is uncertain about a new medication that has been prescribed for an older preoperative client with a history of gastrointestinal issues. Which resource should the nurse use **initially** to gain understanding about the medication?
    1. The pharmacist on call
    2. The other nurses on the unit
    3. The prescribing health care provider
    4. The drug reference provided by the unit

20. Which pediatric client is at **greatest** risk for medication toxicity?
    1. A 1-year-old diagnosed with a heart valve problem
    2. A 6-year-old being treated for first-degree burns
    3. A 10-year-old recovering from an appendectomy
    4. A 15-year-old diagnosed with exercise-induced asthma

21. Which nursing assessment question will provide the **most** relevant information concerning an older adult client's risk for medication adverse effects and toxicity? Select all that apply.
    1. "How old are you?"
    2. "What is your height and weight?"
    3. "Do you have difficulty swallowing pills?"
    4. "How many times per week do you eat meat or poultry?"
    5. "Have you ever been diagnosed with a kidney problem?"

22. A client of Asian ethnicity is prescribed a selective serotonin reuptake inhibitor (SSRI). Which information should the nurse provide when educating the client on the prescription?
    1. Many Asian clients develop an allergy to SSRIs.
    2. Asian clients tend to respond especially well to SSRIs.
    3. SSRIs are prescribed in lower dosages for Asian clients.
    4. The SSRI is more likely to cause nausea in Asian clients.

23. Which statement, made by the family of a client who is experiencing withdrawal symptoms from a schedule I narcotic, indicates the need for further education on the topic of medication abuse and addiction?
    1. "Treatment for this type of addiction is available and has been successful."
    2. "Withdrawal can produce some very serious situations that require medical attention."
    3. "Schedule 1 narcotics are only mildly addictive and produce minor withdrawal symptoms."
    4. "This type of narcotic is capable of producing physical and/or psychological withdrawal symptoms."

24. A parent calls the local poison hotline to report that their 3-year-old appears to have drank some liquid detergent. Which nursing assessment question would have the **greatest** impact on determining the method of treatment?

    1.   "Is your child conscious and alert?"

    2.   "When did your child ingest the detergent?"

    3.   "What was the brand name of the detergent?"

    4.   "Has your child been diagnosed with any allergies?"

25. When considering treatment for a medication overdose, the nurse would question the prescription for activated charcoal for a client with which extenuating medical factor?

    1.   Allergy to aspirin (ASA)

    2.   Acute bowel obstruction

    3.   Exercise-induced asthma

    4.   Recent myocardial infarction

2

FLUIDS, ELECTROLYTES, AND HEMATOLOGY MEDICATIONS

BRIEF OVERVIEW OF FLUID, ELECTROLYTE, AND HEMATOLOGIC DISORDERS AND MEDICATIONS

The body requires homeostasis, including a balance between fluid and electrolyte levels, for optimal functioning. There are many reasons for disruptions in fluid and/or electrolyte levels. Hematologic disorders may also result in an imbalance in homeostasis. The nurse must be familiar with laboratory values, common signs and symptoms of imbalance, and the ways to treat these conditions in an effort to restore homeostasis.

- ◆ **Isotonic fluid loss:** Isotonic fluid loss occurs when solute (sodium) and solvent (water) are lost in equal proportions, which occurs during short-term vomiting and/or diarrhea, or improper (high) dosage of diuretic medications. This type of fluid loss is treated with isotonic intravenous fluids (0.9% normal saline).
- ◆ **Hypotonic fluid loss:** Hypotonic fluid loss occurs when more sodium is lost than water, which can occur with chronic renal insufficiency. This type of fluid loss is usually treated with isotonic intravenous fluid (0.9% normal saline).
- ◆ **Hypertonic fluid loss:** Hypertonic fluid loss occurs when more water is lost than sodium, which can occur with excessive sweating. This type of fluid loss is treated with hypotonic intravenous fluid (0.45% normal saline).

SAFETY ALERT! The best indicator of fluid volume status is daily weight.

- ◆ **Electrolyte imbalances:** Electrolyte imbalances occur for a variety of reasons, including malnutrition/starvation, as side effects of medications, and as a result of medical disorders. The goal of treatment is to identify and correct the underlying cause of the imbalance.
- ◆ **Anemia:** Anemia is a decrease in red blood cells, hemoglobin, and hematocrit. It can be caused by a variety of issues, including chronic blood loss or acute blood loss (hemorrhage), inadequate dietary intake of certain vitamins or minerals necessary for red blood cell production, or chronic disorders that directly disrupt the production of red blood cells (cancer, renal disease). Anemia is a symptom, not a disease. The underlying cause of anemia must be identified and corrected to improve red blood cell production and function. For severe anemia, blood products may be administered.
- ◆ **Hemophilia:** Hemophilia is a genetic bleeding disorder most commonly affecting males, with females being carriers of the disorder. The two types of hemophilia are type A and type B, each with a characteristic deficient clotting factor. Type A is caused by a deficiency of clotting factor VIII. Type B is caused by a deficiency of clotting factor IX. Treatment depends on the type and consists of replacement of the deficient clotting factor.

SAFETY ALERT! Remember, medications that promote bleeding (aspirin, heparin, nonsteroidal anti-inflammatory drugs [NSAIDs]) should not be used in patients with hemophilia. Acetaminophen is a good alternative for pain management that will not disrupt clotting.

CLINICAL PEARLS: FLUIDS AND ELECTROLYTES

Fluids

Assessment/Signs and Symptoms

Signs of hypovolemia include tachycardia, hypotension, dry mucous membranes, decreased urinary output, and weight loss. If electrolyte levels are impaired, signs and symptoms will occur based on the electrolyte affected (see Table 2-1). Signs of hypervolemia include weight gain, edema, bounding pulse, and increased blood pressure. Refer to Table 2-1 for pertinent laboratory values.

Diagnostics

Along with signs and symptoms, laboratory values are used to assess for fluid and electrolyte imbalances. Electrolyte levels and serum osmolality help identify the type of fluid loss (isotonic, hypotonic, or hypertonic). The underlying cause of the imbalance must be identified and corrected.

Electrolytes

Assessment/Signs and Symptoms

The signs and symptoms of electrolyte imbalance vary based on the electrolyte(s) affected.

Diagnostics

It is critical for nurses to know reference ranges for serum electrolyte levels. Table 2-2 lists these values.

CLINICAL PEARLS: HEMATOLOGY

Anemia

Assessment/Signs and Symptoms

Signs and symptoms vary depending on the severity of the anemia and its underlying cause. Fatigue is the most common symptom. It is important to note that anemia is a symptom of an underlying problem, not a disease itself. The goal of treating anemia is to identify and correct the underlying cause. Other signs and symptoms include tachycardia, hypotension, pallor, cool extremities, shortness of breath, and impaired activity intolerance.

Diagnostics

Laboratory values are used to diagnose anemia. More invasive testing may be required to identify the source of blood loss, including endoscopy and/or colonoscopy, because the gastrointestinal tract is a common source of blood loss secondary to disorders such as peptic ulcer disease.

Table 2-1

Signs and Symptoms of Electrolyte Imbalances

Imbalance	Level	Causes	Symptoms	Treatment	Nursing Interventions
Hyperkalemia	>5 mEq/L (5 mmol/L)	Excessive intake of potassium-containing foods or supplements	Muscle weakness	Insulin	Cardiac monitoring
		Potassium-sparing diuretics and ACE inhibitors	Tall, peaked T waves on EKG	Kayexalate	Restrict dietary sources of potassium
		Renal failure	Ventricular dysrhythmias	Loop diuretics (furosemide)	
				Hemodialysis	
Hypokalemia	<3.5 mEq/L (3.5 mmol/L)	Poor dietary intake	Fatigue	Increase dietary intake of potassium	Cardiac monitoring
		Vomiting and/or diarrhea	Muscle cramps	Oral or IV supplementation	Administer IV potassium slowly (10 mEq/hr)—never push
		Potassium-wasting diuretics	Flat T waves on EKG		Ensure adequate renal function prior to administering
Hypernatremia	>145 mEq/L (145 mmol/L)	Dehydration	CNS disturbances (hallucinations, confusion, seizures)	Sodium restriction	Initiate seizure precautions
		Burns		Increase water or hypotonic fluid intake	Monitor fluid volume status (I&O, daily weight)
		Vomiting and/or diarrhea			
Hyponatremia	<135 mEq/L (135 mmol/L)	Excessive water intake	CNS disturbances (headache, confusion, seizures)	Sodium replacement via diet, oral or IV supplements	Monitor fluid volume status
		Decreased sodium intake	Edema		Hypertonic IV solutions only for severe cases due to risk of cerebral edema
		Excessive sweating			
Hypercalcemia	>10.2 mg/dL (2.55 mmol/L)	Excess vitamin D	Decreased reflexes, bone pain, kidney stones, dehydration, cardiac dysrhythmias	Loop diuretics, mediations to decrease calcium levels (calcium chelators)	Monitor cardiac rhythm, encourage ambulation/mobility
		Hyperparathyroidism			
		Bone cancer			
		Excessive dietary intake of calcium			

Condition	Lab value	Causes	Signs/Symptoms	Treatment	Nursing considerations
Hypocalcemia	<8.6 mg/dL (2.05 mmol/L)	Deficient vitamin D; Hypoparathyroidism; Poor dietary intake; Alcohol abuse	Tetany, cramps; Positive Trousseau and Chvostek signs; Seizures	Calcium and vitamin D replacement via dietary intake, oral or IV supplements	Seizure precautions
Hypermagnesemia	>2.5 mEq/L (2.5 mmol/L)	Renal failure; Excess intake	Bradycardia, decreased reflexes, cardiac arrest	Medications to reduce levels: loop diuretics and IV calcium gluconate	Monitor vital signs, cardiac rhythm, and reflexes
Hypomagnesemia	<1.5 mEq/L (1.5 mmol/L)	Alcohol abuse; Poor dietary intake; Diuretics; Laxative abuse	Hypertension, hyperactive reflexes, dysrhythmias, seizures	Supplementation of magnesium in diet and/or with oral or IV magnesium	Monitor cardiac rhythm, seizure precautions
Hyperphosphatemia	>4.4 mg/dL (1/52 mmol/L)	Renal failure; Excess intake; Pancreatitis	Tetany, paresthesias, dysrhythmias	Diuretics, restrict intake, dialysis	Monitor diet
Hypophosphatemia	<2.4 mg/dL (0.74 mmol/L)	Vitamin D deficiency; Excessive loss of body fluids; Antacid abuse	Weakness, bone pain, confusion, seizures	Oral or IV replacement, increase dietary intake	Seizure precautions

ACE, angiotensin–converting enzyme; CNS, central nervous system; EKG, electrocardiography; I&O, input and output; IV, intravenous.

Table 2-2

Normal Laboratory Values for Serum Electrolytes

Potassium	3.5–5 mEq/L (3.5–5 mmol/L)
Sodium	135–145 mEq/L (135–145 mmol/L)
Chloride	96–106 mEq/L (96–106 mmol/L)
Calcium	8.6–10.2 mg/dL (2.05–2.55 mmol/L)
Magnesium	1.5–2.5 mEq/L (0.65–1.05 mmol/L)
Phosphorus	2.4–4.4 mg/dL/ (0.74–1.52 mmol/L)

Pertinent Laboratory Values

Red blood cell count, hemoglobin, and hematocrit will be decreased. Other lab values such as the ferritin level, vitamin B_{12}, and folic acid levels will be altered depending on the underlying cause of the anemia. Red blood cell indices help identify the type of deficiency based on the size and color of the red blood cell.

Hemophilia

Assessment/Signs and Symptoms

The deficiency of clotting factors leads to prolonged and/or uncontrollable bleeding. This may present as heavy menses, frequent nosebleeds, hematuria, excessive bruising, and/or anemia.

Diagnostics

Hemophilia is diagnosed through laboratory values that indicate a deficiency of clotting factor VIII or IX, as well as prolonged bleeding times.

Pertinent Laboratory Values

Elevate activated partial thromboplastin time (aPTT) and decreased factor VIII or IX. The prothrombin time (PT) and platelet levels are normal.

MEDICATION OVERVIEW

Fluid Replacement

Fluid deficit can be treated with oral and/or intravenous (IV) fluid volume replacement (see Table 2-3) and should be guided by the type of fluid loss. With all IV fluids, there is a risk of fluid volume overload. Monitoring intake and output, and for signs and symptoms of hypervolemia, is vital when administering IV fluids.

Electrolyte Replacement

Dietary sources can provide electrolyte replacement when the imbalance is not severe (see Fig. 2-1). If dietary supplementation does not produce the desired replacement, the use of specific electrolytes may be necessary (see Table 2-4).

Table 2-3

Types of Intravenous Fluids

Type of Intravenous Fluid	Prototype	Indications
Isotonic fluid	0.9% sodium chloride "Normal saline"	Isotonic and mild–moderate hypotonic fluid loss
Hypotonic fluid	0.45% sodium chloride "Half normal saline"	Hypertonic fluid loss
Hypertonic fluid	3% sodium chloride	Severe hypotonic fluid loss

Electrolyte	Food
Potassium	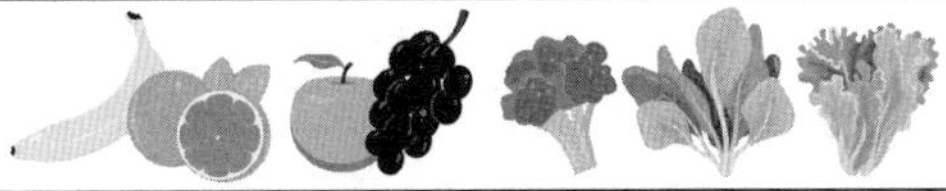
Sodium	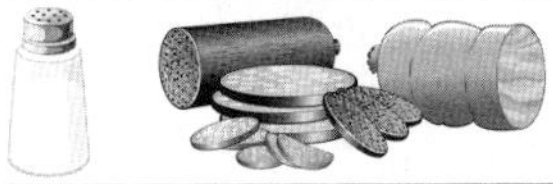
Chloride	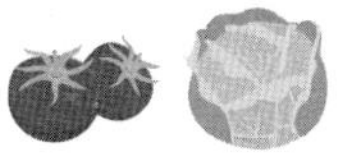
Calcium	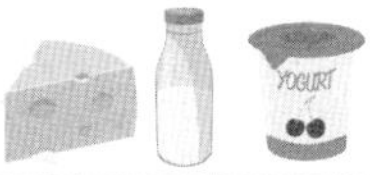
Magnesium	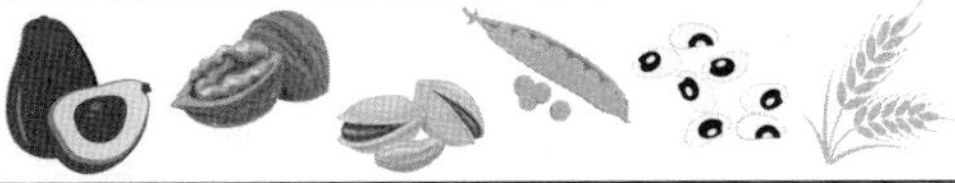
Phosphorus	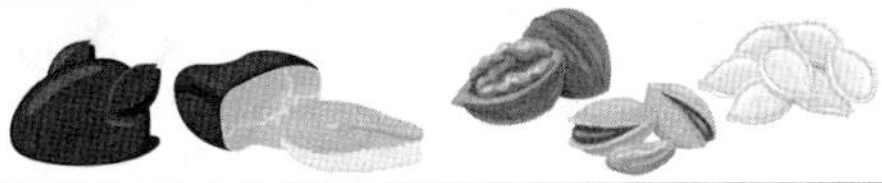

Figure 2-1 Dietary sources of electrolytes.

Table 2-4

Specific Substances Used in Electrolyte Replacement

Class	Prototype	Major Side and Adverse Effects	Critical Information	Indications
Electrolyte	Oral/IV: potassium chloride	Nausea, vomiting, diarrhea IV site reactions (phlebitis) Hyperkalemia	Never push IV potassium; max hourly dose is 40 mEq/hr (40 mmol/L)	Hypokalemia
Electrolyte	Hypertonic saline	Excess sodium may lead to cerebral edema	For use with severe hyponatremia (sodium <125 mEq/L [125 mmol/L]), slow infusion	Hyponatremia

(continued)

Table 2-4

Specific Substances Used in Electrolyte Replacement *(continued)*

Class	Prototype	Major Side and Adverse Effects	Critical Information	Indications
Electrolyte	Oral: calcium chloride IV: calcium gluconate	Hypercalcemia, kidney stones, constipation, hypomagnesemia IV administration can lead to dysrhythmias, syncope	IV: administer over 10 minutes Be sure IV site is flushing properly, as IV calcium can lead to necrosis of tissue	Hypocalcemia Adjunct treatment for hypermagnesemia and hyperphosphatemia
Electrolyte	Oral: magnesium oxide IV: magnesium sulfate	Oral: diarrhea, nausea, vomiting IV: serious reactions can occur, such as fatal dysrhythmias, paralysis of respiratory muscles, and pulmonary edema Common side effects include flushing, suppression of deep tendon reflexes, hypocalcemia, and hypophosphatemia	IV dose administered 1–2 g over 1 hour	Hypomagnesemia, dysrhythmias, suppression of uterine contractions, prevention and/ or treatment of seizures caused by preeclampsia
Electrolyte	Oral/IV: sodium phosphate/ potassium phosphate	Oral/IV: nausea, vomiting, diarrhea Serious reactions include hyperkalemia and arrhythmias	IV phosphorus should be used with caution, because it can lead to hypocalcemia Review potassium levels and kidney function prior to administering potassium-containing phosphorus Oral: should be given with 8 oz water and meal IV dose should be decreased by half with kidney disease	Hypophosphatemia

IV, intravenous.

Anemias

Table 2-5 provides an outline of the various medications to treat anemias.

> **BLACK BOX WARNING:** Iron dextran administered intravenously can cause potentially fatal anaphylactic reactions. Be sure to administer a small test dose and have epinephrine at the bedside.

Table 2-5

Drugs Used in the Treatment of Anemia

Class	Prototype	Mechanism of Action	Major Side and Adverse Effects	Critical Information	Indications
Iron	Oral: ferrous sulfate	Replacement of iron, which is critical for hemoglobin function	Oral: nausea, vomiting, constipation, dark stools (harmless)	Oral: take iron with vitamin C source (e.g., orange juice)—ascorbic acid helps improve absorption of ferrous sulfate	Iron deficiency anemia, diet supplementation
	IV: iron dextran		IV: nausea, vomiting, headache, injection site reactions (phlebitis)	IV: must begin with a small test dose, keep epinephrine on hand in the event of anaphylaxis	
Vitamin B$_{12}$	Oral, IM/SC, nasal: cyanocobalamin	Replacement of vitamin B$_{12}$ (cyanocobalamin)	Common side effects: headache, nausea, diarrhea	If underlying cause has not yet been identified (B$_{12}$ vs. folic acid deficiency), cyanocobalamin should be administered to avoid permanent neurologic damage	Vitamin B$_{12}$ anemia/deficiency, diet supplementation, replacement for those with gastric surgery or absence of intrinsic factor
			Serious adverse reactions: anaphylaxis, hypokalemia, and pulmonary edema		
				Available as oral tablet, oral disintegrating tablet, IM/SC administration, and nasal spray	
Folic acid	Folic acid	Replacement of folic acid	Nausea, flatulence, rash	If client unable to absorb via GI tract, may administer via SC, IM, or IV route	Folic acid anemia, diet supplementation
Hematopoietic agents	Erythropoietin alfa	Stimulates the production of red blood cells by the kidneys	Hypertension	Monitor hemoglobin and hematocrit, may be administered IV or subcutaneously	Anemia caused by deficient erythropoietin production (kidney disease, chemotherapy)
				Do not administer if hemoglobin is over 8 g/dL (80 g/L), as this increases the risk of clotting	

GI, gastrointestinal; IM, intramuscular; IV, intravenous; SC, subcutaneous.

> **BLACK BOX WARNING:** Erythropoietin alfa has three black box warnings. First, it can increase the risk of potentially fatal cardiac events. Second, erythropoietin alfa has been shown to increase the rate of tumor progression of certain cancers. Third, erythropoietin alfa can increase the risk of deep vein thrombosis in clients after surgery. This medication should be used only when the benefit outweighs this risk, at the lowest dose for the shortest duration.

Hemophilia

Both types of hemophilia are treated using medications to reduce the risk of bleeding, as discussed in Table 2-6.

Administration of Blood Products

In situations such as hemorrhage, severe anemia, and impaired oxygen-carrying capacity that can worsen comorbid cardiac and respiratory conditions, blood transfusions may be required. There are several different types of blood products (see Table 2-7). The most commonly used are packed red blood cells. Regardless of the type of blood product, prior to administration, these

Table 2-6

Drugs Used in the Treatment of Hemophilia

Class	Prototype	Mechanism of Action	Major Side and Adverse Effects	Critical Information	Indications
Coagulation factor; antihemophilic factor	Factor VIII	Replete lost clotting factor caused by destruction through disease process	Side effects include headache, dizziness, flushing	Dose depends on degree of bleeding risk or actual bleeding present	Type A hemophilia
Coagulation factor	Factor IX	Replete lost clotting factor caused by destruction through disease process	Thromboembolism is a potential adverse effect Injection site reactions are common (redness, pain)	Dose depends on degree of bleeding risk or actual bleeding present	Type B hemophilia
Synthetic vasopressin	Desmopressin	Increases blood levels of factor VIII	Blood clots are a potentially fatal adverse effect Common side effects: flushing, hypotension, and headache	Can be used intranasally or parenterally To prevent excess bleeding during surgery, administer 30 min prior to the procedure	Mild type A or B hemophilia

Table 2-7

Use of Blood Products

Blood Product	Infusion Time	Uses	Possible Adverse Reactions
Whole blood	4 hr maximum	Hemorrhage, surgery	Allergic, hemolytic, anaphylactic
Packed red blood cells	4 hr maximum	Anemia	Allergic, hemolytic, hypervolemia
Platelets	30 min maximum	Thrombocytopenia	Febrile
Fresh frozen plasma	60 min maximum	Replace clotting factors: warfarin overdose, DIC, hemorrhage	Febrile, allergic, anaphylactic
Albumin	Varies	Decreased albumin levels, burns, expansion of fluid volume	Pulmonary edema, hypervolemia

DIC, disseminated intravascular coagulation.

products must be verified as correct by two registered nurses and the infusion must begin within 30 minutes of the blood product arriving to the unit. In addition, vital signs are required before, 15 minutes into, and immediately after administration. The nurse should remain with the client for the first 15 minutes of the transfusion in the event that a transfusion reaction occurs. If a reaction occurs, the transfusion should be stopped immediately, 0.9% normal saline should be infused, and the provider must be notified. The addition of excess volume with any transfusion can result in fluid volume excess. Monitor for signs of hypervolemia, such as hypertension, bounding pulse, peripheral edema, jugular vein distention, or crackles in the lungs.

Practice Questions and Rationales

1.   A client is prescribed potassium chloride 10 mEq/(10 mmol)/100 mL 0.9% normal saline to be infused over 1 hour. Prior to administration, the nurse notes that the client's urine output has been 15 mL/hr for the past 3 hours. What is the **priority** action by the nurse?
     1.   Administer the medication over 30 minutes.
     2.   Administer the medication via the oral route.
     3.   Increase oral intake of fluids for the next 2 hours.
     4.   Hold the medication and notify the prescriber.

2.   The nurse is reviewing the client's laboratory values from this morning's laboratory blood draw. Based on the values, what is the **priority** action of the nurse?

Sodium	146 mEq/L (146 mmol/L)
Potassium	3.3 mEq/L (3.3 mmol/L)
Calcium	8.4 mg/dL (2.10 mmol/L)
Magnesium	0.7 mEq/L (0.35 mmol/L)
Phosphorus	3 mg/dL (0.97 mmol/L)

     1.   Place the client on the cardiac monitor.
     2.   Initiate seizure precautions.
     3.   Increase dietary intake of calcium-containing foods.
     4.   Prepare for intravenous magnesium supplementation.

3.   A client presents to the emergency department with reports of nausea, vomiting, and diarrhea for the past 4 days and the following laboratory data. Which of the prescribed interventions should the nurse perform **first**?

Sodium	148 mEq/L (148 mmol/L)
Potassium	3.3 mEq/L (3.3 mmol/L)
Serum osmolality	320 mOsm/kg (320 mmol/kg)

     1.   Administer prescribed ondansetron 4 mg intravenously (IV).
     2.   Increase the rate of 0.45% normal saline infusion to 200 mL/hr.
     3.   Insert nasogastric (NG) tube and begin low intermittent wall suction.
     4.   Bring the client for ordered abdominal computed tomography (CT) scan.

4.   A client with chronic kidney disease and anemia has been prescribed erythropoietin alfa for a current hemoglobin level of 13 mg/dL (130 g/L). What is the **priority** action of the nurse?
     1.   Question the order.
     2.   Administer the medication as prescribed.
     3.   Contact the provider for an order for packed red blood cells.
     4.   Determine the client's allergy history.

5.   A client with hemophilia A reports increased frequency of epistaxis over the past several days. What are the **priority** actions by the nurse? Select all that apply.
     1.   Review the client's prothrombin time (PT) and international normalized ratio (INR).
     2.   Obtain a complete medication list.

   3. Consult the prescriber for an order for factor IX.

   4. Prepare the client for a blood transfusion.

   5. Request an order to obtain an activated partial thromboplastin time (aPTT) level.

6. The client is prescribed 1 unit of packed red blood cells in 250 mL for infusion over 2 hours. How many milliliters per hour should the nurse program the pump to infuse? Record the answer using a whole number.

        _____ mL/hr

7. A client has been receiving a unit of whole blood and suddenly develops shortness of breath and bibasilar crackles. What is the **priority** action of the nurse?

   1. Stop the infusion.

   2. Give 2 L of oxygen via nasal cannula.

   3. Notify the prescriber.

   4. Elevate the head of the bed to 90°.

8. A client has been admitted to the unit with a serum sodium level of 127 mEq/L (127 mmol/L) and anxiety. What are the **priority** nursing action(s) based on these data? Select all that apply.

   1. Place the client on telemetry.

   2. Put up side rail pads on the client's bed.

   3. Prepare suction at the bedside.

   4. Obtain an order for lorazepam as needed.

   5. Obtain intravenous (IV) access.

9. A client is receiving potassium chloride 10 mEq/(10 mmol)/L in 100 mL 0.9% normal saline. On assessment, the client reports pain at the infusion site. The nurse notes that the site is warm and erythematous. What is the **best** action for the nurse to take?

   1. Slow the rate of the infusion.

   2. Apply a warm pack to the site.

   3. Stop the infusion and restart at another site.

   4. Request an order for an oral form of potassium.

10. A client has a serum potassium level of 3.2 mEq/L (3.2 mmol/L). What foods will the nurse suggest the client eat to help improve the serum potassium level? Select all that apply.

   1. Carrots

   2. Potatoes

   3. Strawberries

   4. Spinach

   5. Yogurt

   6. Legumes

11. Which laboratory value of a client taking milk of magnesia (MOM) would alert the nurse to notify the prescriber?

   1. Serum potassium 5.3 mEq/L (5.3 mmol/L)

   2. Glomerular filtration rate (GFR) 45 mL/min

3. Blood urea nitrogen (BUN) 4 mmol/L
4. Serum sodium 130 mEq/L (130 mmol/L)

12. Which medication(s) would the nurse anticipate administering to a client with hyperkalemia? Select all that apply.

1. Regular insulin
2. Magnesium sulfate
3. Furosemide
4. Sodium polystyrene sulfonate
5. Spironolactone

13. A client with a history of electrolyte imbalances reports right-sided flank pain and hematuria. The nurse suspects the client may be experiencing which electrolyte imbalance?

1. Hyponatremia
2. Hyperphosphatemia
3. Hypercalcemia
4. Hypokalemia

14. A client is prescribed 2 L of 0.45% normal saline intravenous infusion to infuse over the next 12 hours. What is the drip rate (gtt/min) using tubing with a drop factor of 10 gtt/mL? Round answer to the nearest whole number.

_____ gtt/min

15. A client receiving a transfusion of whole blood has the following vital signs. What is the **priority** action by the nurse?

	Baseline Vital Signs	**15-Minute Vital Signs**
Blood pressure	132/78 mm Hg	124/62 mm Hg
Pulse	72	88
Temperature	98.2°F (36.8°C)	100.2°F (37.9°C)
Respirations	18	22
Oxygen saturation	98%	96%

1. Slow the rate of the transfusion.
2. Give 2 L oxygen via nasal cannula.
3. Stop the infusion and notify the prescriber.
4. Administer prescribed acetaminophen 650 mg by mouth.

3

CARDIAC MEDICATIONS

BRIEF OVERVIEW OF CARDIAC DISORDERS

Cardiac disorders vary in both chronicity and complexity. While many of the disorders of the cardiac system are preventable (e.g., hypertension and heart failure), cardiac disorders are some of the most frequently treated conditions around the world. Many of the medications in this chapter overlap, as they can be used for a variety of cardiac-related conditions.

◆ *Hypertension (HTN):* A chronic elevation in blood pressure (BP) >120/80 mm Hg. The diagnosis of hypertension is based on at least two separate readings on separate days above 120/80 mm Hg. Hypertension can be mixed, where both the systolic and diastolic readings are elevated or isolated, where either the systolic or diastolic reading is elevated. Hypertension is also classified as either primary or secondary. Primary hypertension is most common, affecting about 90% of all clients with hypertension. Primary hypertension, also known as essential hypertension, has no single underlying cause. Secondary hypertension is much less common and occurs as a result of an identifiable underlying cause (e.g., pheochromocytoma, an epinephrine-secreting tumor on an adrenal gland that causes an increase in BP). Treatment of primary hypertension involves lifestyle changes, such as reduction of weight/body mass index; increasing aerobic physical activity to at least 30 minutes, 5 days per week; and limiting sodium intake. In addition to lifestyle changes, pharmacologic therapy is instituted if BP does not decrease after 6 months of lifestyle management. Secondary hypertension treatment focuses on identification and correction of the underlying cause. Hypertension is known as the "silent killer," as there are no obvious signs or symptoms of the disorder until target organ damage has occurred. The major organs affected by hypertension include the kidneys, brain, eyes, and heart.

◆ *Heart failure (HF):* A progressively worsening disorder in which cardiac output is decreased, leading to a decline in systemic perfusion. Alterations in pumping ability of the heart can be caused from a variety of conditions, including hypertension, coronary artery disease, myocardial infarction, and cardiac valve disorders. As the disease progresses, the heart's ability to pump effectively declines, leading to symptoms such as shortness of breath, fluid overload, fatigue, and cardiac dysrhythmias. Decreased perfusion to vital organs also contributes to organ dysfunction, such as renal insufficiency. The goals of treatment include improving quality of life and ability to perform activities of daily living, and reduction of symptoms. There is no cure for heart failure.

◆ *Dysrhythmias:* An abnormality in cardiac rate and/or rhythm that can impair cardiac output. Dysrhythmias can be atrial or ventricular, bradycardic or tachycardic. Atrial dysrhythmias are more common, while ventricular dysrhythmias are more dangerous. The goal of treatment is to restore adequate cardiac output and systemic perfusion and identification of the underlying cause.

◆ *Clotting disorders:* An abnormality in coagulation that can occur for a variety of reasons. Regardless of the underlying cause, the end result is the formation of clots or thrombi, which can lead to vessel occlusion and emboli. Medications used to treat coagulation disorders can work to decrease platelet aggregation, alter coagulation pathways, or breakdown existing clots that have formed. Regardless of the mechanism of action, since these medications interfere with coagulation, a major adverse effect is bleeding.

◆ *Hyperlipidemia:* An elevation of blood cholesterol, which can occur in various ways and results from lifestyle habits and/or genetic factors. Low-density lipoproteins (LDLs) are the primary cause of atherosclerosis. In addition, very-low-density lipoproteins (VLDLs), such as triglycerides, are also responsible for plaque accumulation in arteries. High-density lipoproteins (HDLs) are a protective form of cholesterol that work to decrease cardiac risk that occurs with elevated LDLs and/or VLDLs. Lifestyle changes are a cornerstone of therapy for hyperlipidemia, such as increasing aerobic exercise, decreasing dietary intake of saturated fats, decreasing weight/body mass index, and quitting smoking.

◆ *Angina and myocardial infarction (MI):* Angina, also known as chest pain, is a symptom of underlying cardiac disease. There are various types of angina, including stable/chronic, unstable, and variant/vasospastic/Prinzmetal angina. Stable angina is caused by coronary artery disease, is predictable in nature, and is treated with a variety of medications. Variant angina may occur with or without coronary artery disease with the goal of treatment to prevent or decrease the occurrence of coronary artery vasospasm using calcium channel blockers and/or vasodilators. Unstable angina is a medical emergency that can progress to MI. Treatment revolves around the relief of chest pain and prevention of further obstruction of oxygen to the myocardial tissue using a combination of an antiplatelet, vasodilator, and afterload reducers (beta-blockers, angiotensin-converting enzyme [ACE] inhibitors). MI is a marked decrease in oxygen supply with an increase in oxygen demand, causing cell death. MI usually presents as chest pain that has lasted for longer than 30 minutes, unrelieved by rest and/or nitroglycerin. The goal of treatment is immediate reperfusion to decrease the degree of cell death and myocardial muscle damage.

CLINICAL PEARLS—CARDIAC DISORDERS

Hypertension

Assessment/Signs and Symptoms
Frequently, hypertension has no symptoms. When the BP is elevated chronically over a long span of time, the client may develop symptoms related to target organ damage such as visual changes, headache, peripheral vascular disease, and renal dysfunction.

Diagnostics
Diagnosis of hypertension is based upon two or more readings of BP elevation >120 mm Hg and/or 80 mm Hg more than 2 weeks apart. An electrocardiogram (ECG) and chest x-ray (CXR) are frequently completed to evaluate for left ventricular hypertrophy as a result of hypertension and an increased workload on the heart.

Pertinent Laboratory Values
Laboratory testing helps to identify possible underlying causes if secondary hypertension is suspected. Otherwise, laboratory testing is used to evaluate the presence and degree of target organ

damage caused by long-standing under or uncontrolled hypertension. The major organs impacted by hypertension are the eyes, brain, heart, and kidneys.

Heart Failure

Assessment/Signs and Symptoms
Signs and symptoms depend upon the type of heart failure (systolic or diastolic, left or right sided; Fig. 3-1).

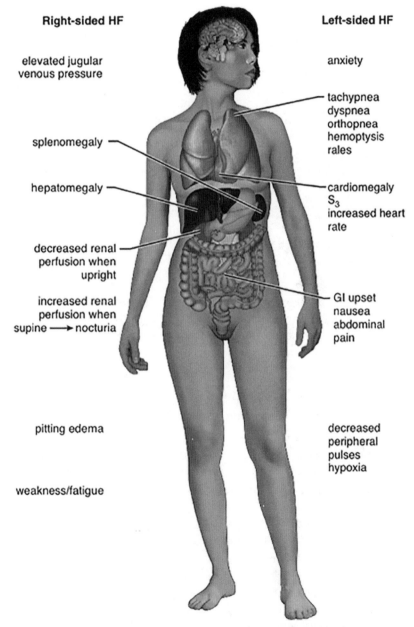

Right-sided HF

elevated jugular
venous pressure

splenomegaly

hepatomegaly

decreased renal
perfusion when
upright

increased renal
perfusion when
supine ⟶ nocturia

pitting edema

weakness/fatigue

Left-sided HF

anxiety

tachypnea
dyspnea
orthopnea
hemoptysis
rales

cardiomegaly
S_3
increased heart
rate

GI upset
nausea
abdominal
pain

decreased
peripheral
pulses
hypoxia

Figure 3-1 Signs and symptoms of heart failure. (Reprinted with permission from Karch, A. *Focus on Nursing Pharmacology*, 5th edition. Philadelphia: Wolters Kluwer Health, 2009.)

Diagnostics

Diagnosis of heart failure is obtained through an echocardiogram, which evaluates valvular function, ventricular and atrial pumping (systolic) and relaxing (diastolic) ability, and the left ventricle's ejection fraction (EF), which is the percent of blood ejected by the left ventricle with each beat.

Pertinent Laboratory Values

The elevation of brain natriuretic peptide >100 pg/mL (100 ng/L) is indicative of heart failure.

Dysrhythmias

Assessment/Signs and Symptoms

Symptoms vary based upon the severity and location of the dysrhythmia. Atrial dysrhythmias (atrial fibrillation and atrial flutter) frequently present with palpitations, light-headedness, and decreased BP. Ventricular dysrhythmias (pulseless ventricular tachycardia and fibrillation) present with pulselessness and loss of consciousness related to significantly diminished or absent cardiac output. Ventricular tachycardia can also present with a pulse where the client may have no symptoms or report palpitations, feelings of light-headedness or weakness as the cardiac output begins to become impaired. Bradycardia can be asymptomatic or can cause symptoms such as weakness, light-headedness, or fatigue. Tachycardia can also be asymptomatic or can present with palpitations and anxiety.

Diagnostics

The initial identification of the dysrhythmia is by ECG.

Pertinent Laboratory Values

Electrolyte imbalance (potassium or magnesium) can cause dysrhythmias. Damage to cardiac muscle during unstable angina, MI, or cardiogenic shock can also cause dysrhythmias, which can be assessed by measuring cardiac-specific troponin levels. Anemia can lead to dysrhythmias, represented by decreased hemoglobin and hematocrit levels.

Clotting Disorders

Assessment/Signs and Symptoms

A clot, also known as a thrombus, can develop in veins or arteries. Symptoms are dependent on the size and location of the clot. Clots that form in or travel to the arteries of the heart or brain lead to symptoms of heart attack or stroke, respectively. Venous thrombi are most commonly located in the lower extremities, although they can also occur in the upper extremities. Symptoms of venous thrombi include redness, unilateral swelling, pain, and warmth. If a portion of the clot breaks off and travels to another region, this is known as an embolus. A risk of venous thrombi is pulmonary emboli, which occurs when a portion of a venous clot breaks off and travels to the pulmonary vasculature. Signs and symptoms of a pulmonary embolus include shortness of breath, tachypnea, cough, chest pain, and decreased oxygen saturation levels. Arterial clots can lead to emboli that travel to the brain, causing ischemic stroke. Frequently, this is the result of untreated atrial fibrillation, when the pooling of blood in the atria form clots that travel to the brain.

Diagnostics

Diagnosis of clots is completed by obtaining a thorough history and physical examination. If a clot is suspected in an extremity, Doppler ultrasound is performed to detect the size and location of the clot. Pulmonary emboli are detected using imaging, such as computed tomography (CT) scans or ventilation/perfusion scans. More invasively, pulmonary angiogram can be performed. Coronary angiogram is used to identify clots within coronary arteries. A noncontrast head CT is used to detect alterations in hemostasis within the brain that would be indicative of an ischemic stroke caused by a thrombus.

Pertinent Laboratory Values

The D-dimer is a blood test that can be used to screen for clot formation. Levels equal to or <500 ng/mL fibrinogen equivalent units (FEUs) can help to exclude the presence of a clot. Higher levels (>500 ng/mL FEU) indicate the presence of a pulmonary embolism or deep vein thrombosis; however, it is not specific and does not identify the location of the clot.

Hyperlipidemia

Assessment/Signs and Symptoms

High cholesterol, especially LDLs, is known to lead to the development of atherosclerosis, or plaque build-up in arteries. The build-up of plaque is responsible for the signs and symptoms that correspond to hyperlipidemia. For example, when plaque build-up occurs in the coronary arteries, there is decreased perfusion to the heart, which can lead to heart failure and/or MI. Atherosclerosis of the arteries of the brain may result in ischemic strokes and/or transient ischemic attacks.

Diagnostics

Screening for elevated cholesterol levels may occur as early as age 9, due to the rise of adolescent obesity. In addition to blood testing, screening of organs affected by atherosclerosis may also occur, including ECG, carotid artery ultrasound, and lower extremity examinations that may indicate decreased arterial perfusion (e.g., ankle–brachial index measurements).

Pertinent Laboratory Values (Table 3-1)

Cholesterol levels should be measured with the client fasting (nothing to eat or drink 8 hours prior to the blood test). Total cholesterol levels as well as individual lipoprotein levels are measured.

Angina and Myocardial Infarction (MI)

Assessment/Signs and Symptoms

Signs and symptoms of angina vary based on the type of angina. All types result in chest pain that may radiate to other regions of the body (arm, shoulder, back). Stable angina is chest pain that occurs with exertion and is relieved by rest; it is predictable in nature. Prinzmetal or vasospastic angina occurs with or without exertion and is relieved by nitroglycerin and/or calcium channel blockers. Unstable angina is chest pain that occurs at rest, is unpredictable, and/or is more severe

Table 3-1

Laboratory Values Measured to Check for Hyperlipidemia

Serum Laboratory Measurement	Normal Range
Total cholesterol	<200 mg/dL (5.18 mmol/L)
Low-density lipoprotein (LDL)	<100 mg/dL (2.59 mmol/L)
	<70 mg/dL if concurrent diabetes (1.81 mmol/L)
High-density lipoprotein (HDL)	≥40 mg/dL for men (1.04 mmol/L)
	≥50 mg/dL for women (1.29 mmol/L)
Triglycerides/very-low-density lipoprotein (TG/VLDL)	<150 mg/dL (3.88 mmol/L)

than stable angina. Unstable angina is a medical emergency and may progress to necrosis of the heart muscle and MI.

MI is severe chest pain or pressure that is unpredictable and not relieved by rest. It typically causes additional symptoms such as diaphoresis, shortness of breath, nausea, an impending sense of doom, and radiating pain to the jaw, left arm, and/or back. In women, symptoms of MI are more vague and tend to include fatigue, shortness of breath, and nausea.

Diagnostics

The first component of diagnosing angina or MI is an ECG. Stable or unstable angina may result in T-wave inversion and ST-segment depression. MI can cause ST-segment elevation and/or changes in cardiac biomarker levels, depending on the degree of artery occlusion. See Figure 3-2 for additional information.

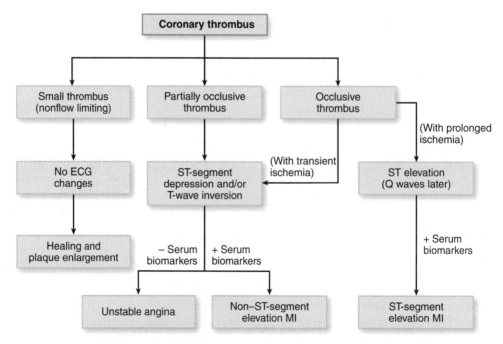

Figure 3-2 Consequences of coronary thrombosis. (Reprinted with permission from Lilly, L. *Pathophysiology of Heart Disease*, 6th edition. Philadelphia: Wolters Kluwer Health, 2015.)

Pertinent Laboratory Values

Cardiac biomarkers are the cornerstone of laboratory testing to screen for MI. Cardiac-specific troponin levels are the most sensitive laboratory values for MI.

MEDICATION OVERVIEW

In HTN, medications are used to reduce BP and slow the progression of target organ damage. In HF, medications are used to reduce symptoms and improve quality of life. In angina and MI, medications are used to relieve chest pain, decrease myocardial oxygen demand, increase myocardial oxygen supply, and reduce the risk of permanent cardiac damage. Diuretics work in various parts of the nephron, the functional unit of the kidney. The earlier in the nephron the diuretic works, the more diuresis will be produced (Fig. 3-3). Within cardiac disorders, diuretics are used to treat HTN and HF (Table 3-2).

> **BLACK BOX WARNING:** ACE inhibitors and ARBs can cause a potentially fatal adverse reaction known as angioedema. This causes swelling of the tongue and lips and may cause respiratory distress. Angioedema is a medical emergency. The medication that caused the angioedema should be stopped immediately and never restarted.

Dysrhythmias

Medications are used to convert the dysrhythmia back into a normal sinus rhythm, prevent a dysrhythmia from reoccurring, or controlling the heart rate for a current tachydysrhythmia. Antidysrhythmic medications are grouped by classes, classes I to IV, called the Vaughan Williams classification and a fifth category that includes miscellaneous antidysrhythmics digoxin and adenosine. It is important to remember that all antidysrhythmic medications can also cause dysrhythmias, so they are used with caution and when the benefit outweighs the risk. See Table 3-3 for a description of antidysrhythmic agents.

> **BLACK BOX WARNING:** There are several black box warnings for amiodarone, including potentially fatal pulmonary toxicity, hepatic failure, and worsening of dysrhythmias.

Clotting Disorders

Medications are used to prevent clots from forming, limit the size of an existing clot, or break down a clot. Medications in the treatment of clotting disorders act within various parts of the clotting cascade to decrease clot formation or dissolve existing clots (Table 3-4). Figure 3-4 depicts the various steps and clotting factors within the clotting cascade.

> **SAFETY ALERT!** All medications for clotting disorders carry a risk of bleeding or hemorrhage. Clients should be monitored for signs and symptoms of bleeding such as petechiae, epistaxis, melena, hematuria, and an increased duration, and/or amount of menses.

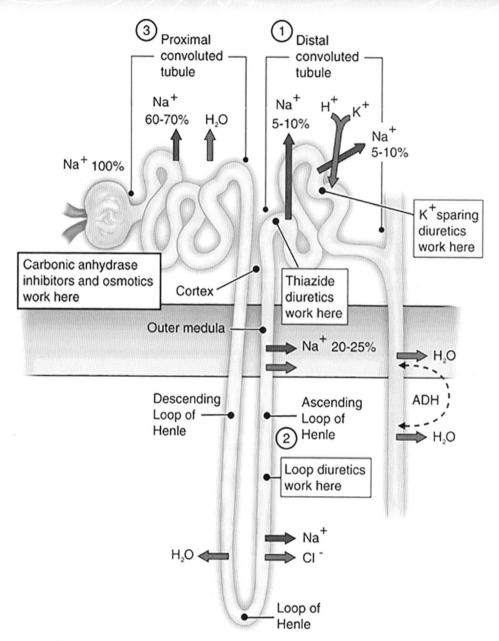

Figure 3-3 Diuretics in the nephron. (Reprinted with permission from Aschenbrenner, D., Venable, S. *Drug Therapy in Nursing*, 4th edition. Philadelphia: Wolters Kluwer Health, 2012.)

SAFETY ALERT! Utilize nursing measures to reduce the risk of bleeding, including avoiding IM injections and unnecessary venipuncture, use of soft-bristle toothbrush and electric razor, avoid other medications that promote bleeding, placing the client on fall precautions, and instructing the client to avoid straining.

Table 3-2

Drugs Used to Treat Hypertension, Heart Failure, Angina, and Myocardial Infarction

Class	Prototype	Mechanism of Action	Major Side and Adverse Effects	Critical Information	Indications
Loop diuretic	Furosemide	Block sodium and water reabsorption in the ascending loop of Henle	Side effects are related to the loss of water and electrolytes, including dehydration, hypokalemia, hypomagnesemia, hyponatremia, and hypochloremia Dehydration can lead to potentially dangerous hypotension Loop diuretics may increase uric acid levels, which can worsen gout in clients with a history of that disorder	Potassium wasting Use caution if using this medication with other ototoxic drugs (such as gentamicin), as the combination may lead to hearing loss NSAIDs reduce the effectiveness of loop diuretics Alterations in sodium and potassium may lead to toxic levels of lithium and digoxin BP should be monitored frequently Monitor for signs and symptoms of electrolyte imbalance(s)	Edema, HTN, HF, short-term treatment of hyperkalemia
Thiazide diuretic	Hydrochlorothiazide (HCTZ)	Block sodium and water reabsorption in the distal convoluted tubule	Side effects are related to the loss of water and electrolytes, including dehydration, hypokalemia, hypomagnesemia, hyponatremia, and hypochloremia Dehydration can lead to potentially dangerous hypotension Loop diuretics may increase uric acid levels, which can worsen gout in clients with a history of that disorder	Potassium wasting Cannot be used if renal function is impaired NSAIDs reduce the effectiveness of loop diuretics Alterations in sodium and potassium may lead to toxic levels of lithium and digoxin BP should be monitored frequently Monitor for signs and symptoms of electrolyte imbalance(s)	Edema, HTN, diabetes insipidus

(continued)

Table 3-2

Drugs Used to Treat Hypertension, Heart Failure, Angina, and Myocardial Infarction *(continued)*

Class	Prototype	Mechanism of Action	Major Side and Adverse Effects	Critical Information	Indications
Potassium-sparing diuretic	Spironolactone	Increases sodium and water loss by blocking aldosterone in the distal portion of the nephron	Hyperkalemia, as blocking aldosterone prevents excretion of potassium by the kidneys Other side effects are related to endocrine effects, including hirsutism, voice deepening, and gynecomastia	Potassium sparing Use caution when administering this medication with other drugs that increase potassium levels (ACE inhibitors, ARBs) Instruct clients that endocrine side effects will resolve when the medication is stopped	Edema, HTN, HF
Angiotensin-converting enzyme (ACE) inhibitors	Lisinopril "pril"	Inhibits ACE, the enzyme that converts angiotensin I to angiotensin II and causes vasoconstriction Inhibition of ACE also decreases cardiac remodeling through decreased angiotensin II Decreased angiotensin II decreased pressure in glomeruli, which can decrease the rate of nephropathy in clients with diabetes	Hypotension, which is worse with the first dose due to vasodilation Increased bradykinin leads to cough (nonproductive) Other side effects include hyperkalemia and worsening of renal function Adverse effects include fetal harm and angioedema	Dose reduction is required for clients with renal dysfunction Change positions slowly, fall precautions when first initiated If cough develops, client may switch to an ARB Never use an ACE inhibitor if a client has a history of angioedema from an ACE inhibitor or an ARB Avoid in pregnancy	HTN, HF, MI, nephropathy
Angiotensin II receptor blockers (ARBs)	Losartan "artan"	Block receptors for angiotensin II	Side effects include hypotension, hyperkalemia, and worsening of renal function Adverse effects include fetal harm and angioedema	Dose reduction is required for clients with renal dysfunction Never use an ARB if a client has a history of angioedema from an ACE inhibitor or an ARB Less risk of cough with ARBs Avoid in pregnancy	HTN, HF, MI, nephropathy

Class	Drug	Action	Side effects/Adverse effects	Nursing considerations	Indication
Direct renin inhibitor	Aliskiren	Inhibits renin, which then blocks the production of angiotensin I by preventing its conversion from angiotensinogen	Usually well tolerated. Side effects include diarrhea and cough (rare)	Avoid in pregnancy. May increase potassium levels if used with other medications that may cause hyperkalemia (spironolactone, ACE inhibitors)	HTN
Calcium channel blocker (benzothiazepine family)	Diltiazem	Block calcium channels in the vessels, which causes vasodilation and improves perfusion of coronary arteries. Blockage of calcium channels in the heart decreases heart rate, conduction velocity from the atria to the ventricle, and reduces contractility	Well tolerated, constipation is the most common side effect. Hypotension, bradycardia, atrioventricular (AV) blockade, and decreased contractility are potential adverse effects that may be harmful for clients with cardiac disease	Increase fiber and fluids to ease constipation. Check BP and HR prior to administering and hold for HR <60/min, and/or systolic BP <90 mm Hg. Avoid use in clients with second- or third-degree AV block or bradycardic dysrhythmias. Beta-blockers have similar effects on arteries and the heart; avoid concurrent use. Monitor for AV blockade if combined with digoxin. Overdose treated with calcium gluconate	HTN, angina, atrial tachydysrhythmias
Calcium channel blocker (dihydropyridine family)	Nifedipine	Block calcium channels in the blood vessels, which causes vasodilation and improves perfusion of coronary arteries	Side effects include hypotension, flushing, and headache. Decreasing BP leads to triggering of the baroreceptor reflex, which increased HR and contractility of the heart, causing a common side effect of reflex tachycardia	Nifedipine does not block calcium channels in the heart. Usually combined with a beta-blocker to treat reflex tachycardia	HTN, stable, variant angina

(continued)

Table 3-2

Drugs Used to Treat Hypertension, Heart Failure, Angina, and Myocardial Infarction (continued)

Class	Prototype	Mechanism of Action	Major Side and Adverse Effects	Critical Information	Indications
Arterial vasodilator	Hydralazine	Dilation of arteries	Common side effects include headache and fatigue	Combined with beta-blocker to treat reflex tachycardia	HTN, HF, hypertensive crisis
			Trigger of baroreceptors leads to reflex tachycardia	Combined with loop diuretic to treat increased fluid volume	
			Sodium and water retention may occur as a response to decreased BP	Discontinue for SLE-like symptoms	
			Systemic lupus erythematosus (SLE)-like symptoms can occur, such as joint pain, fever, rash		
Venous vasodilator	Nitroglycerin	Dilation of veins through the conversion of nitrate to nitric oxide	Side effects occur as the result of venous vasodilation: headache, flushing, reflex tachycardia, and hypotension	Lipid soluble, high first-pass effect, so cannot be given orally	Stable, unstable, and variant angina, MI
		Decreases oxygen demand (stable angina), decreases coronary spasm (variant angina)		Monitor BP	
				May administer 1 tablet sublingually every 5 min × 3 doses	
				If chest pain not relieved after 1 dose, client should call 911	
				Use caution when used with other medications that lower BP	
				Discontinue use of patches or ointment slowly to prevent rebound angina	
				Contraindicated in clients who have taken a phosphodiasterase-5 inhibitor (e.g, sildenafil) within the last 24 hours due to severe hypotension when the two medications are combined	

		Action	Side/Adverse effects	Nursing considerations	Indication
Venous and arterial vasodilator	Sodium nitroprusside	Dilation of veins and arteries via nitric acid, which is produced as a by-product of nitroprusside	Adverse effects include severe hypotension and cyanide poisoning	Use with caution in clients with liver disease Avoid rapid infusion Normally this medication is brown in color Medication must be protected from light IV administration only	Hypertensive emergencies
Selective alpha-1 blocker/alpha adrenergic antagonist	Prazosin	Blocks alpha-1 receptors, causing dilation of arteries and veins	Side effects include dizziness, hypotension, nasal congestion, and reflex tachycardia as a result of vasodilation and alpha-1 blockade	First-dose loss of consciousness may occur—clients should take this medication at bedtime Avoid potentially dangerous activities (driving, drinking alcohol, taking a bath) for 24 hr after the first dose Instruct clients on safety to prevent falls secondary to orthostatic hypotension	HTN
Nonselective beta-blocker/beta adrenergic antagonist	Propranolol "lol"	Blocks beta-1 and beta-2 adrenergic receptors, reducing heart rate, AV node conduction, and contractility	Side effects of beta-1 blockade include bradycardia and AV node blocks, hyperglycemia Side effects of beta-2 blockade include bronchospasm Adverse effects include AV heart block, asthma exacerbation, and HF exacerbation	Avoid in clients with HF, as this medication may worsen symptoms related to decreased contractility Avoid in clients with asthma Inform clients with diabetes of the impact of beta-blockers on blood sugar as well as the effect of beta-blockers on HR Tachycardia is usually the first sign of hypoglycemia for clients, which may not occur when beta-1 blockade is in place Do not use with calcium channel blockers Discontinue slowly to avoid rebound tachycardia and angina	HTN, angina, MI, dysrhythmias

(continued)

Table 3-2

Drugs Used to Treat Hypertension, Heart Failure, Angina, and Myocardial Infarction (continued)

Class	Prototype	Mechanism of Action	Major Side and Adverse Effects	Critical Information	Indications
Cardioselective beta-blocker/ beta adrenergic antagonist	Metoprolol "lol"	Blocks beta-1 receptors, reducing heart rate, AV node conduction, and contractility	Side effects of beta-1 blockade include bradycardia and AV node blocks, hyperglycemia Adverse effects include AV heart block and exacerbation of HF	At very high doses, this medication can lose selectivity and cause bronchospasm Do not use in clients with AV heart block Use with caution in clients with HF; monitor for worsening signs and symptoms	HTN, HF, MI, stable, and unstable angina
Cardiac glycoside	Digoxin	Inhibits sodium–potassium ATPase enzyme, which causes calcium to accumulate within the heart Increased calcium increases cardiac contractility Digoxin also increases the heart's response to acetylcholine	Side effects include: nausea, headache, diarrhea, bradycardia Adverse reactions include cardiac dysrhythmias such as AV block and/or ventricular fibrillation and thrombocytopenia Symptoms of toxicity include vomiting, fatigue, and yellow halos around objects	Narrow therapeutic range, risk of toxicity Normal range = 0.8–2 ng/mL (1.02–2.56 nmol/L) Check apical pulse for one full minute prior to administering; if HR <60 beats/min, do not administer Review serum potassium levels prior to administration Use caution when combined with medications that alter potassium levels (loop and thiazide diuretics, ACE inhibitors and ARBs) May shorten life span in women with HF Teach clients symptoms of toxicity and to report them immediately	Symptom relief of HF, treatment of atrial tachydysrhythmias

Sympathomimetic	Dobutamine	Activates beta-1 adrenergic receptors to increase cardiac contractility and cardiac output	Side effects include nausea, headache, and phlebitis Adverse effects include tachycardia, which can increase cardiac workload in HF, hypotension, and bronchospasm	Must be administered intravenously	Acute HF
Opioid	Morphine	Binds to opioid receptors to decrease pain Also improves coronary blood flow and decrease oxygen demand through vasodilatory properties	Common side effects include constipation, central nervous system depression Adverse effects include respiratory depression and arrest that is potentially fatal	Do not administer if respiratory rate <10 breaths/min Monitor level of consciousness, BP Administer naloxone in the event of overdose	Pain of MI
Antianginal	Ranolazine	Unknown, reduces frequency of angina	Common side effects include headache and constipation Adverse effects include prolonged QT interval that can result in a potentially fatal dysrhythmia known as torsades de pointes and increased BP	Monitor BP Avoid in clients with prolonged QT interval Prepare to administer IV magnesium sulfate if torsades de pointes occurs	Angina

HF, heart failure; HTN, hypertension; MI, myocardial infarction; NSAID, nonsteroidal anti-inflammatory drug.

Table 3-3

Drugs Used to Treat Dysrhythmias

Class	Prototype	Mechanism of Action	Major Side and Adverse Effects	Critical Information	Indications
IB: Sodium channel blocker	Lidocaine	Block sodium channels in the heart to decrease conduction from the atria to the ventricle, shortens action potential, and decreases automaticity	Usually well tolerated Lidocaine crosses the blood–brain barrier and can cause central nervous system effects such as confusion Toxic doses can lead to respiratory arrest and seizures	Reduced dosing with liver dysfunction to decrease the risk of toxicity Must continuously monitor BP and cardiac rhythm IV route only	Ventricular dysrhythmias
II: Beta-blockers	Propranolol	Blockade of beta-1 and beta-2 adrenergic receptors, which decreases heart rate, AV node conduction velocity, and cardiac contractility	Usually well tolerated Side effects include fatigue, impotence, dizziness, exercise intolerance Blockade of beta-1 receptors can result in bradycardia, AV blocks, and worsening of heart failure by decreasing contractility Blockade of beta-2 receptors can cause bronchospasm in clients with asthma	Avoid in clients with asthma Do not discontinue abruptly Monitor for signs and symptoms of heart failure	Atrial and ventricular tachydysrhythmias

Class	Drug	Action	Side/Adverse effects	Nursing considerations	Use
III: Delay repolarization	Amiodarone	Delay repolarization of fast action potentials by blocking potassium channels Blockade of sodium and calcium channels causes decreases in automaticity and contractility	Common side effects include fatigue, dizziness, corneal deposits, and photosensitivity Central nervous system side effects include changes in mood and hallucinations There are many adverse effects caused by amiodarone, especially organ-specific toxicities Pulmonary toxicity: pulmonary fibrosis Cardiac toxicity: dysrhythmias and worsening of HF Thyroid toxicity: hypo- or hyperthyroidism Liver toxicity: liver dysfunction and possible liver failure Eye effects: optic neuritis or neuropathy Skin effects: photosensitivity, alteration in skin color if prolonged sun exposure	Obtain baseline and frequent testing to monitor for toxicities including chest x-ray, pulmonary function tests, thyroid function, liver function tests, eye exams Avoid in pregnancy and breast-feeding Wear sunscreen, avoid prolonged times in the sun Very long half-life of amiodarone results in long duration of side and adverse effects IV administration can cause severe hypotension and bradycardia	Atrial and ventricular dysrhythmias
IV: Calcium channel blockers	Verapamil	Blockade of calcium channels in the heart that causes decreased heart rate, slowed AV node conduction, and decreased cardiac contractility	Well tolerated, constipation is the most common side effect Hypotension, bradycardia, atrioventricular (AV) blockade, and decreased contractility are potential adverse effects that may be harmful for clients with cardiac disease	Monitor for signs and symptoms of HF Calcium channel blockers can increase risk of digoxin toxicity Avoid use in combination with beta-blockers due to potentiative effects	Atrial tachydysrhythmias

(continued)

Table 3-3

Drugs Used to Treat Dysrhythmias *(continued)*

Class	Prototype	Mechanism of Action	Major Side and Adverse Effects	Critical Information	Indications
Cardiac glycoside	Digoxin	Inhibits sodium–potassium ATPase enzyme, which causes decreased AV node conduction speed and decreased automaticity	Side effects include nausea, headache, diarrhea, bradycardia Adverse reactions include cardiac dysrhythmias such as AV block and/or ventricular fibrillation and thrombocytopenia Symptoms of toxicity include vomiting, fatigue, and yellow halos around objects	Narrow therapeutic range, risk of toxicity Normal range = 0.8–2 ng/mL (1.02–2.56 nmol/L) Check apical pulse for one full minute prior to administering; if HR < 60 beats/min, do not administer Review serum potassium levels prior to administration Use caution when combined with medications that alter potassium levels (loop and thiazide diuretics, ACE inhibitors, and ARBs) Teach clients symptoms of toxicity and to report them immediately	Atrial tachydysrhythmias
Other antidysrhythmic	Adenosine	Activates adenosine receptors to slow AV node conduction and improve blood flow of coronary arteries via vasodilation	Common side effects include flushing, chest discomfort, and light-headedness Adverse effects include cardiac arrest, hypotension, severe bradycardia	Very short half-life (10 seconds), side effects are short lasting Be sure to have emergency cardiac resuscitation equipment available at the bedside Infuse rapidly at IV site closest to the heart followed by rapid saline flush May administer 3 doses	Supraventricular tachycardia

ACE, angiotensin-converting enzyme; ARB, angiotensin II receptor blocker; HF, heart failure; HR, heart rate; HTN, hypertension; IV, intravenous.

Table 3-4

Drugs Used to Treat Clotting Disorders

Class	Prototype	Mechanism of Action	Major Side and Adverse Effects	Critical Information	Indications
Anticoagulant: antithrombin activators	Heparin Enoxaparin	Inactivates clotting factors thrombin and factor Xa through the increased activity of antithrombin Enoxaparin effects factor Xa more than thrombin	The most critical adverse effect of heparin and enoxaparin is hemorrhage Heparin-induced thrombocytopenia is an allergic reaction causing decreased platelet counts Other allergic reactions may occur, causing urticaria, fever, or anaphylaxis Common side effects include injection site reactions (pain, bruising, redness)	Cannot be used orally Heparin is administered IV or subcutaneously Enoxaparin is weight-based dosing and administered subcutaneously Heparin requires frequent monitoring of activated partial thromboplastin (aPTT) levels Enoxaparin does not require laboratory monitoring of levels Platelet levels should be monitored with heparin and the medication should be stopped for platelet levels <100,000/mm^3 Use caution with heparin or enoxaparin in clients with recent spinal surgery, epidural or spinal catheters Use caution with other medications that promote bleeding (warfarin, aspirin, NSAIDs) Contraindicated in clients with bleeding disorders (hemophilia, thrombocytopenia) or risk of bleeding such as uncontrolled hypertension or presence of aneurysm Treatment of overdose or hemorrhage caused by heparin or enoxaparin is with IV protamine sulfate Normal aPTT level for client on heparin is 60–80 seconds	Hypercoagulation during pregnancy, treatment or prevention of DVT, and/or PE, adjunct therapy during MI

(continued)

Table 3-4

Drugs Used to Treat Clotting Disorders (continued)

Class	Prototype	Mechanism of Action	Major Side and Adverse Effects	Critical Information	Indications
Anticoagulant: vitamin K antagonist	Warfarin	Decreases the formation of the vitamin K–dependent clotting factors VII, IX, X, and prothrombin through the inhibition of the enzyme vitamin K epoxide reductase	Common side effects include: nausea, vomiting, diarrhea, bruising, headache, and alopecia The most critical adverse effect of warfarin is hemorrhage Other adverse effects include necrosis of the skin and osteoporosis with long-term use	Avoid in pregnancy or breast-feeding Frequent monitoring of bleeding times required with prothrombin (PT) and international normalized ratio (INR) levels Educate clients about the consistent intake of vitamin K–containing foods (green leafy vegetables, mayonnaise) Use caution with other medications that promote bleeding (heparin, aspirin, NSAIDs) Contraindicated in clients with bleeding disorders (hemophilia, thrombocytopenia) or risk of bleeding such as uncontrolled hypertension or presence of aneurysm Treatment of overdose/hemorrhage is with vitamin k (phytonadione) orally or IV Normal INR levels for client on warfarin is generally 2–3	Prevention of clot formation Prevention of stroke for clients with atrial fibrillation
Direct thrombin inhibitor	Dabigatran etexilate	Reversible inhibition of thrombin, which prevents the production of fibrin	Side effects include nausea, abdominal pain, reflux symptoms, and gastritis The most critical adverse effect is bleeding. Others include GI hemorrhage and GI ulcers	Stop medication before surgery Store the medication in the bottle dispensed to maintain effectiveness No blood monitoring required	Stroke prevention with atrial fibrillation, prevention and treatment of DVT and/or PE
Direct factor Xa inhibitor	Rivaroxaban	Inhibits clotting factor Xa, which decreases production of thrombin	Bleeding is the most common adverse effect	Avoid if recent spinal puncture Dose should be reduced for clients with renal dysfunction Avoid use in clients with liver dysfunction	Stroke prevention with atrial fibrillation, prevention and/or treatment of DVT and/or PE

Classification	Medication	Action	Side/Adverse Effects	Nursing Considerations	Uses
Antiplatelet: cyclooxygenase inhibitor	Aspirin (ASA)	Suppression of platelet aggregation through irreversible inhibition of cyclooxygenase	Side effects include gastric upset, tinnitus (at higher doses), bruising, and bleeding Adverse effects include hemorrhage, GI bleeding, and hemorrhagic stroke, especially in the setting of uncontrolled hypertension	Lower doses used for prevention Higher doses used for acute problem (MI, unstable angina) Frequently used with proton pump inhibitor to decrease gastric discomfort Use of enteric-coated tablets can also decrease GI irritation	Reduce risk of stroke, transient ischemic attack, primary and secondary prevention of MI Treatment during current episodes of unstable angina and MI Prevent occlusion of cardiac stents
Antiplatelet: P2Y$_{12}$ adenosine diphosphate receptor antagonist	Clopidogrel	Preventing platelet aggregation through the blocking of P2Y$_{12}$ ADP receptors	Side effects include diarrhea and gastric discomfort Adverse effects include bleeding and thrombocytopenia	Always use with aspirin for clients with acute coronary syndrome Monitor platelet levels Use caution when combining with other medications that cause bleeding Take clopidogrel 12 hr apart from proton pump inhibitors	Prevent blockage of cardiac stents, reduce risk of MI and stroke for those at high risk Current episode of unstable angina or MI
Glycoprotein IIb/IIIa receptor antagonist	Abciximab	Block GP IIb/IIIa receptors that stop platelet aggregation	Common side effects include nausea, hypotension, injection site pain Adverse effects include bleeding and thrombocytopenia	Use caution when combining with other medications that cause bleeding	Prevention of clot formation during cardiac catheterization
Thrombolytic	Alteplase	Creates plasmin that breaks up a clot through the binding of alteplase with plasminogen	Common side effects include bleeding The most serious adverse effect is severe bleeding	IV infusion only Consider contraindications to dissolving clots: history of hemorrhagic stroke, internal bleeding, uncontrolled hypertension, pregnancy, recent trauma	Acute MI, ischemic stroke, PE

DVT, deep vein thrombosis; GI, gastrointestinal; IV, intravenous; MI, myocardial infarction; NSAID, nonsteroidal anti-inflammatory drug; PE, pulmonary embolism.

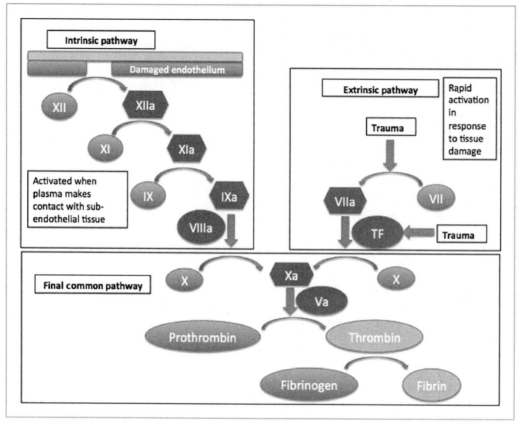

Figure 3-4 Classical clotting cascade. (Reprinted with permission from Bucklin, B., Baysinger, C., Gambling, D. *A Practical Approach to Obstetric Anesthesia*, 2nd edition. Philadelphia: Wolters Kluwer Health, 2016.)

Hyperlipidemia

Certain medications are used to lower LDLs and/or VLDLs, increase HDLs, or prevent atherosclerosis in clients with an increased risk of cardiac disease (e.g., clients with diabetes mellitus). See Table 3-5 for a description of these agents.

Table 3-5

Drugs Used to Treat Hyperlipidemia

Class	Prototype	Mechanism of Action	Major Side and Adverse Effects	Critical Information	Indications
HMG-CoA reductase inhibitor "statins"	Lovastatin	Inhibits HMG-CoA reductase, the enzyme responsible for decreasing LDL receptors in the liver Increasing receptors for LDL synthesis leads to lowered LDL levels	Common side effects include headache, abdominal pain, and diarrhea Statins can cause muscle breakdown that can progress to rhabdomyolysis that can be fatal Hepatotoxicity, memory loss, and new onset of diabetes mellitus can occur	Lowers LDL and total cholesterol Increases HDL Take at bedtime for best effects Avoid use in pregnancy Monitor liver function at baseline and periodically thereafter If muscle pain occurs, creatine kinase levels should be checked There are non–cholesterol-related benefits of statins, including stabilization of atherosclerotic plaques, vasodilation, and increased formation of bone	Elevated cholesterol, primary prevention of MI, angina, and stroke, cardiac risk reduction for clients with diabetes, secondary prevention after MI
Bile acid sequestrant	Colesevelam	Binds bile acids in the GI tract for removal via stool. The decrease in bile acids creates increased LDL receptors in the liver, which reduces circulating LDL	Not systemically absorbed, so side effects occur within the GI tract and not systemically Common side effects include constipation, bloating, and nausea	Lowers LDL cholesterol May bind with other drugs in the GI tract; take this medication 1 hr before or 4 hr after all other medications	Lowering of LDL cholesterol, also used as adjunct treatment of type 2 diabetes mellitus
Cholesterol absorption inhibitor	Ezetimibe	Inhibit dietary cholesterol absorption in the GI tract	Generally well tolerated Common side effects include diarrhea and muscle pain Adverse effects include thrombocytopenia, pancreatitis, and rhabdomyolysis	Lowers LDL, total, and VLDL levels Increased risk of hepatotoxicity if combined with a statin Increased risk of gallstones if used with a bile acid sequestrant	Lowering of LDL and VLDL levels

(continued)

Table 3-5

Drugs Used to Treat Hyperlipidemia *(continued)*

Class	Prototype	Mechanism of Action	Major Side and Adverse Effects	Critical Information	Indications
Fibric acid derivative	Gemfibrozil	Hasten the clearance of VLDLs through the activation of peroxisome proliferator–activated receptor alpha	Well tolerated Side effects include nausea, diarrhea Increased risk of gallstones	Lowers VLDL Increased HDL Teach clients signs and symptoms of gallstones (right upper quadrant abdominal pain, bloating) Increases levels of warfarin, monitor PT/INR levels	Reduction of VLDL levels
Monoclonal antibody	Alirocumab	Binding of LDL receptors to reduce circulating levels through the protein proprotein convertase subtilisin/kexin type 9	Allergic reactions may occur, and injection site reactions are common	Administration is subcutaneous injection every 2 weeks	Very high levels of LDL

GI, gastrointestinal; HDL, high-density lipoprotein; HMG-CoA, 3-hydroxy-3-methyl-glutaryl-coenzyme A; LDL, low-density lipoprotein; MI, myocardial infarction; VLDL, very-low-density lipoprotein.

Practice Questions and Rationales

1. A client prescribed losartan calls the nurse to report muscle weakness and palpitations. What is the **priority** action by the nurse?
   1. Ask the client to check the blood pressure (BP) immediately.
   2. Suggest that the client replace sodium with salt substitutes.
   3. Instruct the client to hold the medication for the next 48 hours.
   4. Tell the client to report to the emergency department for evaluation.

2. A client with heart failure is due for the prescribed digoxin, spironolactone, lisinopril, and furosemide. Over the past 3 days, the client has gained 2 pounds and reports worsening shortness of breath. Physical assessment reveals jugular vein distention of 5cm, 2+ pitting edema, and heart rate of 52 beats per minute. What is the **priority** action by the nurse?
   1. Hold the furosemide and contact the provider.
   2. Administer all medications and document assessment findings.
   3. Hold the digoxin and administer all other medications as ordered.
   4. Apply oxygen via nasal cannula and withhold all medications.

3. A client with a deep vein thrombosis (DVT) has been prescribed rivaroxaban. Which statement indicates effective teaching by the nurse?
   1. "I will maintain a consistent intake of canola and vegetable oils."
   2. "My blood levels will need to be checked every week until my DVT is gone."
   3. "I should stop taking this medication when my leg is no longer swollen."
   4. "If my stool becomes darker, I will notify my provider immediately."

4. A client presents to the emergency department with chest pain. The ECG reveals ST-segment elevation. Vital signs are as follows: blood pressure 142/78 mm Hg, pulse 98 beats/min, respiratory rate 18 breaths/min, temperature 100.6°F (38.1°C), and oxygen saturation 98%. The nurse should prepare to perform which actions? Select all that apply.
   1. Administer 2 L oxygen via nasal cannula.
   2. Obtain blood for laboratory testing.
   3. Administer aspirin 325 mg orally.
   4. Prepare to infuse diltiazem intravenously.
   5. Provide the client with three tablets of sublingual nitroglycerin immediately.

5. A client with hyperlipidemia and type 2 diabetes who has been taking metformin is newly prescribed colesevelam. Which statement, if made by the client, would require additional teaching by the nurse?
   1. "I should take this medication an hour before I take my other diabetes medications."
   2. "If I experience constipation, I should increase my water and fiber intake."
   3. "I can expect a slight increase in my blood sugar while taking this medication."
   4. "It is possible that I may need to decrease the dosage of my metformin now."

6. A client recovering from an ST-segment myocardial infarction (STEMI) is newly prescribed high-dose lovastatin. Which assessment finding would require immediate intervention by the nurse?

    1. Ventricular trigeminy on the cardiac monitor

    2. Tea-colored urine

    3. Blood pressure (BP) 100/60 mm Hg

    4. Bilateral crackles in lower lung lobes

7. A client is on a heparin intravenous infusion for the treatment of a pulmonary embolus. The most recent laboratory values indicate an activated partial thromboplastin time (aPTT) of 100 seconds, platelet count of 88,000 × 10³/μL (88 × 10⁹/L), and a hemoglobin of 10 g/dL (100 g/L). Based on these findings, what is the **correct** action by the nurse?

    1. Increase the heparin infusion by 2 units/hr.

    2. Continue the infusion and assess the client for signs of bleeding.

    3. Stop the infusion and notify the prescriber.

    4. Continue the heparin infusion and document the findings.

8. A client with atrial fibrillation and hypertriglyceridemia on warfarin is newly prescribed gemfibrozil. With the first dose of gemfibrozil, the prescriber advises the nurse to administer an increased dose of warfarin. What is the appropriate action by the nurse?

    1. Administer both medications as prescribed.

    2. Review the most recent prothrombin time (PT) and international normalized ratio (INR) levels.

    3. Consult with the prescriber to recommend a decreased dose of warfarin.

    4. Hold gemfibrozil until updated cholesterol levels are obtained.

9. A client with atrial flutter is taking verapamil. Which new finding on the ECG would require the nurse to hold the medication and notify the prescriber?

    1. PR interval 0.3 milliseconds

    2. Ventricular rate 125 beats per minute

    3. Atrial-to-ventricular ratio of 4:1

    4. Occasional premature ventricular contractions (PVCs)

10. A client presents to the emergency department with reports of palpitations, light-headedness, and shortness of breath. The cardiac monitor shows the rhythm below. What are the **priority** actions by the nurse? Select all that apply.

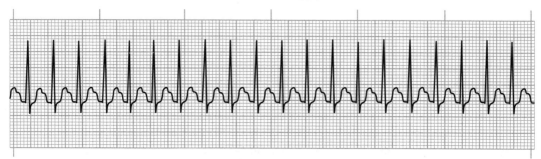

    1. Apply 2 L oxygen via nasal cannula.

    2. Ask the client to perform the Valsalva maneuver.

3. Apply the pacer pads onto the client's chest.
4. Prepare to administer intravenous adenosine.
5. Call the pharmacy to prepare an intravenous infusion of amiodarone.

11. The nurse is caring for a client with an acute exacerbation of heart failure (HF). The client is prescribed spironolactone, losartan, and digoxin. The client reports little improvement of symptoms despite taking all medications as prescribed. Which additional interventions should the nurse recommend? Select all that apply.
    1. Decrease sodium intake to <2 g/day.
    2. Contact the provider to suggest adding furosemide to the medication regimen.
    3. Advise the client to take an additional dose of spironolactone for the next 2 days.
    4. Increase the client's fluid intake to 2.5 L/day.
    5. Increase dietary potassium to improve cardiac function.

12. A client with hypertension has been taking metoprolol for several months. Which assessment finding, if present, would require immediate intervention by the nurse?
    1. Heart rate 62 beats per minute
    2. Bilateral lower extremity edema
    3. Diminished breath sounds in the left lower lung lobe
    4. Serum blood glucose 200 mg/dL (11.1 mmol/L)

13. A client will begin taking prazosin. What is the appropriate action by the nurse?
    1. Administer the medication with food.
    2. Raise all side rails of the hospital bed prior to sleep.
    3. Provide the first dose prior to breakfast.
    4. Offer to take the client to the restroom every 2 hours.

14. Use the heparin protocol below to identify the initial dose of the heparin infusion. Client weight = 168 pounds. Round the answer to the nearest tenth.

PTT (s)	Bolus Dose	Infusion Rate
Initial dose	80 units/kg bolus	Begin infusion at 18 units/kg/hr
aPTT < 35 s	80 units/kg bolus	Increase infusion rate by 4 units/kg/hr
aPTT 35–45 s	40 units/kg bolus	Increase infusion rate by 2 units/kg/hr
aPTT > 45–60	No bolus	Increase infusion rate by 2 units/kg/hr
aPTT > 60–80	No bolus	No change
aPTT > 80–90	No bolus	Decrease infusion rate by 2 units/kg/hr
aPTT > 90	No bolus	Hold infusion for 1 hr then restart and decrease infusion rate by 3 units/kg/hr

_____units/hr

15. Heparin is premixed 25,000 units in 500 mL normal saline. How many milliliters per hour will the nurse administer based on the calculations in question 14? Round the answer to the nearest tenth.

16. Which finding would require the nurse to hold the administration of furosemide?

    1.   Hyperkalemia

    2.   Hyponatremia

    3.   Hyperchloremia

    4.   Hypoxia

17. Which statement compares the difference between nifedipine and hydralazine?

    1.   Nifedipine causes vasodilatation and improves perfusion of coronary arteries.

    2.   Hydralazine causes vasoconstriction and improves blood flow to the organs.

    3.   Both agents affect dilation of veins and arteries.

    4.   Both agents are used to assist with decreasing blood pressure in congestive heart failure.

18. A nurse is teaching a client about the addition of hydrochlorothiazide for a diagnosis of hypertension. Which statement by the nurse is included in the teaching plan?

    1.   "At times, you may experience palpitations and dizziness."

    2.   "Monitoring your food and fluid intake is important."

    3.   "Use NSAIDs such as ibuprofen infrequently."

    4.   "Weigh yourself once a week."

19. Which meal is appropriate for a client taking spironolactone?

    1.   Bacon, eggs, coffee, and banana

    2.   Turkey sandwich, low-sodium chips, and water

    3.   Spinach salad with strawberries and nuts, crackers, and seltzer soda

    4.   A small cherry pastry, low-fat yogurt, and cup of orange juice

20. A nurse is caring for client who was prescribed lisinopril. The client tells the nurse that they are experiencing a cough. Which medication does the nurse anticipate the prescriber to prescribe as an alternative to lisinopril?

    1.   Losartan

    2.   Hydralazine

    3.   Furosemide

    4.   Verapamil

21. Which medications are safe for a pregnant client who has hypertension? Select all that apply.

    1.   Hydralazine

    2.   Lisinopril

    3.   Losartan

    4.   Furosemide

    5.   Verapamil

22. A nurse is caring for a client who has been prescribed diltiazem. Which statement is used in teaching the client about the medication?

    1.   "You should check your blood pressure (BP) and heart rate three times a day."

    2.   "Weigh yourself every week to monitor for weight loss."

3. "The medication should be taken early in the morning to avoid a cough."
4. "Increase your fluids and fiber to prevent constipation."

23. A nurse is caring for a client who has been prescribed digoxin. Which laboratory value would indicate that the nurse should hold the medication?

    1. WBC count 12,000/µL (12 x 10⁹/L)
    2. Potassium level of 3.6 mEq/L (3.6 mmol/L)
    3. Serum digoxin level of 3 ng/mL (3.84 nmol/L)
    4. Blood urea nitrogen of 18 mg/dL (6.43 mmol/L)

24. Which statement by the client receiving digoxin should warrant additional instruction?

    1. "If I experience any nausea, I should call provider."
    2. "I will check my heart rate before I take this medication."
    3. "This medication will slow down my heart rate."
    4. "I will hold this medication if my blood pressure (BP) is >100 mm Hg."

25. Which medications are used for a client who is experiencing an acute myocardial infarction (MI)? Select all that apply.

    1. Morphine
    2. Nitroglycerin
    3. Lisinopril
    4. Metoprolol
    5. Warfarin

26. A nurse is caring for a client who was prescribed gemfibrozil. Which laboratory value indicates the medication is working?

    1. Triglyceride level < 150 mg/dL (1.69 mmol/L)
    2. HDL > 30 mg/dL (0.78 mmol/L)
    3. LDL > 100 mg/dL (2.59 mmol/L)
    4. Total cholesterol < 200 mg/dL (5.18 mmol/L)

27. A client with an extensive cardiac history is prescribed omeprazole. The nurse reviews the medication history and the client is also prescribed clopidogrel, metoprolol, and furosemide. Which instruction should the nurse provide to the client regarding the medications?

    1. "Take all medications with food in the morning."
    2. "Clopidogrel, metoprolol, and furosemide can be taken together, but the omeprazole needs to be taken 4 hours after the other medications."
    3. "Clopidogrel should be taken 12 hours apart from the omeprazole."
    4. "Furosemide is taken in the morning, and the metoprolol is taken at night."

28. A nurse is teaching a client about dabigatran. Which instruction is warranted?

    1. "Use a soft-bristle toothbrush."
    2. "You should take a daily dose of aspirin."
    3. "Use the bedside commode for urinating and defecating."
    4. "You should prepare your family for your discharge tomorrow."

29. A nurse is caring for a client who is prescribed lovastatin. Which instruction is correct regarding the medication?

    1. "Take this medication at night."
    2. "Please check your blood pressure (BP) prior to taking the medication."
    3. "Weigh yourself daily and record it."
    4. "The medication may make you feel tired."

30. A client presents with chronic renal failure with dialysis. The client's blood pressure (BP) is 180/110 mm Hg. The prescriber orders an intravenous line to be placed and administration of sodium nitroprusside. Which statement is included in the instruction to the client about the medication?

    1. "The medication will assist to bring down your blood pressure."
    2. "You should feel less pain with this medication."
    3. "Be prepared to feel more relaxed and have a sense of relief."
    4. "The medication will decrease your oxygen demand and decrease coronary spasm."

4

RESPIRATORY MEDICATIONS

BRIEF OVERVIEW OF RESPIRATORY DISORDERS

The respiratory system performs several crucial functions within the body. The main responsibility of this system is delivering oxygen to the cardiovascular system for distribution throughout the body while removing carbon dioxide from the body. This gas exchange takes place in the alveoli of the lungs. Many of the medications used to treat respiratory disorders can be delivered via inhalation.

◆ **Asthma:** Asthma is a chronic inflammatory disorder of the airways that results in an obstruction of the airway. Asthma involves airway inflammation and bronchoconstriction as TREATMENT for asthma involves medications that both decrease inflammation and open the airways.

◆ **Chronic obstructive pulmonary disease (COPD):** COPD is defined as airflow obstruction caused by emphysema, chronic bronchitis, or a combination of the two. Treatment is mainly based on symptomatic management and is noncurative. Newer classes of medications may help to delay disease progression but cannot reverse the damage done.

◆ **Allergies:** Allergic rhinitis is the most common allergic disorder. It can be triggered by a number of indoor and/or outdoor allergens, and treatment is focused on a symptomatic approach. Intranasal glucocorticoids remain the gold standard of treatment.

◆ **Colds:** The common cold in an acute viral upper respiratory infection and presents with a combination of symptoms. It is self-limiting and usually resolves within 10 to 14 days. Since there is no cure, treatment is based upon symptom management.

CLINICAL PEARLS: RESPIRATORY DISORDERS

◆ Although corticosteroid use does slow growth in children temporarily, it does not reduce their overall final adult height.

◆ Asthma triggers can be environmental or physiologic and may even be related to certain medications or food additives.

◆ Most drugs for asthma are administered via inhalation. This both increases the therapeutic effect by delivering the drug as directly as possible to the action site (lungs) and reduces systemic effects by decreasing the amount of the drug circulating in the blood.

◆ Acute asthma exacerbations require immediate intervention, and full recovery may take weeks.

Asthma

Assessment

- ◆ It is important to assess the client's environment for triggers and allergens as part of the overall treatment plan.
- ◆ Asthma treatment entails a stepwise approach based on factors such as current symptoms, lung function tests, and frequency of quick-relief medication use.
- ◆ Ways to prevent adverse effects of inhalation using glucocorticoids therapy include the following:
  - ● Dysphonia/oropharyngeal candidiasis: Gargle after each administration, and use a spacer device. Candidiasis typically requires medical treatment.
  - ● Bone loss: Use the lowest dose possible, ensure adequate intake of calcium and vitamin D, and encourage regular participation in weight-bearing exercise.

Signs and Symptoms

- ◆ The signs and symptoms of asthma include breathlessness, cough, shortness of breath, chest tightness, wheezing and/or crackles in the lungs, decreased or absent lung sounds, use of accessory muscles for breathing, tachycardia, and tachypnea.

Diagnostics

- ◆ Decreased oxygen saturation rates ($SaO_2 < 95\%$)
- ◆ Pulmonary function tests
  - ● Spirometry
    - ▶ FEV_1 can range from normal to <60% of predicted value.
    - ▶ FEV_1/FVC can range from normal to a >5% change from predicted value.
  - ● Methacholine challenge test: Performed in cases where other lab values are not definitive for a diagnosis of asthma. The test determines if the client has a response to increasing amounts of methacholine (will cause airway to spasm and narrow if client has asthma). A test is considered positive if lung function drops by at least 20%.

> **SAFETY ALERT!** When giving a client a methacholine challenge test, always have a broncho-dilator on hand to reverse the effects of methacholine at the end of the test.

COPD

Assessment/Signs and Symptoms

- ◆ COPD is a noncurative diagnosis. Therefore, treatment goals are to reduce symptoms and maintain client health status.
- ◆ Signs and symptoms may include cough, exertional dyspnea, wheezing and crackles in the lungs, barrel chest appearance (if emphysema is present), use of accessory muscles for breathing, prolonged expiration, and orthopnea.

Diagnostics

◆ Chest x-ray to assess for the presence of congestion and hyperinflation
◆ Arterial blood gases to assess for respiratory acidosis and hypoxemia
◆ Decreased oxygen saturation rates
◆ Pulmonary function tests
  ● Spirometry
    ▸ FEV_1 can range from normal to <50% of predicted value.
    ▸ FEV_1/FVC < 70% from predicted value.

SAFETY ALERT! A client may require lesser amounts of supplemental oxygen than antici-pated related to the hypoxic drive to breathe in some clients with COPD. Monitoring PaO_2 levels will help determine which clients fall into this category.

Allergies

Assessment/Signs and Symptoms

◆ Allergies can be seasonal or perennial. Seasonal allergies are usually triggered by outdoor allergens such as pollen or mold, while perennial allergies are characterized by how fre-quently they occur, usually defined as at least 1 hour a day on most days throughout the year. Perennial allergies typically occur in response to animal dander, dust mites, smoke, and mold.
◆ Signs and symptoms may include sneezing, rhinorrhea, pruritus, and nasal congestion.

Diagnostics

◆ Allergies are typically treated based on symptom report. However, in severe cases, testing for allergy triggers can be performed.
  ● Type 1 immunoglobulin E (IgE) testing can be done via skin or blood testing. A posi-tive reaction to an allergen will result in a wheal and flare response where skin was tested.

Colds

Assessment/Signs and Symptoms

◆ The determination of a cold virus versus bacterial infection is often troublesome. Some ways to determine the client is dealing with more than a virus are if the symptoms last longer than 10 to 14 days, a high fever accompanies the symptoms, and if the fever worsens after 3 to 4 days rather than improving.
◆ Signs and symptoms may include rhinorrhea, cough, sneezing, nasal congestion, sore throat, and headache.

Diagnostics

◆ The diagnosis of the cold is based on symptom report. There are no diagnostic testing or labs to consider initially.

◆ If the client does not improve after 10 to 14 days, a reassessment and potential diagnostic imaging or labs may be considered.

MEDICATION OVERVIEW

Asthma

The medications used for asthma can be categorized into rescue (or quick-relief) medications and long-term control medications. (See Table 4-1 for more information on drugs used to treat asthma.) Asthma management and the types of medications needed will largely depend upon the client's age, severity of symptoms, and response to medications. The medications used to treat asthma will likely require adjustments over time and therefore require a close relationship with a client provider to treat this disorder.

◆ Clients should have a respiratory assessment at the start of treatment and periodically thereafter to ensure appropriate medical management.

◆ Peak flow meter should be used frequently to assess for symptom and medication management.

◆ If more than one inhaled medication is prescribed, the bronchodilator (short-acting beta2 agonist) should be given first to open the airways and increase airflow into the lungs, followed by the second inhaled medication 5 minutes later.

COPD

Medication management is a cornerstone of the treatment for COPD. The medications for this disorder are defined as either maintenance medications, which are used to help control and prevent exacerbations, or exacerbation management medications, which are used as needed to treat sudden flares of client symptoms. (See Table 4-2 for more information on drugs used to treat COPD.)

Allergies (Table 4-3)

Although allergies are usually not a curable disorder, there are several medications that can make the symptoms more manageable. Glucocorticoids, antihistamines, and decongestants, as well as combination medications, make up the majority of medications used to treat allergies. (See Table 4-3 for more information on drugs used to treat allergies.)

Colds

There is no cure for the common cold, but there are ways to help relieve some of the discomfort associated with the virus. For nasal congestion, decongestants may help, and for a cough, antitussives or expectorants, may be taken in order to obtain some relief. (See Table 4-4 for more information on drugs used to treat colds.)

Table 4-1

Drugs Used to Treat Asthma

Class	Prototype Medication	Mechanism of Action	Major Side and Adverse Effects	Critical Information	Indications
Beta2-adrenergic agonists (short acting)	Albuterol	Relaxes smooth muscle throughout the airway, allowing better airflow into the lungs	Bronchospasm, tachycardia, palpitations, tremors, and dry mouth	Preferred because of decreased systemic absorption and fewer adverse effects	Symptomatic quick relief for clients with asthma and/or undergoing an acute asthma attack
Beta2-adrenergic agonists (long acting)	Salmeterol	Relaxes smooth muscle throughout the airway, allowing better airflow into the lungs	Bronchospasm, tachycardia, palpitations, tremors, and hypertension	Not used for acute symptom management, but used prophylactically to prevent against asthma attacks	Used in conjunction with anti-inflammatory drugs such as corticosteroids for clients with asthma
Corticosteroids (inhaled)	Beclomethasone	Works by inhibiting the release of anti-inflammatory mediators and is minimally absorbed systemically due to inhaled administration	Hoarseness, oropharyngeal irritation, and oral candidiasis	Clients with diabetes should be closely monitored for hyperglycemia while on this medication	The most effective medication given for long-term treatment of asthma
Corticosteroids (oral)	Prednisone	Works by inhibiting the release of anti-inflammatory mediators and is absorbed systemically	Hyperglycemia, nausea and vomiting, and insomnia	Should be used in the lowest dose and for the shortest time to prevent adverse effects	Reserved for use with clients who have moderate to severe asthma exacerbations
Leukotriene modifiers	Montelukast	Suppresses the effects of leukotrienes, promoting airway dilation	Dizziness, headaches, nausea, vomiting, and cough	Less effective than inhaled glucocorticoids Use cautiously for clients with liver disease	Used for long-term management of asthma for clients with mild to moderate diagnosis

(continued)

Table 4-1

Drugs Used to Treat Asthma *(continued)*

Class	Prototype Medication	Mechanism of Action	Major Side and Adverse Effects	Critical Information	Indications
Methylxanthines	Theophylline	Relaxes the smooth muscle of the bronchi thereby decreasing airway reactivity and relaxing the bronchi	Nausea, vomiting, epigastric pain, abdominal cramping, diarrhea, headaches, restlessness, insomnia, dizziness, tachycardia, palpitations, and arrhythmias	Narrow therapeutic index Was widely used in past but has been replaced by safer and more effective medications Important to periodically draw blood to assess for toxicity High-fat meals can increase risk of theophylline toxicity Client should be encouraged to take with plenty of water to help avoid GI effects Smoking causes the medication to be metabolized faster—smokers may need an increased dose	Can be used to treat chronic stable asthma
Anticholinergics (inhaled)	Ipratropium bromide	Inhibits muscarinic receptors resulting in bronchial dilation	Oropharyngeal irritation and/or infection, trouble breathing, flu-like symptoms, paradoxical bronchospasm, difficulty or pain with voiding, and urinary tract infection	Off-label use for asthma The anticholinergic side effects including oropharyngeal irritation, and urinary retention can be particularly problematic for older adult clients and can result in medication noncompliance	Used as an adjunctive therapy to prevent wheezing and difficulty breathing
Mast cell stabilizers	Cromolyn	Reduces inflammation by preventing mast cells from releasing histamine along with other inflammatory mediators	Oropharyngeal irritation, wheezing, cough, headache, and metallic taste	*Safest* drug for asthma Administered via inhalation	Used for asthma prophylaxis and long-term control

GI, gastrointestinal.

Table 4-2

Drugs Used to Treat Chronic Obstructive Pulmonary Disease (COPD)

Class	Prototype Medication	Mechanism of Action	Major Side and Adverse Effects	Critical Information	Indications
Beta2-adrenergic agonists (short acting)	Albuterol	Relaxes smooth muscle throughout the airway, allowing better airflow into the lungs	Bronchospasm, tachycardia, palpitations, tremors, and dry mouth	Preferred because of decreased systemic absorption and fewer adverse effects	As needed for COPD exacerbations, although some clients are prescribed standing orders (maintenance therapy) for this medication
Beta2-adrenergic agonists (long acting)	Salmeterol	Relaxes smooth muscle throughout the airway, allowing better airflow into the lungs	Bronchospasm, tachycardia, palpitations, tremors, and hypertension		Maintenance therapy to help with lung function and help relieve shortness of breath
Corticosteroids (inhaled)	Beclomethasone	Works by inhibiting the release of anti-inflammatory mediators and reducing the amount of swelling in the airways	Hoarseness, oropharyngeal irritation, and oral candidiasis	Minimally absorbed systemically due to inhaled administration Clients with diabetes should be closely monitored for hyperglycemia while on this medication, although this is more common with oral/systemic steroid preparations	Used to help control COPD symptoms as part of daily maintenance therapy Can also be used during a symptom flare
Anticholinergics (inhaled)	Tiotropium bromide	Inhibits muscarinic receptors resulting in bronchial dilation	Tachycardia, nervousness, dizziness, and headache With high doses, difficulty urinating, constipation, and dry mouth	Off-label use	Frequently used in combination with a short-acting beta2-adrenergic agonist as long-term management, preventing wheezing and difficulty breathing
PDE-4 inhibitors	Roflumilast	Inhibition of the production of PDE-4 enzymes resulting in a strong anti-inflammatory response	Nausea, diarrhea, anorexia with associated weight loss, tremors, pain with urination, headache, dizziness, back pain, insomnia, flu-like symptoms	Contraindicated for clients with liver disease	Maintenance therapy for treatment of severe COPD to reduce the risk of exacerbations and prevent the worsening of symptoms

COPD, chronic obstructive pulmonary disease; PDE-4, phosphodiesterase 4.

Table 4-3

Drugs Used to Treat Allergies

Class	Prototype Medication	Mechanism of Action	Major Side and Adverse Effects	Critical Information	Indications
Glucocorticoids (intranasal)	Fluticasone	Decrease synthesis and release of inflammatory mediators	Drying of nasal mucosa and burning or itching sensation	Approximately 90% of clients respond to treatment Maximal response may take 1–3 weeks to develop	Relieve sneezing, runny nose, nasal congestion, and itching
Antihistamines	First generation: diphenhydramine Second generation: loratadine	Competitively blocks the binding of histamine to H_1 receptors	First generation: sedation, confusion, GI disturbances, dry mouth, constipation, and urinary retention Second generation: headache	Second generation do not cross blood–brain barrier as compared to first generation First generation have a centralized effect on the body and therefore can cause significant sedative effects as well Second generation has significantly fewer side effects when compared to first generation	Relieve sneezing, runny nose, watery eyes, and itching
Decongestants	Pseudoephedrine	Stimulates the alpha1-adrenergic receptors causing vasoconstriction in nasal blood vessels as well as throughout the respiratory tract. Also shrinks the swollen nasal membranes resulting in easier nasal drainage	Rebound congestion, restlessness, insomnia, anxiety, and vasoconstriction	Only relieves nasal congestion Avoid taking with other medications that act as sympathomimetics If taken with MAO inhibitors, severe hypertension or a hypertensive crisis may occur Clients who are hypertensive should not take this medication Caution for clients with diabetes: hyperthyroidism, BPH, glaucoma, and heart disease Rebound congestion can occur with intranasal administration Pseudoephedrine has the potential to be abused, and although it is available without a prescription, clients must purchase with a photo ID and are subject to limits on the amount of medication purchased	Relieves nasal, sinus, and eustachian tube congestion
Mast cell stabilizers (intranasal)	Cromolyn	Reduces inflammation by preventing the mast cells from releasing histamine along with other inflammatory mediators	Oropharyngeal irritation, wheezing, cough, headache, and metallic taste	Maximal response may take 1–2 weeks to develop As effective as antihistamines but less effective than intranasal corticosteroids more effective when taken prior to the onset of symptoms	Relieves runny nose and itchy eyes

BPH, benign prostatic hyperplasia; GI, gastrointestinal; MAO, monoamine oxidase.

Table 4-4

Drugs Used to Treat Colds

Class	Prototype Medication	Mechanism of Action	Major Side and Adverse Effects	Critical Information	Indications
Expectorants	Guaifenesin	Thins out the respiratory tract mucus, allowing it to easily clear the airway and makes cough more productive to expel mucus	Vomiting, diarrhea, nausea, abdominal pain, and hives	N/A	Relief of cough associated with a virus or bacterial infection
Antitussives (opioid)	Codeine	Elevates the cough threshold and suppresses the cough reflex	Sedation, dizziness, and constipation With larger amounts, CNS depression can be seen (lethargy, respiratory depression, coma)	Do not take with other CNS depressants Avoid driving or drinking alcohol Encourage client to take deep breaths	Severe, nonresponsive cough
Antitussives (nonopioid)	Dextromethorphan	Elevates the cough threshold and suppresses the cough reflex	Very minimal and are rare: sedation, dizziness, and constipation	N/A	Treatment of nonproductive cough that interferes with client's sleep and/or ADLs
Decongestants	Pseudoephedrine	Stimulates the alpha1-adrenergic receptors causing vasoconstriction in nasal blood vessels. Also shrinks the swollen nasal membranes resulting in easier nasal drainage	Restlessness, insomnia, anxiety, palpitations, tachycardia, urinary retention, and hypertension	Only relieves nasal congestion Avoid taking with other medications that act as sympathomimetics If taken with MAO inhibitors, severe hypertension or a hypertensive crisis may occur Clients who are hypertensive should not take this medication Caution for clients with diabetes, hyperthyroidism, BPH, glaucoma, and heart disease Rebound congestion can occur with intranasal administration Pseudoephedrine has the potential to be abused, and although it is available, clients must purchase with a photo ID and are subject to limits placed on the amount of medication purchased	For the treatment of allergic rhinitis, sinusitis, and the common cold

ADLs, activities of daily living; BPH, benign prostatic hyperplasia; CNS, central nervous system; MAO, monoamine oxidase.

Practice Questions and Rationales

1. A client is newly diagnosed with asthma. While learning to use a metered-dose inhaler (MDI) for delivery of a short-term beta agonist, the client asks if a spacer is appropriate to use with this device. What is the nurse's **best** response?
    1. "Yes, a spacer is recommended because it increases the amount of medication that is delivered to the lungs."
    2. "Yes, a spacer is recommended because it enables the MDI to function as a nebulizer."
    3. "No, a spacer is not recommended because it can increase the risk of developing oropharyngeal candidiasis."
    4. "No, a spacer is not recommended because it increases the amount of hand–mouth coordination needed to administer."

2. An adolescent client is diagnosed with mild persistent asthma and is prescribed a low-dose inhaled glucocorticoid to be taken daily. The client's parents express concern about receiving a daily glucocorticoid and how that will affect their child. Which statement indicates the parents and client need further education?
    1. "Inhaled glucocorticoids slow how fast my child grows, but they will still be as tall as they would have been without the medication as an adult."
    2. "Our child needs to take supplements of calcium and vitamin D and perform regular exercise to ensure the bones remain strong. Loss of bone mass may occur when inhaled corticosteroids are used over long periods of time."
    3. "We understand that long-term use of inhaled glucocorticoids may increase the risk of eye problems such as cataracts and glaucoma."
    4. "Oral thrush and a hoarse voice are unavoidable side effects when using inhaled glucocorticoids."

3. When providing discharge teaching regarding beta agonists for a client newly diagnosed with asthma, which information is the **most** important to give to the client?
    1. "It is essential that you contact your health care provider should you find yourself needing to use a short-acting beta2-agonist rescue inhaler more than twice weekly."
    2. "Oral beta2 agonists can be used for short-term relief of an ongoing asthma attack as well long-term control."
    3. "You may be prescribed a long-acting inhaled beta2 agonist to be taken on an as needed basis."
    4. "Quick relief of asthma symptoms can be achieved via inhaled or oral doses of a short-acting beta2 agonist."

4. A client with moderate persistent asthma has been taking an oral glucocorticoid for several years. Because of a new diagnosis of renal impairment, the prescriber writes a prescription to discontinue the oral glucocorticoid and start taking inhaled glucocorticoids instead. What is the **priority** action of the nurse?
    1. Assess the client for hyperglycemia, a sign of glucocorticoid withdrawal syndrome.
    2. Ask the prescriber to place an order to taper the oral glucocorticoids.

3. Ensure the client is aware that the risk of adrenal suppression will last for 2 to 3 weeks after stopping the oral glucocorticoid.
4. Monitor the client for signs and symptoms of hypertension, a sign of glucocorticoid withdrawal syndrome.

5. The nurse is preparing to educate the client on a new diagnosis of chronic obstructive pulmonary disease (COPD). After teaching, the nurse knows the client understands the material by which statement?
   1. "It is likely that I will develop other illnesses along with COPD; however, a complete recovery is possible."
   2. "Mild to moderate COPD may be treated with long-acting bronchodilators for management of COPD, however, when my COPD becomes severe, it will not respond to long-acting bronchodilator use."
   3. "The treatment goals of COPD are to reduce my symptoms, prevent progression of the disease, and prevent exacerbations of COPD."
   4. "Systemic glucocorticoids do not help when used for COPD exacerbations."

6. A client with severe, chronic obstructive pulmonary disease (COPD) is taking a phosphodiesterase 4 (PED-4) type inhibitor. Which assessment findings would alert the nurse that the client is experiencing a side effect of the medication? Select all that apply.
   1. Diarrhea
   2. Weight loss
   3. Hypertension
   4. Cough
   5. Insomnia

7. A client has been prescribed ipratropium bromide to help treat stable chronic obstructive pulmonary disease (COPD). What discharge instructions will the nurse provide to reduce the risk of side effects?
   1. "Expect that this medication will cause an increase in urination."
   2. "Take this medication 1 hour before meals or 2 hours after to decrease risk of gastric upset."
   3. "Move positions slowly as this medication may cause a quick drop in blood pressure when you stand up."
   4. "Increase your fluid intake and use sugar-free gum to help with decreased salivation."

8. A client is resistant to taking the prescribed intranasal glucocorticoids to treat seasonal allergies and asks why an over-the-counter pill was not prescribed instead. What is the **best** response by the nurse?
   1. "Over-the-counter oral antihistamines, intranasal sympathomimetics, and intranasal glucocorticoids all work equally as well when treating allergies. We can speak to the provider about changing your prescription to any of these."
   2. "Oral antihistamines, such as pseudoephedrine, can relieve nasal stuffiness, rhinorrhea, and sneezing related to allergies. We can speak with the provider about changing your prescription."

3. "Intranasal glucocorticoids, such as fluticasone, are the most effective drugs for the treatment of allergies. You should give this medication a try before exploring other options."
4. "Oral antihistamines cannot be taken preventively, whereas intranasal glucocorticoids can."

9. The nurse is providing client education regarding the use of medications to treat seasonal allergies. Which statement by the client shows a need for further teaching?
    1. "I should avoid driving after taking a first-generation antihistamine like diphenhydramine."
    2. "Diphenhydramine and loratadine can cause side effects like dry mouth, constipation, and urinary retention."
    3. "Second-generation antihistamines such as loratadine do not cause sedation."
    4. "It doesn't matter which second-generation antihistamines I take, they all work equally as well."

10. The client has been prescribed pseudoephedrine 60 mg orally four times a day. What is the nurse's **priority**?
    1. Instructing the client to take the medication for up to 3 days because of the risk of rebound congestion
    2. Reassuring the client that sympathomimetics cannot be abused
    3. Assessing the client's blood pressure and cardiac history before giving medication
    4. Assessing the client's mental status and psychiatric history prior to administration

11. A client asks about the possibility of taking a combination over-the-counter medication to treat cold symptoms. What is the **best** response by the nurse?
    1. "Combination over-the-counter cold remedies are safe to use for clients of any age."
    2. "No single drug can help relieve all symptoms of a cold. Choose a product that only treats the symptoms you are currently experiencing."
    3. "Antihistamines are frequently added to combination over-the-counter cold remedies in case the client also has seasonal or perennial allergies."
    4. "Combination over-the-counter products can be quite effective in curing a cold."

12. A client with a chronic nonproductive cough is prescribed codeine 15 mg by mouth four times a day. The liquid suspension available is 30 mg/5 mL. How many milliliters will the nurse administer for each dose? Record your answer using one decimal place.

    _____ mL

13. A client was prescribed intranasal oxymetazoline 2 to 3 sprays every 12 hours. The client calls the office 8 days later to say that symptoms were improving but now seem much worse with increased nasal congestion. What is the correct action by the nurse?
    1. The client should stop taking oxymetazoline, because the symptoms are likely related to rebound congestion.
    2. Request an order from the provider to increase the client's dose of oxymetazoline.

3. Request an additional order for an intranasal glucocorticoid.
4. Reassure the client that this is an expected side effect and to continue the medication as prescribed.

14. The client is prescribed an albuterol inhaler to be used four times a day to treat asthma. Which condition in the client's past medical history is **most** likely to be a contraindication to taking this medication?

1. Chickenpox
2. Glaucoma
3. Bradycardia
4. Gout

15. A client is receiving prednisone to treat an acute asthma exacerbation in the hospital.
Order: prednisone 40 mg orally every 8 hours × 48 hours.
On hand: 20-mg tablets
How many tablet(s) will the nurse give the client for each dose? Record your answer using a whole number.

_____ tablet(s).

5

PAIN AND ANTI-INFLAMMATORY MEDICATIONS

BRIEF PRINCIPLES OF PAIN AND ITS MANAGEMENT

Pain can be classified in many different ways, and understanding the type of pain to be managed is a key component in treating clients experiencing pain. Pain can be described as acute or chronic, nociceptive or neuropathic, postoperative, migraine-related, musculoskeletal, or cancer-related pain. Each type of pain requires an individualized treatment plan and a commitment by both the client and the health care providers to be actively engaged in the diagnosis, treatment, and follow-up care.

A multimodal pain management strategy uses nonopioids, anti-inflammatories, opioids, and nonpharmacologic measures. The medications vary drastically with regard to their efficacy for particular types of pain as well as by their side and adverse effects. Combining a variety of strategies allows for optimal analgesia with the lowest incidence of side effects and rapid recovery. Nurses should be involved in the team approach of caring for the client experiencing pain.

CLINICAL PEARLS—PAIN AND ANTI-INFLAMMATORY MEDICATIONS

SAFETY ALERT! Use caution when administering aspirin to certain populations. In children, use of aspirin may result in Reye syndrome; clients undergoing surgery should discuss the need to discontinue use of high-dose aspirin up to a week prior to surgery with their provider due to the risk of bleeding. In clients with asthma, the use of aspirin results in a greater risk for adverse effects such as bronchospasm, angioedema, and urticaria.

SAFETY ALERT! Many pain and anti-inflammatory medications are given in extended dose or enteric-coated tablets. Be sure not to crush these medications!

Assessment/Signs and Symptoms

◆ The assessment of pain is crucial to both correctly diagnose a client and to ensure that the most efficacious treatment plan is developed for the client in pain. This assessment must include an evaluation of the following pain parameters:
  ● Chronicity
  ● Severity
  ● Quality
  ● Contributing/associated factors
  ● Location/distribution
  ● Etiology of pain, if identifiable
  ● Mechanism of injury, if applicable
  ● Barriers to pain assessment
  ● Alleviating factors

There are many pain scales that are available for use to aid in the pain assessment, including ones that are single dimensional (self-reported measures of pain intensity) as well as multidimensional (measuring the intensity, location, impact on client's functionality, etc.). It is also important to consider the age and functional status of the client when assessing for pain. For many clients, a verbal discussion of pain may be most appropriate; however, in children less than 4 years of age or for functionally or neurologically impaired adults, it may be necessary to use a scale that relies on behavioral and physiologic measurements to assess the client's pain.

◆ As mentioned above, there are many different types of pain, and each one tends to present itself slightly differently. The client assessment should help to identify the differences in the types of pain, which typically present in the following ways:

- Nociceptive pain: This type of pain is related to tissue damage and may cause symptoms of an ache, sharp-stabbing pain, or a throbbing pain at the affected site. The pain may "come and go" or it may be a constant pain. The pain may worsen when the client moves, coughs, or laughs, and even a deep breath can intensify the pain depending on location. Somatic pain can be from damage to the tissue, bone, soft tissue, or organs. It can be classified as acute pain (sports injuries) or chronic (chronic headaches, arthritis). Visceral pain results from injury to visceral organs such as the small intestine. The pain itself may be felt in regions remote from the actual site of injury (referred pain), and the client may feel a deep ache or pain, tenderness, and muscle contractions of the abdomen. Both forms of nociceptive pain respond well to nonopioids (anti-inflammatories and centrally acting agents) and opioids.

- Neuropathic pain: This type of pain is caused by an injury to the nerve and typically results in a burning or shooting pain along the nerve affected. Many clients report this type of pain to feel like a stabbing pain or like "pins and needles." Many clients are very sensitive to temperature changes or touching the affected site. Type of pain is usually chronic. This pain does not respond to opioids but to adjuvant analgesics such as anti-inflammatories, nerve stabilizers, and/or antidepressants. Opioids are used as a last resort.

Diagnostics

◆ While assessment and a physical examination are the cornerstone for a pain treatment plan, depending on the type of pain and assessment findings, further diagnostic studies may be required to most effectively manage a client's pain.

◆ These tests may include an x-ray, MRI, CT scan, ultrasound, nerve blocks, electromyogram (EMG), and, for back pain, myelograms or discography.

◆ For the most part, blood tests will not help with the diagnosis or treatment of acute pain; however, for chronic pain conditions, such as rheumatoid arthritis, blood tests may be ordered to achieve a diagnosis.

◆ Assessment of a client's psychological processes is important to consider such as social support, coping abilities, adaptation, disability, and other physical comorbidities. It is important to note if a client is experiencing anxiety, depression, anger, or fear, as these may contribute to the subjective perception of pain.

MEDICATION OVERVIEW

Anti-Inflammatory Medications

Anti-inflammatory medications are used to relieve pain and reduce inflammation and represent some of the most commonly used medications by clients. Many of these medications can be purchased without a prescription and can be administered topically as well as orally. Anti-inflammatories work by inhibiting cyclooxygenase (COX) enzymes and are either nonselective (inhibiting COX-1 and COX-2 enzymes) or selective (COX-2 inhibitors). They can be used to treat many different types of pain ranging from soft tissue injuries to rheumatoid arthritis. It should be noted that nonsteroidal anti-inflammatory drugs (NSAIDs) as well as COX-2 inhibitors can be combined with a proton pump inhibitor for clients at risk for developing gastrointestinal distress or ulcers. In addition, recent evidence has shown that aspirin and other NSAIDs may decrease the client's response to vaccinations and should not be administered following a vaccination for pain relief or fever reduction. See Table 5-1 for additional information.

> **BLACK BOX WARNING:** Due to increased risk of myocardial infarction and stroke in cyclooxygenase (COX) inhibitors (particularly COX-2 inhibitors), the American Heart Association recommends a stepwise approach for treatment of chronic pain with COX inhibitors. This stepwise approach starts with nondrug measures, and if medications are added, they are used in the lowest dose necessary and with the shortest duration possible. The risk increases the longer the client takes the medication, and clients with existing cardiac risk factors are at greater risk.

Opioid Analgesics

Opioids have been used for hundreds of years for pain management and are one of the most common pharmacologic agents used for the treatment of moderate to severe pain. When properly prescribed and managed, these medications can be used safely and effectively; however, it is essential for both the client and the prescriber to fully understand the risks and benefits associated with the medications in this class. See Table 5-2 for additional information.

> **SAFETY ALERT!** Respiratory depression and/or respiratory arrest in clients who are taking opioid agonists is a very real risk. Clients should be monitored for level of consciousness, respiratory rate, and oxygen saturation, and the medication should be held and provider notified if the client experiences a decrease in the level of consciousness or a respiratory rate <12 breaths per minute.

Nonopioid Centrally Acting Analgesics

Nonopioid centrally acting analgesics relieve pain by activating opioid and nonopioid receptors. While they are used for moderate to severe pain relief, they have fewer side effects and do not cause respiratory depression or have abuse potential. The medications are not regulated under the Controlled Substance Act and are available by prescription only. See Table 5-3 for additional information.

Local Anesthetics

Local anesthetics: Local anesthetics provide the pain relief or the prevention of an anticipated pain in a specific area of the body. They can be delivered topically or via injection (subcutaneously, nerve blocking, epidural, spinal and/or intravenously) and are used for pain relief when other forms of analgesia cannot treat the pain effectively. Additionally, local anesthetics can be used to prevent pain during medical procedures Whenever possible, they are used in place of general anesthesia for clients at an increased risk for receiving general anesthesia, such as the elderly or clients with respiratory disorders. See Table 5-4 for additional information.

Table 5-1

Anti-inflammatory Drugs and Related Agents Used to Manage Pain

Class	Prototype	Mechanism of Action	Major Side and Adverse Effects	Critical Information	Indications
Nonsteroidal anti inflammatory drugs (NSAIDs)—first generation	Aspirin; ibuprofen	Irreversible inhibition of both cyclooxygenase (COX)-1 and COX-2 (aspirin is the only irreversible inhibitor in the class. All other NSAIDs are reversible inhibitors)	Side effects are rare with low doses for pain or fever relief. More common when taken in high doses for anti-inflammatory effects Heartburn, nausea, bleeding, renal damage, and salicylism; Reye syndrome (pediatric clients); anaphylaxis	Protection of MI and stroke (only aspirin; all other NSAIDs **increase** the risk of MI and stroke) Use with caution for clients who have peptic ulcer disease or a bleeding disorder Closely monitor clients with hypertension, edema, renal disease, or heart failure Contraindicated for use during pregnancy due to the potential for the premature closure of the ductus arteriosus in fetus	Mild to moderate pain relief Fever suppression Prevention of thrombotic disorders Anti-inflammatory conditions such as rheumatoid arthritis
Nonsteroidal anti-inflammatory drugs (NSAIDs)—second generation	Celecoxib	Selectively inhibits only COX-2, thereby decreasing prostaglandin synthesis	Headache, hypertension, dyspepsia, abdominal pain Elevated risk of MI or stroke Renal impairment	Closely monitor clients with hypertension, edema, renal disease, or heart failure while taking this medication Contraindicated for clients with a sulfa allergy Contraindicated for use during pregnancy due to the potential for the premature closure of the ductus arteriosus in fetus	Mild to moderate pain relief Dysmenorrhea Arthritis (including ankylosing spondylitis, rheumatoid arthritis, and osteoarthritis) Off-label use: familial adenomatous polyposis

(continued)

Table 5-1

Anti-inflammatory Drugs and Related Agents Used to Manage Pain (continued)

Class	Prototype	Mechanism of Action	Major Side and Adverse Effects	Critical Information	Indications
Centrally-acting non-opioid analgesic	Acetaminophen	Acts on hypothalamus to reduce fever Decreases prostaglandin synthesis in the central nervous system to decrease pain	Rare, but serious: anaphylaxis, Steven-Johnson syndrome, acute generalized exanthematous pustulosis (AGEP), and toxic epidermal necrolysis (TEN)	Side effects are relatively rare at therapeutic doses May be an association between daily use of acetaminophen and onset of hypertension. Use cautiously with clients at risk for hypertension Contraindicated for clients with a history of hypersensitivity or liver disease Risk of injury to the liver exists in clients who take more than the recommended amount of the medication or taking recommended doses while drinking alcohol	Mild to moderate pain relief Fever suppression

MI, myocardial infarction.

Table 5-2

Opioids Used to Manage Pain

Class	Prototype	Mechanism of Action	Major Side and Adverse Effects	Critical Information	Indications
Opioid agonists	Morphine	Opiate receptor agonist, inhibiting pain pathways, and producing pain relief, respiratory depression, euphoria, and sedation	Hypotension, constipation, hypotension, urinary retention, pruritus, cough suppression, vomiting, elevation of intracranial pressure, sedation, euphoria, and miosis	Caution should be exercised for clients with respiratory disorders, a head injury, benign prostatic hyperplasia, hypotension, liver disorders, and inflammatory bowel disease	Moderate to severe pain relief
				Tolerance develops to pain relief, euphoria, sedation, and respiratory depression. Little to no tolerance develops with constipation and miosis	
			Respiratory depression	Constipation during use of opioids can be helped by giving stool softeners and other medications to combat against constipation prophylactically	
				Use in labor and birth is not advised due to respiratory depression in the newborn	
				Use during pregnancy significantly increases risk of birth defects	
				Concurrent use with other CNS-depressant medications is contraindicated	
				Abstinence syndrome occurs in clients who are physically dependent on opioid agonists, and the severity is directly related to both the individual drug's half-life and the length of time the medication has been taken. Symptoms can be severe but are generally not dangerous. They include yawning, rhinorrhea, and sweating and can escalate into abdominal cramping, diarrhea, tremors, and pain	

(continued)

Table 5-2

Opioids Used to Manage Pain (continued)

Class	Prototype	Mechanism of Action	Major Side and Adverse Effects	Critical Information	Indications
Mixed opioid agonist–antagonists	Pentazocine	Acts as an agonist at some opiate receptor sites (producing pain relief, sedation, and respiratory depression) and as an antagonist at others (producing an antagonistic effect when given to a client taking opioid agonists)	Nausea, vomiting, diarrhea, pruritus, sedation, tachycardia, and sleep disturbances Respiratory depression	Respiratory depression may occur but is limited as opposed to opioid agonists, and euphoria does not occur At elevated doses, anxiety, hallucinations, and nightmares can occur Although the medication provides pain relief, antagonistic effects can occur resulting in withdrawal symptoms when given to a client currently dependent on opioid agonists Physical dependence can occur, although withdrawal symptoms are more mild than with opioid agonists	Mild to moderate pain relief
Opioid antagonists	Naloxone	Competitive opioid antagonist reversing the effects of opioid agonists including respiratory depression, sedation, and pain relief	Precipitation of withdrawal from opioid agonists resulting in nausea, vomiting, tachycardia, sweating, and tremors	Caution should be used for clients with a history of cardiac disease and seizure disorders Acute opioid withdrawal may occur, and clients should be monitored accordingly Abrupt withdrawal in newborns can occur when their mother has been using opioid agonists. Early identification of clients at risk for withdrawal should be done	Provides complete or partial reversal of opioid agonist effects including pain relief, respiratory depression, sedation, and euphoria

Table 5-3

Nonpioid Centrally Acting Analgesics Used to Manage Pain

Class	Prototype	Mechanism of Action	Major Side and Adverse Effects	Critical Information	Indications
Nonopioid centrally acting analgesics	Tramadol	Inhibiting pain pathways and producing pain relief	Sedation, dizziness, headache, dry mouth, and constipation	Caution with other central nervous system depressants such as alcohol or benzodiazepines Should not be given to clients with a history of drug abuse Constipation during use of opioids can be helped by giving stool softeners and other medications to combat against constipation prophylactically Risk of suicide with clients who are suicidal or addiction prone and caution with those who have depression, taking antidepressants, or prone to alcohol use	Moderate to severe pain relief
	Clonidine	Acts by blocking pain signals to the brain	Hypotension, bradycardia, rebound hypertension, dry mouth, sedation	Risk for severe hypotension and bradycardia and should not be used for hemodynamically unstable clients, obstetrics, postpartum, or surgical clients	Moderate to severe pain relief

Table 5-4

Local Anesthetics Used to Manage Pain

Class	Prototype	Mechanism of Action	Major Side and Adverse Effects	Critical Information	Indications
Amide drugs	Lidocaine	Inhibit the axonal conduction by interfering with the sodium channels in the nerve membrane. The action potential is not spread along as the threshold level is not reached Amide-type drugs are metabolized via hepatic enzymes	Local effects at the site of injection may include pain, hematoma, bruising, and infection Systemic effects may include allergic reaction and systemic toxicity (early signs include tinnitus, circumoral numbness, diplopia, and a metallic taste in the mouth and may progress to nystagmus, slurred speech, and eventually seizures, respiratory depression, and coma if left untreated) Cardiac effects may also be seen with high rates of systemic absorption including bradycardia, heart block, and cardiac arrest Allergic reaction (increased risk with ester-type drugs)	Systemic effects may occur if the concentration of local anesthetic reaches toxic levels in the blood Can be administered topically or via injection Anesthesia is more rapid, intense, and prolonged than with procaine Metabolism is greatly reduced for clients taking medications that inhibit the cytochrome P-450 system Use during labor and birth may prolong labor by decreasing uterine contractility and may also result in bradycardia and central nervous system depression in neonate	Pain relief prior to surgical procedures May also be used to treat dysrhythmias Topical: pain relief for skin conditions including minor burns, eczema, hemorrhoids
Ester drugs	Procaine	Inhibit the axonal conduction by interfering with the sodium channels in the nerve membrane. The action potential is not spread along as the threshold level is not reached Ester-type drugs are metabolized through plasma esterases	Local effects at the site of injection may include pain, hematoma, bruising, and infection Systemic effects may include allergic reaction and systemic toxicity (early signs include tinnitus, circumoral numbness, diplopia, and a metallic taste in the mouth and may progress to nystagmus, slurred speech, and eventually seizures, respiratory depression, and coma if left untreated) Cardiac effects may also be seen with high rates of systemic absorption including bradycardia, heart block, and cardiac arrest Allergic reaction (increased risk with ester-type drugs)	Systemic absorption is very rare as drug is rapidly converted to an inactive, nontoxic form. However, use with epinephrine (a vasoconstrictor) delays absorption and further reduces the risk of systemic absorption Must be given by injection Risk of allergic reactions is uncommon overall but more likely for ester-type drugs than amide-type drugs Use during labor and birth may prolong labor by decreasing uterine contractility and may also result in bradycardia and central nervous system depression in neonate	Pain relief prior to surgical procedures Used for oral procedures/surgeries to numb the area

Practice Questions and Rationales

1. A client given lidocaine as a local anesthetic agent for a surgical procedure reports tinnitus and a metallic taste in the mouth. What is the **appropriate** action of the nurse?

    1. Recognize the symptoms of systemic toxicity, notify the prescriber, and prepare to provide airway support if needed.
    2. Reassure the client that these are expected side effects that will diminish quickly.
    3. Recognize the symptoms of an allergic reaction, notify the prescriber, and prepare to administer epinephrine.
    4. Reassure the client that because they received a topical dose of the medication, they are not as risk for systemic toxicity or allergic reaction.

2. The client is prescribed morphine to be taken postoperatively. Which condition in the client's past medical history might be a contraindication to taking this medication?

    1. Hypertension
    2. Renal disease
    3. Gout
    4. Emphysema

3. A client with chronic pain is taking morphine to help manage symptoms. Which client education is appropriate for the nurse to review with the client at a routine, follow-up visit?

    1. "The long-term use of opioids can result in a nonproductive cough. You may take an over-the-counter cough suppressant to minimize this adverse reaction."
    2. "The concurrent use of central nervous system depressants, including alcohol, can result in profound sedation and respiratory depression. Use of alcohol while taking an opiate should be avoided."
    3. "The use of morphine is acceptable for use until the third trimester of pregnancy. If you plan to become pregnant, you do not need to discontinue this medication."
    4. "The combination of opioids with antihistamines may result in severe diarrhea. If you plan to take the two medications together, please consult with your provider prior to starting."

4. A client is receiving morphine to treat postoperative pain.
    Order: morphine 12.5 mg IV push every 4 hours
    On hand: morphine 10 mg/mL
    How many milliliters will the nurse give for each dose? Do not round answer.

    _____ mL.

5. A client was newly prescribed an opioid to treat chronic pain. The client calls the office to report that he or she is experiencing nausea and vomiting after taking the medication for the past 2 days. Which is the **correct** response by the nurse?

    1. "You need to make an appointment to be seen to ensure you are not experiencing an allergic reaction to the medication."
    2. "Initially, opioids may cause nausea and vomiting, but these symptoms should subside soon. We can consult with your prescriber to order an antiemetic to help with the symptoms."

3. "Tolerance to nausea and vomiting does not occur. You will need to take an antiemetic for the entire duration of your opioid treatment to help with these side effects."
4. "Nausea and vomiting are signs of an opioid overdose. You will need to seek emergency treatment immediately."

6. The client asks the nurse what the main benefits are for prescribing pentazocine, over morphine, for mild to moderate pain. Which response by the nurse is appropriate?
    1. "Respiratory depression is limited and abuse liability is low with the use of pentazocine, whereas both are major concerns for clients taking morphine."
    2. "Pentazocine is cardioprotective and provides more effective relief of pain after a myocardial infarction."
    3. "Clients who become physically dependent to morphine can be quickly transitioned over to pentazocine without the risk of adverse effects."
    4. "Unlike morphine, pentazocine can be given via many different routes, both enterally and parenterally."

7. Naloxone reverses which effects when given to a client experiencing an opioid overdose? Select all that apply.
    1. Sedation
    2. Kuphoria
    3. Respiratory depression
    4. Pain relief
    5. Abdominal cramping

8. Which client is exhibiting signs of opioid tolerance?
    1. A client who has been taking 30 mg of morphine daily with continued therapeutic effects over the last month
    2. A client who has stopped experiencing constipation while continuing to take opioids for chronic pain
    3. A client taking oxycodone and experiences significant sedation when drinking alcohol
    4. A client who requires increased doses of an opioid to provide the same level of pain relief over time

9. A 10-year-old client with a recent diagnosis of chickenpox presents to urgent care with vomiting, confusion, reports of hallucinations, lethargy, and a decreased level of consciousness. The parents report administering 325 mg of aspirin by mouth 3 hours prior to treat a fever of 100.7°F (38.1°C). Which action by the nurse is correct?
    1. Ensure that the client cardiac and respiratory statuses are stable and request an order to draw labs for electrolytes and liver function.
    2. Reassure the client that these symptoms are characteristic of a client with chickenpox.
    3. Recognize symptoms are signs of salicylism, and request an order to check aspirin levels in blood.
    4. Recognize the symptoms of a hypersensitivity reaction, and educate the client and family of the symptoms of aspirin allergy.

10. The client is prescribed aspirin. Which conditions would contraindicate the use of aspirin? Select all that apply.
    1. Peptic ulcer disease
    2. Hemophilia
    3. Hepatic cirrhosis
    4. Asthma
    5. Gout

11. Which client would be recommended to start a proton pump inhibitor along with the prescription for a nonsteroidal anti-inflammatory drug (NSAID)?
    1. A client with a history of rheumatoid arthritis
    2. A client currently taking glucocorticoids
    3. A client with a history of myocardial infarction
    4. A client currently taking metformin for diabetes mellitus

12. A client asks why they should not give their 10-month-old child ibuprofen after receiving vaccinations. Which response by the nurse is correct?
    1. "Ibuprofen is not effective in a 10-month-old due to their immature liver and inability to metabolize the drug. Acetaminophen is a more effective choice to give."
    2. "Ibuprofen must be given intramuscularly to treat vaccination related side effects, which adds more pain for the child."
    3. "Ibuprofen and other NSAIDs blunt the effect of the vaccination by decreasing the production of antibodies necessary to mount the immune response desired by the vaccination."
    4. "Ibuprofen is not recommended for use related to the risk of Reye syndrome."

13. The client asks the nurse why COX-2 inhibitors should be used in the lowest dose possible for the shortest amount of time. Which response by the nurse provides an accurate explanation?
    1. "COX-2 inhibitors are converted into toxic metabolites that may accumulate if the medication is taken over a long period."
    2. "Long-term use of COX-2 inhibitors is associated with increased risk of bleeding."
    3. "Elevated liver enzymes and resulting liver damage can be seen with the long-term use of COX-2 inhibitors."
    4. "COX-2 inhibitors increase the risk of myocardial infarction, stroke, and other cardiovascular events."

14. A client taking acetaminophen for a soft tissue injury states that they realized they were taking double his or her prescribed dose for the past 2 days and as a result took 4,800 mg a day for the past 2 days. Upon further questioning, the client did experience nausea, diarrhea, and abdominal pain. What is the **correct** response by the nurse?
    1. "As long as you return to your prescribed dose, the nausea, diarrhea, and abdominal pain will diminish and no further issues should occur."
    2. "The abdominal pain may persist. You should take the medication with food for the remainder of the treatment."

3. "You may be experiencing early signs of poisoning, which can progress into liver damage if not treated. You need to seek immediate medical attention."
4. "The symptoms you are describing may be Stevens-Johnson syndrome for which you should seek immediate medical attention."

15. A client is experiencing acute pain after ankle surgery. The prescriber has ordered acetaminophen every 4 hours for 48 hours. The client is stating that the pain is constant and rates it a 10 on a 1–10 scale. Using SBAR (Situation, Background, Assessment, Recommendation), which additional medication should the nurse suggest to the health care provider?

1. Morphine
2. Aspirin
3. Ketorolac
4. Pregabalin

16. An older adult with hypertension and diabetes mellitus reports experiencing pain in the feet that feels like "pins and needles" when resting at night. Which medication does the nurse expect to be prescribed for the client?

1. Hydromorphone
2. Fentanyl
3. Melatonin
4. Celecoxib

6

INFECTIOUS DISEASE AND IMMUNE SYSTEM MEDICATIONS

BRIEF OVERVIEW OF INFECTIOUS DISEASE AND IMMUNE SYSTEM DYSFUNCTION

Infectious diseases are illness resulting from the invasion of a microorganism, such as a virus, bacteria, parasite, or fungi. The infection can be mild to life threatening and can affect any part of the body. The medications in this class are directly associated with the type of microorganism involved and the site of the infection. The focus of immune system dysfunction in this chapter is related to immunosuppression secondary to organ transplantation or as related to autoimmune diseases.

◆ **Bacterial infections:** Bacterial infections occur when harmful bacteria multiply and disrupt the normal, healthy functions of the body. Bacteria can be both "good" and "bad." Bacterial infections occurs when the harmful bacteria outweighs the beneficial bacteria. When treating a bacterial infection, it is crucial to know what type of bacteria is present. Once the site of infection is cultured and the bacteria is identified, the susceptibility to various antibiotics can be determined. Since this process can take up to 48 hours, in many cases, a broad-spectrum antibiotic is started after the culture is obtained and replaced by a more appropriate narrow-spectrum antibiotic after culture and sensitivity results are back.

SAFETY ALERT! Bacterial resistance: The use of antibiotics without regard to their spectrum of activity or appropriateness for use has led to the increase of antibiotic resistance. Currently, there are a significant number of resistant bacteria strains, and it is even more important for providers to ensure their clients are using the best antibiotic for the infection and in a high enough dose for a long enough time to eradicate the bacteria.

◆ **Tuberculosis:** Tuberculosis is a serious lung infection that can be spread through the air via droplet transmission. The infection can be latent, where no symptoms are present, or active, where symptoms are present. It is important to treat both latent and active tuberculosis as latent tuberculosis can become active if not managed. Tuberculosis can be resistant to treatment, and strains with increasing resistance are seen. Thus, clients need to be treated with several different antibiotics at the same time to help ensure eradication of the bacteria. In addition, clients who are particularly at risk of contracting tuberculosis (including people with HIV/AIDS, intravenous drug users, those in contact with infected individuals, and health care workers who treat people with a high risk of tuberculosis as defined by the Centers for Disease Control and Prevention) should be periodically tested for latent tuberculosis.

◆ **Viral infections:** A virus is a very small particle that enters a living cell (the host) to replicate, taking over the cell and then reproducing itself over and over. Traditionally, viral infections have been difficult to treat. Many advances have been made; however, treatments available for these infections remain limited. It is difficult to stop viral cells from replicating and spreading, and because they use the host's cells to do so, it is extremely difficult to destroy the viral particles without harming the host (human) cells as well.

◆ **Immunosuppressants:** Immunosuppressants work by suppressing the body's immune system and are used to treat autoimmune diseases as well as to make it less likely for the client's body to reject a transplant. Immunosuppressants needed to be taken for life if taken for an organ transplant; however, the dosage may be decreased over time as the risk for organ rejection diminishes.

◆ **Fungal infections:** Fungal infections may result from (1) exposure to fungal spores that develop on the surface of the skin or (2) inhalation of spores that develop in the airway and/or lungs. Fungal infections can be classified as either being opportunistic or primary infections and are further broken down as either local or systemic. Local fungal infections typically involve the skin, mouth, and/or vagina and are treated topically, whereas systemic infections are much less common and are much more severe. Systemic infections manifest as pneumonia or fungemia and are treated with systemic antifungal medications. Clients who are immunocompromised are at a much higher risk for more severe infections, including opportunistic infections, and the complications resulting from the infection and the treatment.

◆ **Immunizations:** Vaccinations work by encouraging the body to make antibodies against bacteria and viruses. Vaccines can be killed (inactive) vaccines, live vaccines, toxoid vaccines, or biosynthetic vaccines. Live vaccines use a weakened form of the virus; killed vaccines are taken from a nonactive part of the vaccine, and biosynthetic vaccines are created in the laboratory (synthetic substances that are similar to the virus or bacteria itself). Toxoid vaccines work by giving the client immunity to the harmful effects of the bacteria or virus by providing a small amount of the toxin or chemical made by the bacteria or virus itself.

CLINICAL PEARLS: INFECTIOUS DISEASES AND IMMUNE SYSTEM DYSFUNCTION

Bacterial Infections (Antibiotics)

Assessment/Signs and Symptoms

◆ It is often difficult to ascertain between a bacterial infection and a viral infection. Site of infection should be considered for treatment selection. Diagnostic indicators may be necessary to determine the presence of a bacterial infection.

◆ Common signs and symptoms of bacterial infection include fever and presence of symptoms for >10 to 14 days.

Diagnostics

◆ Culture and sensitivity via blood, wound, sputum, or urine specimen.

Tuberculosis

Assessment/Signs and Symptoms

◆ Latent tuberculosis: The bacteria is present but in an inactive state, no signs or symptoms are present. Client is not contagious, but this can turn into active tuberculosis if not treated.

◆ Active tuberculosis: Symptoms can occur weeks to years after becoming infected with the bacteria and may include persistent coughing, coughing up blood (hemoptysis), chest pain, unintentional weight loss, fever, fatigue, night sweats, and loss of appetite. Bronchial lung sounds and/or crackles in the lungs may be present. Presence of lymph node swelling should be assessed.

Diagnostics

◆ A skin test, known as the purified protein derivative (PPD), can indicate the presence of tuberculosis bacteria. If the test is positive, the client will be referred for a chest x-ray for further diagnostic evidence of the disease. However, the PPD test takes 48 to 72 hours to show results, so if a client presents with active symptoms, he or she is frequently sent for a chest x-ray immediately.

◆ A chest x-ray or CT scan may show infiltrates or cavities in the lungs from the tuberculosis.

◆ Sputum sample: Sputum is collected for the presence of tuberculosis bacteria and can also be used for culture and sensitivity of the bacteria to ensure the correct medications are used for treatment.

◆ Blood tests: These rapid tests can be used to diagnose latent or active tuberculosis by measuring the immune response to tuberculosis bacteria. These may be particularly useful for someone who has minor symptoms and a negative PPD test.

Viral Infections (Antivirals)

Assessment/Signs and Symptoms

◆ The client's past medical history and history of current symptoms are very important to the assessment of a virus.

◆ Signs and symptoms are dependent on type of virus present.

Diagnostics

◆ In some instances, viruses occur in clusters of individuals, and the provider can diagnose disease on the basis of the presence of other individuals with similar symptoms.

◆ Blood tests and/or cultures may be indicated for certain viruses.

Immunosuppressants

Assessment
Organ Transplant

◆ Clients will be assessed for ongoing organ function and quality of life.

◆ Organ-specific focused examinations will be performed.

◆ Clients will be assessed for the presence of opportunistic infections such as cytomegalovirus, Epstein-Barr virus, fungal infections, herpes viruses, pneumocystis, and tuberculosis.

Autoimmune Diseases

◆ Symptom history and complete physical examination should be performed to assess client status.

◆ Genetic aspects (race, gender, and ethnicity) will be considered as part of assessment. Family history is also important to assess.

Signs and Symptoms

◆ Common signs and symptoms of a transplant rejection/failure of immunosuppressant therapy
  ● Decline of organ function
  ● General discomfort, unease, or ill feeling
  ● Pain or swelling at site of organ transplant (rare)
  ● Fever
  ● Flu-like symptoms
◆ Common signs and symptoms of an autoimmune disease
  ● Fatigue
  ● Joint pain and swelling
  ● Abdominal pain
  ● Fever
  ● Swollen glands
  ● Skin rashes

Diagnostics

Organ Transplants

◆ Blood work is performed periodically to assess for effectiveness of immunosuppressant therapy.

◆ For those with organ transplants, periodic blood work assesses for transplant rejection marker.

◆ Organ biopsy can be performed to ensure adequate function of transplanted organ.

Autoimmune Diseases

◆ Diagnosis is symptom based, and there are no clear-cut parameters for diagnosis.

◆ The antinuclear antibody blood test may be completed to test for the presence of an auto-immune disease.

Fungal Infections

Assessment/Signs and Symptoms

◆ If a fungal infection is suspected, a thorough travel history should be assessed to rule out endemic mycoses.

◆ Signs and symptoms are dependent on type and location of infection.
  ● Common signs and symptoms of localized fungal infection on the skin
    ▶ Peeling and cracking of the skin and/or nails
    ▶ Redness and/or blistering of skin
    ▶ Itching and/or burning of skin at site of infection

- Common signs and symptoms of systemic fungal infection
  - ► Fever
  - ► Cough
  - ► Fatigue

Diagnostics

◆ Microscopic examinations using potassium hydroxide (KOH) preparation or calcofluor white stain may help diagnose a superficial fungal infection.

◆ A fungal culture and susceptibility is often necessary to confirm diagnosis and appropriate treatment for infection.

◆ Pulmonary fungal infections can be difficult to diagnose. Sputum samples should be obtained, and if necessary, bronchial lavage, or a needle biopsy may be needed for diagnosis.

Immunizations

Assessment

◆ Clients should be assessed for previous reactions to vaccinations prior to receiving one.

◆ Immunocompromised individuals and pregnant women should not receive live vaccinations.

◆ Clients should be assessed for history of thrombocytopenia, or allergies to eggs, gelatin, or neomycin because some vaccinations are contraindicated or used cautiously in the presence of such allergies/conditions.

◆ A vaccination schedule is frequently used and recommended to help ensure clients have received all vaccinations within a series in the appropriate time frame.

Diagnostics

◆ If it is unclear whether or not a client has already received a vaccination, an antibody titer can be drawn in many instances to see if the client already has the antibodies in the blood.

SAFETY ALERT! The practice of giving analgesics for pain and fever relief both prior to and after receiving vaccinations was quite common until 2009. Research now show that the presence of analgesic/antipyretics medications such as acetaminophen and ibuprofen in the bloodstream can reduce the client's immune response to vaccinations. In most instances, these medications should be avoided for use before and immediately after vaccinations.

MEDICATION OVERVIEW

Bacterial Infections

Antibacterial drugs (antibiotics) are either bactericidal or bacteriostatic, meaning that they either kill bacteria or inhibit its growth. Bacteriostatic drugs require the host's immune system to eliminate the bacteria from the body; therefore, the host (client) must be healthy enough to mount an immune response and eliminate the bacteria. Antibiotics have many mechanisms of action some of the main mechanisms of action are: interference with the cell wall of the bacteria, inhibition of protein synthesis, or interruption of folic acid synthesis. See Table 6-1 for information about specific antibacterial agents.

Table 6-1

Drugs Used to Treat Bacterial Infections

Class	Prototype	Mechanism of Action	Major Side and Adverse Effects	Critical Information	Indications
Penicillins	Penicillin G	Bactericidal; act by binding to the penicillin-binding proteins, weaken the cell wall, which allows excessive water to enter cell and lyses cell	Allergic reaction Hyperkalemia (may be seen with high dose IV administration)	Most common cause of drug allergies Decreased doses may be required for older adult clients (particularly those with renal dysfunction) Can inactivate aminoglycosides. Do not mix in same IV if giving concurrently	Bacterial infections in infants, children, and adults.
Cephalosporins	Cephalexin	Bactericidal; act by binding to the penicillin-binding proteins, weaken the cell wall, which allows excessive water to enter cell and lyses cell	Overall very safe; serious adverse effects are rare Allergic reactions most common adverse effect (cross sensitivity for those allergic to penicillin is 1%) Hemolytic anemia rarely occurs Rare occurrence of pseudo-membranous colitis	Grouped into five generations based on entry into market and clinical use Should not be given to clients with a severe penicillin allergy due to potential for fatal reaction Ceftriaxone and cefotetan both pose in increased risk of bleeding. Use cautiously for clients with a history of bleeding disorder Cefditoren contains milk protein, clients with milk protein allergy should avoid this A disulfiram-like reaction can occur with cefazolin, and cefotetan is used with alcohol	Broad spectrum

Tetracyclines	Tetracycline	Bacteriostatic; inhibit bacterial protein synthesis	GI distress: epigastric burning, nausea, vomiting, diarrhea, and cramping	GI side effects can be minimized by giving with meals (in as small amounts as possible since food decreases the medication absorption)
			Superinfection may occur, either CDAD or a fungal infection (*Candida*). CDAD may be life threatening	Avoid giving to children under 8 and pregnant women as permanent staining (brown or yellow discoloration) of the child's teeth or developing fetus' teeth may occur
			Hepatotoxicity	Pregnant women and clients with kidney disease are at greatest risk for hepatotoxicity
			Renal toxicity	Clients with renal disease should not be given tetracyclines
			Photosensitivity	Clients should avoid prolonged exposure to sun related to photosensitivity
				Medication should not be given at the same time as any 2+ cations (calcium, iron, magnesium, aluminum, or zinc). Tetracyclines should be administered at least 1 hour before or 2 hours after a 2+ cation-containing food, medication, or supplement
				Broad spectrum
				Mostly used as second-line treatment options
Lincosamides	Clindamycin	Usually bacteriostatic but can be bactericidal in certain situations; inhibit bacterial protein synthesis	Most severe risk: suprainfection— CDAD	Can result in severe CDAD and may be fatal. If occurs, discontinue medication immediately
			Most common: diarrhea (unrelated to CDAD)	Give slowly via IV. Too quick an infusion may result in ECG changes, hypotension, and cardiac arrest
			Allergic reactions	Limited use related to CDAD risk
			Rare: hepatotoxicity, blood dyscrasias	

(continued)

Table 6-1

Drugs Used to Treat Bacterial Infections *(continued)*

Class	Prototype	Mechanism of Action	Major Side and Adverse Effects	Critical Information	Indications
Macrolides	Erythromycin	Bacteriostatic; inhibit bacterial protein synthesis	Most common: GI effects (epigastric pain, nausea, vomiting, diarrhea) Rare and small risk of sudden cardiac death (QT prolongation) Suprainfection of bowel can occur Transient hearing loss with high-dose therapy Thrombophlebitis	Can reduce GI effects by administering with meals Inhibition of cytochrome P-450 drug-metabolizing enzymes; caution used with other medications affected by cytochrome P-450 system Ensure enteric coated form of erythromycin is used if medication is needed to be given with food	Broad spectrum
Glycopeptides	Vancomycin	Bactericidal; acts by weakening the cell wall, allowing water to enter the cell and lyse cell	Common: thrombophlebitis Most serious: renal failure, red man syndrome Rare: ototoxicity, immune-related thrombocytopenia	Renal failure is a large concern (dose related) and increased risk when taken with other nephrotoxic medications Blood levels, specifically trough levels are drawn to minimize risk of renal toxicity If ototoxicity occurs, it is usually reversible. Increased risk related to longer treatment, history of renal disease, and the use of other ototoxic medications Thrombophlebitis risk can be decreased by changing infusion site frequently and diluting the concentration given via IV Not absorbed well from GI tract, given IV for most indications Oral use of medication is limited to treat CDAD Discontinue infusion if Red Man Syndrome Develops	Can treat CDAD, MRSA Reserved for use with serious infections Alternative option for clients with penicillin allergy

Class	Drug	Action	Adverse Effects	Nursing Considerations	Uses
Carbapenems	Imipenem	Bactericidal; act by weakening the cell wall, allowing excessive water to enter cell and lyse cell	GI effects: nausea vomiting, diarrhea Seizures may occur in rare instances Allergic reactions may occur (cross sensitivity for those allergic to penicillin is 1%)	Not absorbed well from GI tract, must be given IV	Very broad spectrum Used to treat infections that are combination of bacteria due to broad spectrum Pregnancy risk category B
Aminoglycosides	Gentamicin	Bactericidal; inhibit bacterial protein synthesis	Ototoxicity, nephrotoxicity, thrombocytopenia, and agranulocytosis can occur	Poorly absorbed from GI tract, most given parenterally Peak and trough levels must be monitored to prevent toxicity Clients should be encouraged to drink plenty of fluids to help prevent nephrotoxicity	Serious infections Prevention of endocarditis during GI surgery
Monobactams	Aztreonam	Bactericidal; inhibits cell wall synthesis	Hypotension, nausea, vomiting, diarrhea Elevated liver enzymes may occur	Not absorbed from the GI tract and must be given parenterally	Very narrow spectrum of activity Often used when a client is allergic to penicillins Can treat UTIs, respiratory tract infections, and skin infections
Fluoroquinolones	Ciprofloxacin	Bactericidal; inhibit DNA synthesis of bacteria	GI distress (nausea, vomiting, and diarrhea), dizziness, headache, confusion, phototoxicity Rarely tendon rupture can occur	Cannot be taken with compounds containing cations, including antacids with magnesium or aluminum, calcium, and dairy products. Must administer 6 hours before or 2 hours after antibiotic Increased risk of developing CDAD while taking. Clients should report any persistent diarrhea Take with plenty of water to avoid crystalluria	Broad spectrum of activity Can treat UTIs, respiratory tract infections, as well as bone, skin, and joint infections Drug of choice to treat anthrax

(continued)

Table 6-1

Drugs Used to Treat Bacterial Infections *(continued)*

Class	Prototype	Mechanism of Action	Major Side and Adverse Effects	Critical Information	Indications
Sulfonamides	Sulfamethoxazole	Bacteriostatic; interrupts folic acid synthesis	Hypersensitivity reactions may occur and are often dosage dependent Steven-Johnson syndrome (particularly with topical application) Photosensitivity, hematologic effects, including agranulocytosis, leukopenia, thrombocytopenia, aplastic anemia (rare) Hemolytic anemia can occur in clients with glucose-6-phosphate dehydrogenase deficiency	Take with plenty of water to avoid crystalluria When taken for an extended time frame, periodic blood tests should be performed	Treatment of UTIs
Urinary antiseptic	Nitrofurantoin	Bacteriostatic; may become bactericidal if concentration in urine is high enough and bacteria are susceptible enough Mechanism of action largely unknown, but damages bacterial DNA	GI distress (nausea, vomiting, and diarrhea), hypersensitivity reactions involving lungs, hematologic effects, including agranulocytosis, leukopenia, and thrombocytopenia	Contraindicated for clients with renal impairment: concentration in urine will be too low to be effective and increased risk of systemic toxicity occurs Can given with food to help with GI distress Monitor complete blood count Educate client that medication may turn urine darker in color	Treatment of lower UTIs

CDAD, *Clostridium difficile*–associated diarrhea; ECG, electrocardiographic; GI, gastrointestinal; IV, intravenously; MRSA, methicillin-resistant *Staphylococcus aureus*; UTI, urinary tract infection.

> **BLACK BOX WARNING:** The use of fluoroquinolones increases the risk of tendinitis and tendon rupture. Additionally, the risk is increased further in clients over the age of 60, those who have received a transplant, and for anyone taking corticosteroids concurrently.

Tuberculosis

Medication management is the cornerstone to the treatment of tuberculosis. Medications must be taken for at least 6 months. For active tuberculosis, several drugs at once are required, whereas latent tuberculosis may only require one medication. The medications listed in Table 6-2 are the gold standard of treatment for active tuberculosis.

Viral Infections

Antiviral medications treat a very broad range of viral infections (Table 6-3). In general, the drugs are used to treat systemic infections. Antiviral medications work by interfering with the reproduction of the virus or by strengthening the host's immune response to the virus.

Immunosuppressants

Drugs used to treat immune conditions (see Table 6-4) work by inhibiting the body's immune response with a goal of preventing organ rejection or treating an autoimmune disease. Immunosuppressants can be toxic and have increased risk of infection and an increased risk of developing a neoplasm. Clients taking immunosuppressants must be continuously monitored and evaluated throughout therapy.

Fungal Infections

The treatment of fungal infections can be lengthy and difficult to resolve (see Table 6-5). Most superficial infections will only require a topical antifungal medication to treat; however, more resistant cases may need oral therapy. Clients with systemic fungal infections will require oral or IV therapy. The length of time to treat will depend on type of infection, location, and client status.

Immunizations

Vaccinations result in an active immunity that develops over several weeks and will then last for years. In general, vaccinations are considered to be very safe. However, it is common for mild reactions to occur, and in rare instances, serious reactions can occur (see Table 6-6). Clients who have had a previous allergic reaction to a vaccine should not receive that vaccine again.

Table 6-2

Drugs Used to Treat Tuberculosis

Medication	Mechanism of Action	Major Side and Adverse Effects	Critical Information	Indications
Isoniazid	Bactericidal to mycobacteria that are in division stage; bacteriostatic to mycobacteria in resting stage Exact mechanism of action unknown, does inhibit development of cell wall	Most common: peripheral neuropathy (dose dependent) Most severe: hepatotoxicity Optic neuritis, seizures, dizziness, ataxia, anemia, GI distress, urinary retention, and dry mouth can also occur	Alcohol intake will increase risk of hepatotoxicity. Clients should limit or avoid alcohol use Liver function tests should be done at baseline and regularly thereafter Periodic eye exams should be performed	Primary medication for both treatment and prophylaxis of tuberculosis
Rifampin	Bactericidal; inhibits protein synthesis	Most common: hepatitis Most severe: hepatotoxicity GI distress, flushing, itching, rashes, discoloration of body fluids	Drug resistance can develop quickly to this medication; always given with at least one other medication to treat tuberculosis Liver function tests should be done at baseline and regularly thereafter Clients should be instructed that body fluids (urine, sweat, tears, and saliva) may turn reddish-orange, a harmless side effect	Primary medication for treatment of tuberculosis
Pyrazinamide	Bactericidal; mechanism of action unknown	Most common: polyarthralgias Most severe: hepatotoxicity Polyarthralgias, GI distress, photosensitivity, rash, and rarely, hyperuricemia can occur	Contraindicated for clients with preexisting liver disease	Used in conjunction with other medications to treat active tuberculosis. May be used to treat latent tuberculosis as well (with other medications)
Ethambutol	Bacteriostatic; impacts cell wall, but exact mechanism in unknown	Most severe: optic neuritis Asymptomatic hyperuricemia occurs frequently Dermatitis, pruritus, GI distress, and confusion can occur Rarely, peripheral neuropathy, thrombocytopenia, and renal damage can occur	Baseline and periodic eye exams should be performed to assess for dose-related neuritis	Part of multidrug regimen to treat tuberculosis

GI, gastrointestinal.

Table 6-3

Drugs Used to Treat Viral Infections

Class	Prototype	Mechanism of Action	Major Side and Adverse Effects	Critical Information	Indications
Antiviral	Acyclovir	Inhibits synthesis of viral DNA	Most common (oral): nausea, vomiting, diarrhea, headache Most common (IV): phlebitis and inflammation at IV site Most serious (IV): reversible nephrotoxicity, neurologic toxicity, including agitation, delirium, and hallucinations	Can be administered orally, topically, or IV Dosage should be reduced for clients with impaired kidney function Nephrotoxicity can be avoided by ensuring clients are well hydrated and infusion is slow (over 1 hour) Serious adverse effects primarily seen with IV treatment; rare with oral therapy	Herpes simplex virus Herpes zoster virus (shingles)
Antiviral	Ganciclovir	Inhibits viral DNA replication	Most serious: bone marrow suppression (granulocytopenia, thrombocytopenia) Can also cause infertility and/or sterility in both males and females Most common: nausea, fever, rash, confusion	Serious adverse effects, should be used with close monitoring Reduced dosages for clients with kidney disease Monitoring of complete blood counts related to reversible bone marrow suppression Treatment discontinued with neutrophils or platelets fall Contraindicated during pregnancy, should wait at least 90 days after therapy to become pregnant	Cytomegalovirus in immunocompromised clients
Alpha interferons	Interferon alpha	Suppresses protein synthesis of virus by destroying RNA within the cell	Common: flu-like symptoms, neutropenia, fatigue, depression	Given subcutaneously Most effective for hepatitis B virus, however, are expensive and not well tolerated Long duration of treatment due to increased risk of relapse	Hepatitis B virus, hepatitis C virus

(continued)

Table 6-3

Drugs Used to Treat Viral Infections (continued)

Class	Prototype	Mechanism of Action	Major Side and Adverse Effects	Critical Information	Indications
Protease inhibitors	Boceprevir	Suppress viral enzymes necessary for replication	Common: fatigue, nausea insomnia, vomiting, anemia, and neutropenia. Altered taste may also occur	Highly effective but expensive, extensive drug interactions, and intolerable adverse effects Always used in conjunction with other antivirals, never alone Administered orally Complete blood counts should be done at baseline and periodically thereafter related to risk of anemia and neutropenia Many drug interactions (substrate for CYP3A4)	Hepatitis C virus
Nucleoside analogs	Ribavirin	Suppresses virus replication, mechanism of action largely unknown	Common (oral): anemia	Can be given via inhalation or oral Benefits are minimal, and medication is expensive Inhalation therapy has minimal systemic toxicity Pregnancy category X; female clients should be using two effective forms of contraception to avoid pregnancy (also dangerous for female to become pregnant if male partner is taking medication)	Hepatitis, respiratory syncytial virus infection

IV, intravenously.

Table 6-4

Drugs Used to Treat Immune Conditions

Class	Prototype	Mechanism of Action	Major Side and Adverse Effects	Critical Information	Indications
Calcineurin inhibitors	Cyclosporine	Inhibit calcineurin to suppress production of helper T cells	Most common and most serious: nephrotoxicity Other common adverse effects: increased risk of infection, hypertension May also see hyperkalemia, hepatotoxicity, lymphomas, and nausea and vomiting	Given concurrently with a glucocorticoid Given orally or intravenously Blood levels must be monitored at regular intervals to help prevent toxicity Medication is highly protein bound and is metabolized by cytochrome P-450 system Risk of malignancies increases when combined with another immunosuppressant Clients should be educated to avoid grapefruit juice	Organ transplant rejection for allogenic kidney, liver, and heart transplant recipients Also used to treat psoriasis and rheumatoid arthritis
Glucocorticoids	Prednisone	Suppression of lymphocyte production Lysis of lymphocytes and a reduction of response to interleukin-1 by the T lymphocytes	Increased risk of infection, osteoporosis with increased risk for fractures, thinning of the skin, adrenal suppression	Large doses of medication must be given for immunosuppressant actions	Organ transplant rejection for allogenic recipients Treatment of autoimmune diseases such as rheumatoid arthritis, systemic lupus, and multiple sclerosis

Table 6-5

Drugs Used to Treat Fungal Infections

Class	Prototype	Mechanism of Action	Major Side and Adverse Effects	Critical Information	Indications
Polyene antibiotics	Amphotericin B	Can be fungistatic or fungicidal Binds to fungal cell membrane, enabling permeability of cell and contents "leak out"	Infusion related: fever, chills, rigors, nausea, and headache Common and severe: nephrotoxicity, hypokalemia Bone marrow suppression, delirium, hypotension, hypertension, wheezing, hypoxia, seizures, anaphylaxis, and acute liver failure may occur	Highly toxic; therefore, it is crucial to ensure clients have a definitive diagnosis before treatment is initiated IV administration is needed, and treatment is usually at least 6–8 weeks long Clients are closely monitored while taking medication, frequent vital signs and assessments IV fluids are recommended to be given with infusions to help decrease impact on kidneys Diphenhydramine can be given prior to treatment to help decrease infusion reactions Blood tests particularly potassium creatinine, and hematocrit levels should be monitored frequently	Severe systemic fungal infections
Azoles	Itraconazole	Inhibits synthesis of fungal cell membrane resulting in increased permeability of membrane and "leakage" of cellular content	Most serious: cardiosuppression, liver injury Most common: GI distress (nausea, vomiting, and diarrhea) Rash, headache, and dizziness may also occur	Hepatic cytochrome P-450 enzyme inhibitor resulting in many drug–drug interactions Given orally	Systemic fungal infections (alternative to polyenes) Can also be used for superficial fungal infections
Echinocandins	Caspofungin	Inhibits synthesis of fungal cell wall	Most common: fever and phlebitis at site of infusion Paresthesia, tachycardia, tachypnea, headache, rash, nausea, vomiting, and allergic reactions (rash, facial flushing, and pruritus) may also occur	Given IV, narrow-spectrum range for treatment Highly protein bound Cytochrome P-450 inducers may lower caspofungin levels, resulting in a need for an increase in the caspofungin dose Assess client for histamine-mediated reactions Dosage may need to be decreased for clients with hepatic impairment	Used to treat systemic aspergillosis or *Candida* infections when other therapies have failed

Table 6-6

Commonly Available Immunizations

Immunizations	Type	Route	Side Effects	Critical Information
Measles, mumps, and rubella vaccine (MMR)	Live virus	Subcutaneous (SubQ)	Mild: rash, fever, swollen glands in the neck and face Moderate: pain, stiffness and swelling at joints, seizure related to fever, temporary low platelet counts Severe (rare): allergic reactions, deafness, long-term seizures, coma, permanent brain damage	2 doses Clients with a life-threatening reaction to neomycin or a previous dose of MMR should not receive vaccine Pregnant women should not receive vaccine Immunocompromised clients may have vaccine delayed/contraindicated
Diphtheria, tetanus, and acellular pertussis vaccine (DTaP)	Toxoids (diphtheria and tetanus) Killed (inactivated pertussis)	IM	Mild: fever, redness, or swelling at injection site; soreness at injection site; fussiness; poor appetite; vomiting Moderate: seizure, nonstop crying for 3 or more hours, high fever (>105°F) Severe (rare): allergic reaction, long-term seizures, encephalopathy	5 doses Given to clients 7 years of age or younger (if older see Tdap below) Clients with a minor cold may receive vaccine; however, those moderately or severely ill should wait until symptom free to receive vaccine It is more common to see side effects at 4th or 5th dose Contraindicated if previous allergic reaction to DTaP, encephalopathy within 7 days of receiving prior DTaP, inconsolable crying for longer than 3 hours after previous DTaP, or seizures occurring within 3 days of last DTaP
Tetanus, diphtheria, and acellular pertussis (Tdap)	Toxoids (diphtheria and tetanus) Killed (inactivated pertussis)	IM	Mild: pain, redness, or swelling at injection site; low-grade fever; headache; fatigue; GI distress (nausea, vomiting, and fever); chills; body aches Moderate: fever above 102°F or 38.9°C, swelling of entire limb where injection was given Severe (rare): allergic reaction, swelling, severe pain, bleeding, and redness in limb where injection was given	1 dose at greater than age 7 Clients with history of Guillain-Barré syndrome should be given vaccination with caution Contraindicated if previous allergic reaction to DTaP, encephalopathy within 7 days of receiving prior DTaP, inconsolable crying for longer than 3 hours after previous DTaP, or seizures occurring within 3 days of last DTaP

(continued)

Table 6-6

Commonly Available Immunizations *(continued)*

Immunizations	Type	Route	Side Effects	Critical Information
Hepatitis B vaccine	Killed (inactivated)	IM	Mild: soreness at injection site, mild fever Severe: allergic reaction	3 doses given
Rotavirus vaccine	Live	Oral	Mild: irritability, diarrhea (mild), vomiting Severe (rare): intussusception, allergic reaction	2 doses; first dose given before 15 weeks of age and the second dose by 8 months of age Contraindicated for clients with severe combined immunodeficiency (SCID) or history of intussusception Vaccine should be delayed if client is moderately or severely ill
Haemophilus influenzae type b vaccine (Hib)	Biosynthetic	IM	Mild: redness, warmth, or swelling at injection site; fever Severe (rare): allergic reaction	3 or 4 doses; not given to those younger than 6 weeks of age
Pneumococcal conjugate vaccine (PCV13)	Biosynthetic	IM	Mild: drowsiness, poor appetite, redness or soreness at injection site, mild fever, irritability Severe (rare): allergic reaction	4 doses
Inactivated poliovirus vaccine (IPV)	Killed (inactivated)	SubQ	Mild: soreness at injection site Severe (rare): allergic reaction	4 doses Clients with an allergy to neomycin, streptomycin, or bacitracin should be closely monitored when receiving vaccine
Influenza vaccine	Killed (inactivated)	IM	Mild: soreness, redness, or swelling at injection site; hoarseness; itchy eyes; cough; fever; aches; headache; fatigue Severe (rare): allergic reaction, increased risk of developing Guillain-Barré syndrome after vaccine (1–2 people out of a million)	Annual vaccination Protection against influenza begins 1–2 weeks after receiving vaccine Not given under 6 months of age Clients with a history of Guillain-Barré syndrome should not receive this vaccine Increased risk of seizures when combined with pneumococcal vaccine and/or DTaP vaccine Vaccines should not be given at same visit

Vaccine	Type	Route	Adverse effects	Considerations
Varicella vaccine	Live	SubQ	Mild: soreness or swelling at injection site, fever, mild rash Moderate: seizure caused by fever Severe (rare): allergic reaction, pneumonia	2 doses Clients with a previous allergic reaction to the varicella vaccine, gelatin, or neomycin should not receive vaccination Pregnant women should not receive vaccination Side effects are more likely after the first dose than the second
Hepatitis A vaccine (Hep A)	Killed (inactivated)	IM	Mild: soreness or redness at injection site, low-grade fever, headache, fatigue Severe (rare): allergic reaction	2 doses now routinely given between 12 and 23 months of age
Human papillomavirus vaccine (HPV)	Biosynthetic	IM	Mild: dizziness; nausea; headache; pain, redness, or swelling at injection site Moderate: fainting Severe (rare): allergic reaction, slight increased risk of developing Guillain-Barré syndrome after vaccine	2–3 doses starting at the age of 9 and can be given until the age of 26 Pregnant women should not receive this vaccine
Meningococcal vaccine	Biosynthetic	IM	Mild: pain, redness, or swelling at injection site; headache; fatigue; low-grade fever Severe (rare): allergic reaction	2 doses given at as part of routine vaccination at age 10 or above Can be given as young as age 2 for those clients with increased risk of exposure or with an injured spleen or certain immune disorders

IM, intramuscular; SCID, severe combined immunodeficiency; SubQ, subcutaneous.

Practice Questions and Rationales

1. Which statement, made by a client prescribed metronidazole, would require the nurse to intervene?
    1. "My urine has been a bit darker than normal lately."
    2. "I enjoy having a small glass of wine with dinner at night."
    3. "I've been nauseous for the past several days."
    4. "I've increased my intake of green leafy vegetables this week."

2. A client is prescribed penicillin V potassium for a bacterial infection. Which assessment finding would require the nurse to notify the health care provider **immediately**?
    1. White blood cell (WBC) count of 16,000/µL (16 × 10⁹/L)
    2. Tall, peaked T waves on the electrocardiogram (ECG)
    3. Hypoactive bowel sounds in all four quadrants
    4. Absolute neutrophil count (ANC) of 4,500/µL (4.5 × 10⁹/L)

3. The nurse is administering the first dose of vancomycin intravenously when a client develops intense generalized itching and redness. What is the **priority** action of the nurse at this time?
    1. Stop the infusion immediately.
    2. Administer epinephrine intravenously.
    3. Decrease the rate of the intravenous infusion.
    4. Administer diphenhydramine intramuscularly.

4. A client prescribed clindamycin calls the clinic to report several episodes of diarrhea over the past 2 days. Based on this information, what is the **best** response by the nurse?
    1. "Diarrhea is a common side effect of this medication. Increase fiber in your diet to help with this side effect."
    2. "This may be a symptom of your infection. Please bring a stool sample to the clinic for culture."
    3. "Decrease your dose by half starting today. Call the clinic if your diarrhea does not improve."
    4. "This may be a serious effect of the medication. Stop the medication immediately and come to the clinic for evaluation."

5. A client has been diagnosed with onychomycosis. The client reports disliking the yellow discoloration of their toenails and requests an oral form of ketoconazole to "get rid of the discoloration quickly." What is the correct response by the nurse?
    1. "I will contact your provider to arrange for this formulation for you."
    2. "Ketoconazole is used to treat viral infections."
    3. "Ketoconazole taken orally has a higher risk of liver injury."
    4. "The discoloration will subside without treatment in the next several days."

6. A client who was prescribed nitrofurantoin for a urinary tract infection 1 week ago calls to report that the symptoms have returned. What is the most appropriate response by the nurse?
    1. "You need to restart the antibiotic since your symptoms are back."
    2. "Did you complete the full course of the antibiotic as directed?"

3. "It is common for symptoms to return after completing the antibiotic."
4. "It is likely that you have another infection. Do you have a fever?"

7. A client with osteoporosis and a urinary tract infection is prescribed calcium supplements and ciprofloxacin to be administered at 0800. What is the **priority** action by the nurse?
   1. Administer the medications as prescribed at 0800.
   2. Hold the ciprofloxacin and administer the calcium supplement.
   3. Contact the prescriber to change the dosing schedule for the calcium.
   4. Contact the pharmacist to discuss an alternative antibiotic.

8. Based upon current recommendations for the influenza vaccine, which clients should receive the immunization? Select all that apply.
   1. 19-year-old college student
   2. 28-year-old pregnant woman
   3. 32-year-old client with asthma
   4. 45-year-old client on prednisone for rheumatoid arthritis
   5. 58-year-old woman who cares for her husband with cancer

9. Vancomycin is available as 1,500 mg in 250 mL. Normal saline is prescribed to a client to infuse over 2 hours. How many milliliters per hour will the nurse program the intravenous infusion pump? Round the answer to the whole number.

   _____ mL/hr

10. A female client with genital herpes simplex becomes pregnant. What statement made by the client concerning her prescribed acyclovir would indicate that teaching by the nurse has been effective?
    1. "I may continue the acyclovir throughout the course of my pregnancy."
    2. "I need to switch to the topical formulation of this medication now that I am pregnant."
    3. "It is best to discontinue the use of this medication until I deliver the baby."
    4. "I should only take this medication during an active outbreak of my herpes."

11. A client has been prescribed rifampin for the treatment of tuberculosis and calls the nurse reporting orange-tinted tears. What are the correct responses to the client's concern by the nurse? Select all that apply.
    1. "This may be a sign of liver injury that is common with rifampin. Stop the medication immediately."
    2. "You may need to replace your contact lenses, if you wear them."
    3. "This is a harmless effect of the medication. Continue taking the rifampin."
    4. "This is a sign that your tuberculosis has spread outside of your lungs. The dose of the medication will need to be increased."
    5. "Decrease your intake of carrots and other foods high in beta-carotene to reduce future discoloration of your tears."

12. The client diagnosed with latent tuberculosis is prescribed isoniazid. The client asks the nurse why other medications have not been prescribed along with isoniazid. What is the correct response by the nurse?

1. "This is an error, you should also be prescribed rifapentine."
2. "Your tuberculosis is not active, therefore one-drug therapy is prescribed."
3. "Your Gram stain shows that your strain of tuberculosis is sensitive only to isoniazid."
4. "Treatment begins with one drug, and then a second drug is added after you have adjusted to the first drug."

13. A client is scheduled for a dose of ciprofloxacin to be given "stat." The nurse learns that the client has recently been diagnosed with myasthenia gravis. What is the **priority** action of the nurse?
    1. Document the diagnosis in the medical record.
    2. Contact the prescriber to request a higher dose of ciprofloxacin.
    3. Review the client's most recent renal function studies prior to administering the ciprofloxacin.
    4. Hold the medication and notify the prescriber.

14. To reduce the risk of nephrotoxicity caused by amphotericin, the nurse will avoid concurrent administration of which medications? Select all that apply.
    1. Acetaminophen
    2. Fexofenadine
    3. Cyclosporine
    4. Gentamicin
    5. Ibuprofen

15. A client has been diagnosed with chronic hepatitis B and wants to know what medications can be used to treat the disease. Which medications does the nurse include? Select all that apply.
    1. Interferon alfacon-1
    2. Boceprevir
    3. Lamivudine
    4. Ribavirin
    5. Acyclovir

16. A client on antibiotics for a bacterial infection has developed esophageal candidiasis. The nurse instructs the client that this is **most** likely the result of which process?
    1. Superinfection
    2. Immunosuppression
    3. Prolonged hyperglycemia
    4. A second, unrelated bacterial infection

17. A nurse determines that a completed antibiotic regimen for pneumonia was below the minimum bactericidal concentration based upon which assessment finding?
    1. Sterile sputum cultures
    2. Increased tactile fremitus in right lung base
    3. White blood cell count of 4,500/μL (4.5×10^9/L)
    4. Productive cough with thin, clear sputum

18. The provider has prescribed an antibiotic for an immunocompromised client with a fever without a diagnosed cause. What is the **priority** action by the nurse?

    1. Administer the antibiotic as prescribed.
    2. Contact the provider to suggest discontinuing the medication until the cause has been found.
    3. Obtain all ordered cultures prior to administering the antibiotic.
    4. Review the client's white blood cell count prior to administering the antibiotic.

19. A client with atrial fibrillation on warfarin has been prescribed erythromycin for a bacterial infection. The nurse anticipates which adjustment in the current medication regimen?

    1. Increased dose of warfarin
    2. Decreased dose of erythromycin
    3. Decreased dose of warfarin
    4. Increased dose of erythromycin

20. A 64-year-old client with a bacterial infection is prescribed a fluoroquinolone. Which information, if mentioned by the client, would require the nurse to withhold the medication?

    1. The client has recently completed an antibiotic for a urinary tract infection.
    2. The client is completing training for a marathon this month.
    3. The client has a severe allergy to penicillin antibiotics.
    4. The client struggles with medication compliance.

21. After administration of gentamicin, the client reports a headache rated as 3/10 (0 to 10 pain scale). What is the **priority** action by the nurse?

    1. Administer the prescribed acetaminophen.
    2. Review the client's gentamicin trough level.
    3. Administer calcium gluconate "stat."
    4. Notify the prescriber.

22. A client has been prescribed trimethoprim 160 mg for a bacterial skin infection. What is the appropriate action of the nurse?

    1. Contact the provider to request an increase in dose.
    2. Withhold the medication and request an alternate antibiotic.
    3. Administer the medication as prescribed.
    4. Advise the client to take the medication with a full glass of water.

23. A client diagnosed with a urinary tract infection has been prescribed trimethoprim/sulfamethoxazole (TMP/SMZ). Which information in the client's history would alert the nurse to withhold the medication?

    1. Prior urinary tract infection caused by *Escherichia coli*
    2. History of calcium kidney stones
    3. Allergy to furosemide
    4. Recent vaginal child birth

24. A client has been diagnosed with a central nervous system (CNS) bacterial infection. Which antibiotics does the nurse recognize as options for the treatment of a CNS infection? Select all that apply.

    1. Penicillin G orally (PO)

    2. Cefepime intravenously (IV)

    3. Vancomycin PO

    4. Metronidazole IV

    5. Ciprofloxacin

25. Which instruction does the nurse provide to a client taking an antibiotic for suspected streptococcal pharyngitis to reduce the risk of drug resistance?

    1. Stop the antibiotic once your symptoms have completely resolved.

    2. Use an oral probiotic while taking the antibiotic.

    3. Use the lowest dose antibiotic for the shortest duration possible.

    4. If your culture results are negative, discontinue the antibiotic.

26. A child weighing 32 lb is prescribed piperacillin/tazobactam 240 mg/kg/day in three divided doses. Calculate the individual dose. Round the answers to the nearest whole number.

    _____ mg/dose

27. Piperacillin/tazobactam is available as 1,200 mg in 100 mL normal saline. Calculate the drop rate (gtt/min) for this medication on microtubing to be infused over 30 minutes. Round answer to the nearest whole number.

    _____ gtt/min

28. Ethambutol is prescribed for a client with tuberculosis. Which assessment findings would alert the nurse that the client is experiencing adverse effects of this medication? Select all that apply.

    1. Blurred vision

    2. Elevated blood glucose

    3. Nausea

    4. Jaundice

    5. Decreased visual acuity of colors

29. A client has been prescribed amikacin via intramuscular injection to be administered at 0900. At what time will the nurse draw blood to monitor the ordered serum peak amikacin level?

    1. 0915

    2. 0930

    3. 0945

    4. 1000

30. To reduce the risk of adverse effects caused by tetracycline, which instruction will the nurse provide to the adult client?

    1. "Limit direct sunlight exposure to 2 hours per day."

    2. "Avoid alcohol while taking tetracycline."

    3. "Increase your intake of calcium while on this medication."

    4. "Brush your teeth three times per day."

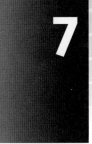

7   ENDOCRINE MEDICATIONS

BRIEF OVERVIEW OF ENDOCRINE DISORDERS AND MEDICATIONS

The endocrine system works in conjunction with the central nervous system to regulate the body's metabolic actions to maintain homeostasis. Therefore, drugs that mimic, stimulate, or suppress hormones make up the medications for these disorders.

- ◆ **Diabetes mellitus (DM):** Diabetes mellitus (DM) is a disorder of the metabolism of carbohydrates, fat and protein due to the absence of insulin or a decrease in its effectiveness. DM is classified by category depending on the underlying cause, such as beta cell destruction (Type 1) or intolerance to glucose during pregnancy (gestational). Diabetes medications (both insulin and oral antidiabetic medicines) are also known as hypoglycemic medications. They work by lowering the blood glucose levels in the body. Glucagon, another medication for diabetes, works by raising the blood glucose levels in the event of hypoglycemia caused by excess use of oral or injectable hypoglycemic medications.

- ◆ **Thyroid disorders:** The thyroid gland plays a major role in metabolism. Thyroid medications used to treat hypothyroidism and hyperthyroidism act to balance thyroid hormone deficiencies or thyroid hormone overstimulation. Hypothyroidism is most commonly an autoimmune disorder resulting in attack and atrophy of the thyroid gland, known as Hashimoto thyroiditis. The treatment for hypothyroidism is the use of exogenous thyroid hormones, usually lifelong. Hyperthyroidism is also most commonly autoimmune in nature, resulting in overactivity of the thyroid gland and overproduction of thyroid hormones, known as Graves disease. The treatment is antithyroid medications, radioactive iodine, and/or partial or complete removal of the thyroid gland. It is important to note that the excessive dosing of antithyroid medications, radioactive iodine, or complete or large portion of gland removed may place the client at risk for hypothyroidism. If this is caused by removal of part or all of the thyroid gland, the client will require lifelong thyroid hormone medication.

- ◆ **Pituitary disorders:** The pituitary gland consists of an anterior and posterior lobe, each responsible for the production of several hormones. The anterior lobe produces hormones vital for various target cells and glands, such as the thyroid gland and is responsible for growth, metabolism, and glucocorticoid levels. The posterior lobe is responsible for the storage and release of antidiuretic hormone (ADH) and oxytocin. Pituitary drugs simulate the hormones produced by the pituitary gland. There are two groups of medications: the anterior pituitary drugs used to control the function of the endocrine glands and the posterior pituitary drugs used to control fluid volume. Posterior pituitary drugs are used to treat conditions such as diabetes insipidus (DI) and syndrome of inappropriate antidiuretic hormone (SIADH). Posterior pituitary drugs can also stimulate smooth muscle contraction.

- ◆ **Adrenal cortex disorders:** The adrenal cortex is responsible for the synthesis of corticosteroids, which are broken down into mineralocorticoids, glucocorticoids, and androgens. Disorders of the adrenal cortex are the result of either excessive or deficient amounts of the corticosteroids. Treatment is targeted at removal of excess corticosteroids or replacing deficient amounts. The primary medications for these disorders are exogenous corticosteroids, particularly prednisone for deficient endogenous steroid production, as seen with Addison disease. Excess steroid administration results in Cushing disease.

CLINICAL PEARLS: ENDOCRINE DISORDERS

Diabetes Mellitus

Assessment Signs and Symptoms

◆ The signs and symptoms of diabetes may have a rapid onset (as with type I diabetes) or a gradual onset (as with type II).

◆ Monitor for short-term complications of diabetes related to hyperglycemia or hypoglycemia.

◆ Signs of hyperglycemia include thirst, headache, frequent urination, weight loss, and fatigue.

◆ Signs of hypoglycemia include tachycardia, diaphoresis, hunger, agitation, and tremors.
   - Clients with diabetes on beta-blockers (e.g., metoprolol) should be advised that beta-blockers mask the first symptom of hypoglycemia (tachycardia). For this reason, be sure clients are aware of the other symptoms of low blood sugar.

◆ Monitor for long-term complications of diabetes related to microvascular and macrovascular disease caused by sustained hyperglycemia.
   - Microvascular disease assessments:
      ▶ Peripheral neuropathy
         - Assess sensation using monofilament testing and vibratory and position sense.
      ▶ Autonomic neuropathy
         - Assess the abdomen for signs of slowed gastric motility (decreased bowel sounds, abdominal distention).
      ▶ Retinopathy
         - Assess vision, inner eye examination via ophthalmoscope.
      ▶ Nephropathy
         - Assess blood urea nitrogen (BUN), creatinine, and perform urinalysis for albuminuria.
   - Macrovascular disease assessments:
      ▶ Neurologic system:
         - Assess for risk factors and signs or symptoms of altered neurologic status (symptoms of transient ischemic attack [TIA], history of cerebrovascular accident [CVA], also known as stroke.
      ▶ Cardiovascular system
         - Blood pressure
            ○ Systolic blood pressure should be <130 mm Hg.
         - Serum cholesterol levels
            ○ Low-density lipoprotein levels should be <70 mg/dL (1.81 mmol/L).
         - Atherosclerosis
            ○ Auscultation of major arteries (carotid, aortic, renal) for the presence of bruits that may indicate atherosclerosis.
      ▶ Peripheral circulation
         - Assess peripheral pulses, skin color, and hair distribution for signs of decreased circulation.

Table 7-1

Characteristics of DKA and HHS

	DKA	HHS
Most likely to affect	Type I diabetes	Type II diabetes
Onset	Rapid	Gradual
Blood sugar (BS)	250 mg/dL (13.9 mmol/L) or greater	600 mg/dL (33.3 mmol/L) or greater
pH	pH ≤ 7.3	pH normal
Presence of ketones	+ketones	−ketones
Odor	+Urine/breath odor	No change
Respiratory status	Hyperventilation (Kussmaul's)	No change

DKA, diabetic ketoacidosis; HHS, hyperosmolar hyperglycemic state.

Diagnostics

◆ A diagnosis of diabetes can be made with one of the following:
  ● Glycated hemoglobin (HbA1c) of 6.5% or higher on two separate occasions
  ● Random blood sugar test of 200 mg/dL (11.1 mmol/L) or greater on two separate occasions
  ● Fasting blood sugar test of 126 mg/dL (6.99 mmol/L) or higher on two separate occasions
  ● Oral glucose tolerance test of 200 mg/dL (11.1 mmol/L) or greater
◆ Short-term complication of diabetes should be monitored closely and can be identified with the following pertinent lab values.
  ● Hyperglycemia
    ▶ Fasting hyperglycemia: 130 mg/dL (7.2 mmol/L) or greater
    ▶ Postprandial hyperglycemia: 180 mg/dL (10 mmol/L) or greater
  ● Hypoglycemia: <70 mg/dL (3.9 mmol/L)
  ● Ketoacidosis (diabetic ketoacidosis [DKA])
    ▶ Blood glucose of 250 mg/dL (13.9 mmol/L) or greater
    ▶ Blood pH < 7.30 and bicarbonate level of 18 mEq/L or less
    ▶ Presence of ketones in blood or urine
  ● Hyperosmolar hyperglycemic state (HHS): blood glucose levels of 600 mg/dL (33.3 mmol/L) or greater (accompanied by dry mouth, fever of 101°F [38.3°C] or greater, sleepiness, and vision loss)
◆ DKA and HHS are two serious acute complications of diabetes. The need for swift diagnosis and treatment is essential. Table 7-1 can help differentiate between the two conditions.

Thyroid Disorders

Assessment/Signs and Symptoms

◆ Hyperthyroidism
  ● Clients may experience tremors; overactive reflexes; protruding eyes; and, on assessment, warm, moist skin; rapid heart rate; and an enlarged thyroid gland. See Table 7-2 for more details.
◆ Hypothyroidism
  ● Clients may experience a number of issues that develop very slowly such as fatigue and weight gain. On assessment the provider may note dry skin, puffy face, bradycardia, and an enlarged thyroid gland. See Table 7-2 for more details.

Table 7-2

Hyperthyroidism Versus Hypothyroidism

Hyperthyroidism = Hypermetabolic	Hypothyroidism = Hypometabolic
Hypertension, tachycardia	Hypotension, bradycardia
Diarrhea	Constipation
Insomnia	Hypersomnia
Weight loss, despite increased appetite	Weight gain
Heat intolerance	Cold intolerance
Exophthalmos	Hair loss of lateral ⅓ of eyebrows
+/- Goiter	+/- Goiter

Diagnostics

◆ Diagnosis is by history and physical exam as well as laboratory results, including thyroid-stimulating hormone (TSH) and free thyroxine (T4). (Refer to Table 7-3 for changes in serum levels.) Treatment is guided based on TSH levels
  ● Normal lab values
    ▶ TSH 0.4 to 4.2 ng/dL (5.15 to 54.06 pmol/L)
    ▶ Free T4 0.8 to 2.7 ng/dL (10.3 to 34.75 pmol/L)
    ▶ Free T3 2.3 to 4.2 pg/mL (3.5 to 6.5 pmol/L)
◆ Radioiodine uptake tests may be done to assess for an elevated uptake of radioiodine indicating Graves disease. A low uptake indicates thyroiditis.

SAFETY ALERT! Clients who have existing cardiac disease/CAD and are taking thyroid hormones should be assessed for any signs or symptoms of coronary insufficiency.

SAFETY ALERT! Clients taking thyroid hormones and anticoagulants should be assessed for increased risk of bleeding (PT, INR, aPTT) and may require reduced dosage of anticoagulants.

Life Span Considerations: Hypothyroidism in infancy is known as cretinism and requires thyroid hormone replacement to prevent delays in growth and mental function.

Life Span Considerations: Hypothyroidism in pregnancy is common and must be treated with thyroid hormone replacement to reduce the risk or neuropsychological defects in the developing fetus.

Table 7-3

Selected Laboratory Values in Two Thyroid Disorders

Lab	Primary Hypothyroidism (Hashimoto Thyroiditis)	Hyperthyroidism (Graves Disease)
TSH (0.4–4.2 ng/dL [5.15–54.06 pmol/L])	High	Low
T3 (0.8–2.7 ng/dL [10.3–34.75 pmol/L])	Low	High
T4 (2.3–4.2 pg/mL [3.5–6.5 pmol/L])	Low	High

T3, triiodothyronine; T4, thyroxine; TSH, thyroid-stimulating hormone.

Pituitary Disorders

Syndrome of Inappropriate Antidiuretic Hormone
Assessment/Signs and Symptoms

- Most commonly a result of small cell lung cancer.
- Largely a diagnosis of exclusion, so ruling out other disorders/disease processes is crucial.
- Signs and symptoms include hypertension, a bounding pulse, crackles in lung bases, and possibly altered mental status.
- An important part of the assessment is to ensure the client is not currently using or has not recently used diuretics.

Diagnostics

- Low serum sodium (dilutional) <135 mEq/L (135 mmol/L)
- Low serum osmolality (hemodilution) <280 mOsm/kg (280 mmol/kg)
- High urine specific gravity (concentrated) >1.025
- Euvolemic
- TSH levels within normal range

Diabetes Insipidus
Assessment/Signs and Symptoms

- Main causes include brain surgery and head trauma: classified as central or neurogenic DI.
- Signs and symptoms include decreased blood pressure, weak/thready pulse, dry mucous membranes, polyuria, nocturia, polydipsia, confusion and/or coma if hypernatremia is not addressed.

Diagnostic Criteria

- Elevated serum osmolality (concentrated) >295 mOsm/kg (295 mmol/kg)
- Elevated serum sodium >145 mEq/L (145 mmol/L)
- Low urine specific gravity (dilute) <1.005
- Excessive diuresis of urine ranging from 5 to 20 L/day

Adrenal Cortex Disorders

Addison Disease
Assessment/Signs and Symptoms

- Clients typically present with both glucocorticoid AND mineralocorticoid deficiency.
- Many clients will first present in an acute crisis brought on by infection, trauma, gastrointestinal illness, or other stress to the body.
- Signs and symptoms include hypotension, a hyperpigmentation of the skin, progressive weakness, fatigue, weight loss, nausea, and vomiting.
- If not treated, and the client is in adrenal crisis, vascular collapse and death may occur.

Diagnostic Criteria

- Decreased serum cortisol levels
- Decreased serum sodium <135 mEq/L (135 mmol/L)
- Elevated serum potassium >5 mEq/L (5 mmol/L)
- Hypoglycemia

Cushing Disease
Assessment/Signs and Symptoms

- Disease results from an excess of corticosteroids, most commonly a result of excessive exogenous steroid doses. Treatment is to decrease or stop exogenous steroid medications.
- Signs and symptoms include a redistribution of adipose tissue away from extremities to central areas (moon faces, buffalo hump, truncal obesity); purplish striae on abdomen; thin, weak skin; hirsutism; and gynecomastia.

Diagnostics

- Elevated cortisol levels in blood or urine

MEDICATION OVERVIEW

Diabetes Mellitus

- Insulins for diabetes mellitus is required for all clients with type I DM and some with type II DM and gestational DM.
- All insulins are clear, except for Novolin N (neutral protamine Hagedorn [NPH]), which is cloudy in appearance. See Table 7-4 for characteristics of the various types of insulins.
- NPH can be mixed with short-duration insulins in one syringe. Draw up clear first and then cloudy (short-duration insulin, followed by NPH).
- Refrigerate insulin if unopened. Once open, multidose vials must be used within 28 days.
- Only short-duration insulin can be administered IV.
- All insulins are given subcutaneously (SC). Rotate injection sites to reduce risk of lipodystrophy.
- Insulin pens and insulin pumps are increasingly used because of their ease of use and ability to have tight blood sugar control.
- When insulin peaks in action, the risk of hypoglycemia is greatest.
- Clients taking insulin should be monitored for hypoglycemia.
- Clients taking oral antidiabetic medications should be monitored for hypoglycemia, especially with regard to drug–drug interactions. See Table 7-5 for further information.
- Clients taking antidiabetic medications (oral or insulin) may require an increased amount during times of stress, both physical (surgery, infection) and emotional.

SAFETY ALERT! The most common side effect of insulin is hypoglycemia. Clients should be educated about all signs and symptoms, wear a medical alert bracelet, and carry an emergency glucagon kit at all times.

Table 7-4

Characteristics of Various Forms of Insulin

Generic Name	Duration	Onset (min)	Peak (hr)	Duration (hr)
Insulin lispro	Short duration, rapid acting	15–30	0.5–2.5	3–6
Insulin aspart	Short duration, rapid acting	10–20	1–3	3–5
Insulin glulisine	Short duration, rapid acting	10–15	1–1.5	3–5
Regular insulin	Short duration, slower acting	30–60	1–5	6–10
NPH insulin	Intermediate duration	60–120	6–14	16–24
Insulin detemir	Intermediate duration	60–120	12–24	Dose dependent from 12–24
Insulin glargine	Long duration	70	No peak	24

(continued)

Table 7-5

Oral and Noninsulin Injectable Medications for Diabetes Mellitus

Class	Prototype Medication	Mechanism of Action	Major Side and Adverse Effects	Critical Information	Indications
Biguanides	Glucophage	Decreases glucose production in liver Increases insulin sensitivity by cells	Diarrhea Lactic acidosis No risk of hypoglycemia	Hold 48 hours before and after IV contrast to reduce renal injury Caution use with renal insufficiency, monitor BUN/creatinine	T2, GD
Sulfonylureas (second generation)	Glipizide Glyburide Glimepiride	Increases insulin released by the pancreas	Hypoglycemia Weight gain	Avoid alcohol: disulfiram-like reaction	T2 only
Alpha-glucosidase inhibitors	Miglitol	Delay of carbohydrate absorption, so decrease postprandial BG	Minimal systemic effects GI: cramps, N/V/D	Can decrease iron absorption; monitor for anemia	T2 only
DPP-4 inhibitors "Gliptins"	Sitagliptin	Increase insulin release and decrease glucagon release	Headache Hypoglycemia Pancreatitis Angioedema SJS	Monitor lipase if symptoms of pancreatitis occur	T2 only
SGLT-2 inhibitors	Canagliflozin	Promotes excretion of glucose by kidneys via urine	Glucosuria (expected)—can lead to UTIs, vaginal infections Ketoacidosis (rare)	Monitor renal functions	T2 only, studies under way for T1

Table 7-5

Oral and Noninsulin Injectable Medications for Diabetes Mellitus (continued)

Class	Prototype Medication	Mechanism of Action	Major Side and Adverse Effects	Critical Information	Indications
Thiazolidinediones	Pioglitazone	Decrease insulin resistance	Headache, muscle aches	Increased risk of bladder cancer; monitor for hematuria	T2 only
		Decrease liver production of glucose		Hepatotoxic; monitor LFTs	
				Fluid retention; avoid if CHF	
				Increased risk of bone fractures with long-term use	
Meglitinides	Repaglinide	Increase insulin release by pancreas	Hypoglycemia	Eat within 30 minutes of taking medication	T2 only
GLP-1 receptor agonists "Incretin mimetics"	Exenatide	Increase insulin release and decrease glucagon release	Hypoglycemia	Take 1–2 hours apart from other medications to avoid changes in absorption	T1 or T2
			N/V/D		Injection
		Slows gastric emptying	Pancreatitis (rare)	Monitor renal function	
		Decreases appetite			
Amylin mimetics	Pramlintide	Slows gastric emptying	Hypoglycemia	Taken with meals and 1–2 hours apart from other medications	T1 or T2
		Decreases glucagon release	Nausea		Injection
Antihypoglycemic agent	Glucagon	Stimulates the production of glucose in the liver	Nausea, vomiting	Ensure client receives carbohydrate to replenish liver glycogen stores once appropriate level of consciousness reached	T1, T2, GD
					Hypoglycemia treatment

CHF, congestive heart failure; GD, gestational diabetes; GI, gastrointestinal; IV, intravenous; LFT, liver function test; N/V/D, nausea, vomiting, and diarrhea; T1 and T2, thyroid hormones; T1 and T2, thyroid hormones; UTI, urinary tract infection.

Thyroid Disorders

There are a variety of drugs to treat thyroid disorders. See Table 7-6 for more information.

Pituitary Disorders

There are a variety of drugs to treat pituitary disorders. See Table 7-7 for more information.

Table 7-6

Drugs Used in the Treatment of Thyroid Disorders

Class	Prototype Medication	Mechanism of Action	Major Side and Adverse Effects	Critical Information	Indications
Synthetic hormone preparation	Levothyroxine	Converts to T3	Well tolerated	Administer alone, in the morning, on empty stomach, due to a decreased absorption when given with medications or food Watch for signs/symptoms of sub- or supratherapeutic dosing Max effect seen in 4–6 weeks This class has a long half-life and a narrow therapeutic index—careful monitoring should be done Minor differences in compounds of medications may affect TSH. For this reason, clients should consistently take the same formulation (brand or generic) to avoid changes in TSH	Hypothyroid, usually required for life Cretinism Hypothyroid in pregnancy
Antithyroid medication	Methimazole	Decreases synthesis of T3/T4	Well tolerated Agranulocytosis; monitor for fever/sore throat Infection symptoms	Not safe for pregnancy/breast-feeding Max effect seen in 12 weeks Can cause hypothyroidism CBC values should be monitored for leukopenia, thrombocytopenia, and agranulocytosis	Hyperthyroid Thyrotoxicosis

(continued)

Table 7-6

Drugs Used in the Treatment of Thyroid Disorders (continued)

Class	Prototype Medication	Mechanism of Action	Major Side and Adverse Effects	Critical Information	Indications
Antithyroid medication	Propylthiouracil (PTU)	Decreases synthesis of T3/T4	Well tolerated Severe liver injury	Multiple daily dosing Monitor LFTs Safer in pregnancy	Hyperthyroid Thyrotoxicosis
Antithyroid medication	Radioactive Iodine-131	Destroys part or all of thyroid tissue		Not safe for children or pregnant or breast-feeding women Can cause lifelong *hypothyroidism* Max effect seen in 8–12 weeks	Hyperthyroid
Beta-blockers	Propranolol	Decrease heart rate associated with hyperthyroid	Bradycardia Hypotension Heart block	Do not use if asthmatic Masks signs of hypoglycemia	Adjunct for hyperthyroid

CBC, complete blood count; T3, triiodothyronine; T4, thyroxine; TSH, thyroid-stimulating hormone.

Table 7-7

Drugs Used in the Treatment of Pituitary Disorders

Class	Prototype Medication	Mechanism of Action	Major Side and Adverse Effects	Critical Information	Indications
Synthetic antidiuretic hormone	Desmopressin acetate	Exerts antidiuretic effects (conserves water) and causes the contraction of both vascular and gastrointestinal smooth muscle	Headache, nausea Hyponatremia, seizures Water intoxication	Daily weights should be taken for all clients taking posterior pituitary drugs Children taking anterior pituitary gland drugs should have their height assessed at regular intervals Monitor renal function Monitor for signs and symptoms of volume overload Monitor serum osmolality, sodium, and urine specific gravity Vasopressin (another drug in this class) can act as a very strong vasoconstrictor; therefore careful attention must be given for severe cardiovascular adverse effects. Gangrene can also result due to this vasoconstriction	Diabetes insipidus

Adrenal Cortex Disorders

There are a variety of drugs to treat adrenal cortex disorders. See Table 7-8 for more information.

Table 7-8

Drugs Used in the Treatment of Adrenal Cortex Disorders

Class	Prototype Medication	Mechanism of Action	Major Side and Adverse Effects	Critical Information	Indications
Corticosteroid	Prednisone		Fluid retention, weight gain, glucose intolerance, elevated blood pressure, hypokalemia	Immune suppression; monitor for signs and symptoms of infection	Corticosteroid deficiency (Addison disease)
			Adrenal insufficiency, hypertension, congestive heart failure, peptic ulcer disease	Monitor BG if client has diabetes Sodium restriction, potassium supplement	
			Long-term use: osteoporosis, cataracts, glaucoma, immune suppression, growth suppression in pediatric clients	Risk reduction with long-term use Taper dose if on for more than 7–10 days Monitor for crisis with subtherapeutic dose (hypotension, shock)	

Practice Questions and Rationales

1. A nurse is reviewing a client's most recent hemoglobin A1c level of 8.7%. What instruction will the nurse provide to the client based upon this finding?
   1. "This test is not a diagnostic measurement of diabetes."
   2. "Your hemoglobin A1c lab value is normal, and no further action needs to be taken at this time."
   3. "The lab value can be altered significantly since you were not fasting. We should repeat this test in 2 weeks."
   4. "This result indicates that your diabetes is not well controlled. Your provider may adjust your medication regimen."

2. A client is newly diagnosed with Type II diabetes mellitus and has been prescribed metformin. The client works overnight as a security guard. What is the appropriate education for the client for this medication regimen?
   1. "Metformin should not be taken if the client is going to skip a meal."
   2. "Metformin can result in hypoglycemia, and blood sugars should be checked daily."
   3. "The client should take the metformin prior to an overnight shift to avoid drops in blood sugar."
   4. "Metformin can be taken without regard to meals, and doses should not be skipped."

3. A client with type I diabetes takes neutral protamine Hagedorn (NPH) insulin, 15 units at 0800 daily. At 1400, the client becomes agitated and confused. What is the **most** appropriate nursing action based on these findings?
   1. Administer an additional 15 units of NPH insulin.
   2. Check the client's oral temperature and urine output.
   3. Provide the client a simple carbohydrate snack.
   4. Assess the capillary blood glucose level.

4. A client with type II diabetes has been prescribed canagliflozin. Which statement made by the client indicates understanding of the teaching provided by the nurse?
   1. "I do not need to worry about hypoglycemia with this medication, since it is not insulin."
   2. "I will monitor for signs and symptoms of urinary tract infections while taking this medication."
   3. "Since I will be urinating more, I can stop taking my diuretic medication."
   4. "I will increase potassium in my diet to counteract side effects of this medication."

5. The nurse is preparing to administer neutral protamine Hagedorn (NPH) insulin 16 units and regular insulin 14 units in the same syringe. Which order of actions below represents the correct steps in combining these medications?
   1. Verify the medication order, inject air into the regular insulin vial, inject air into the NPH vial, draw up 16 units NPH insulin into the syringe, and draw up 14 units regular insulin into the syringe.

2. Verify medication order, inject air into the NPH vial, inject air into the regular insulin vial, draw up 14 units regular insulin into syringe, and draw up 16 units NPH insulin into syringe.

3. Verify medication order, inject air into the regular insulin vial, inject air into the NPH vial, draw up 14 units regular insulin into syringe, and draw up 16 units NPH insulin into syringe.

4. Inject air into the NPH vial, inject air into the regular insulin vial, draw up 14 units regular insulin into syringe, draw up 16 units NPH insulin into syringe, and verify medication order.

6. A client with hypothyroidism has been taking 50 mcg by mouth daily for the past 3 weeks. Which finding, if present, would result in the nurse holding the medication?

   1. Polyuria
   2. Tachycardia
   3. Cold extremities
   4. Pallor

7. A client has been taking levothyroxine for the past 3 months. The nurse would be concerned about toxicity of the medication if which signs or symptoms were discovered? Select all that apply.

   1. Tachydysrhythmias
   2. Constipation
   3. Hypotension
   4. Insomnia
   5. Increased appetite

8. The nurse is reviewing the most recent laboratory results with a client diagnosed with hyperthyroidism. Upon review, the nurse instructs the client to withhold the next dose of the medication based upon which laboratory value?

   1. Platelet count 162,000 × 10^3/µL (162 × 10^9/L)
   2. Thyroid-stimulating hormone (TSH) 2.5 µIU/mL (2.5 mIU/L)
   3. White blood cell count 5,500/µL (5.5 × 10^9/L)
   4. Free thyroxine (T4) 0.2 ng/dL (2.57 pmol/L)

9. A client with Graves disease underwent radioactive iodine therapy 3 months ago. At the most recent clinic visit, the client's thyroid-stimulating hormone (TSH) level was 6.7 µIU/L (6.7 mIU/L) and free thyroxine (T4) was 0.6 ng/dL (7.72 pmol/L). Which treatment will the nurse prepare to administer based on these laboratory data?

   1. No treatment is indicated; these levels are therapeutic.
   2. Give methimazole for continued thyroid suppression.
   3. Give levothyroxine for iatrogenic hypothyroidism.
   4. Repeat radioactive iodine therapy for subtherapeutic response.

10. A client arrives to the emergency department with the following signs/symptoms: blood pressure 186/102, heart rate 144 beats/min, temperature 102.8°F (39.3°C), oxygen saturation 99%. The client, who has a history of hypertension and hyperthyroidism reports

flu-like symptoms for the past week. Which prescribed order is the **priority** nursing action based upon these findings?

    1. Obtain an electrocardiogram.

    2. Apply oxygen via nasal cannula as needed.

    3. Administer propylthiouracil (PTU) 200 mg PO.

    4. Administer propranolol 100 mg PO.

11. A newborn diagnosed with cretinism will begin therapy with levothyroxine. The weight-based dose is 15 mcg/kg/day. The newborn weighs 7 lb (3.175 kg). How many mcg will the nurse administer per dose? Round to the nearest whole number.

    _____ mcg/day

12. A client has been prescribed desmopressin acetate for central (neurogenic) diabetes insipidus (DI). Which assessment finding would alert the nurse to hold the next dose of the medication?

    1. Blood pressure 98/52 mm Hg

    2. Urine specific gravity 1.020

    3. Serum osmolality 250 mOsm/kg (250 mmol/kg)

    4. Serum sodium 155 mEq/L (155 mmol/L)

13. A client newly diagnosed with diabetes insipidus (DI) has been prescribed indomethacin. The nurse verifies that the medication has been effective based upon which assessment findings? Select all that apply.

    1. Decreased joint swelling

    2. Decreased serum osmolality

    3. Decreased blood pressure

    4. Increased serum sodium

    5. Increased urine specific gravity

14. The client with Addison disease has been prescribed prednisone daily during a period of increased psychological stress. The nurse includes which information with regard to the prescribed prednisone therapy?

    1. Monitor for signs/symptoms of hypoglycemia while taking this medication.

    2. Ingest more salt to counteract the hypotension caused by prednisone.

    3. Taper the medication slowly over 7 to 10 days when discontinued.

    4. Increase dietary protein to prevent weight loss while taking prednisone.

15. A client with severe chronic obstructive pulmonary disease has been taking prednisone for several years. Which assessment findings noted by the nurse would indicate an insufficient dose of prednisone? Select all that apply.

    1. Hypotension

    2. Hyponatremia

    3. Tachycardia

    4. 2+ pitting edema

    5. Hyperglycemia

8

GASTROINTESTINAL MEDICATIONS

BRIEF OVERVIEW OF GASTROINTESTINAL DISORDERS AND MEDICATIONS

Gastrointestinal disorders can range from mild to severe and may be acute or chronic. Many of the medications used to treat these disorders focus on symptom management, such as with nausea or diarrhea. Other medications focus on disease management, such as with peptic ulcer disease (PUD). Client education regarding nonpharmacologic management strategies is equally important in the management of gastrointestinal disorders.

◆ **Nausea and vomiting:** Nausea and vomiting are subjective concerns by a client that are symptoms of a disorder. The underlying cause must be determined to treat the symptoms. Nausea can be caused by a variety of problems, such as gastrointestinal disease, endocrine or metabolic disorders, cardiovascular disorders, or as a side effect of medications or noxious stimuli. When nausea occurs, it is the result of receptor activation in the chemoreceptor trigger zone (CTZ) in the brain. The receptors working within the CTZ (serotonin, dopamine, neurokinin) are stimulated. Medications to treat nausea and vomiting are known as antiemetics. These drugs work to block the receptors within the CTZ from being activated, decreasing nausea and vomiting. Nausea usually precedes vomiting. If vomiting is persistent and the nausea is not treated, the client may develop dehydration, metabolic alkalosis, and electrolyte imbalances. Treatment is directed based on the underlying cause. While the cause is being determined, treatment of nausea can include antiemetics as well as nonpharmacologic measures to reduce the symptom. Nonpharmacologic measures to help reduce nausea include small, frequent meals and bland foods that are low in fat and moderate in carbohydrate content. Clients with severe nausea are frequently unable to tolerate anything by mouth. For dehydration, intravenous fluids can be administered.

◆ **Constipation:** Constipation is a disorder leading to hard, infrequent, and painful bowel movements. Constipation is commonly a side effect of medications. Dietary measures to prevent constipation is a daily fiber intake of 25 g/day and fluid intake of 2,000 mL/day if not contraindicated. Frequently, hemorrhoids may develop due to straining. Treatment should first include dietary measures to soften the stool and ease passage and include increased physical activity, if tolerated. Laxatives are classified based on the mechanism of action and onset of action. They should be used for the shortest duration possible to prevent dependency.

SAFETY ALERT! Laxatives should not be used in clients with undiagnosed abdominal pain, because they increase the risk of intestinal rupture in the event of an existing intestinal obstruction.

◆ **Diarrhea:** Diarrhea can be acute or chronic and is most commonly caused by the ingestion of an infectious organism. Diarrhea is a symptom of another problem, which may be food poisoning, drinking of contaminated water, side effects of medications, or an adverse effect of antibiotic therapy (*Clostridium difficile*). Most often, the organism causing diarrhea is *Escherichia coli*. Contaminated food, water, and poor hand hygiene are common ways of *E. coli* transmission. Other causes of diarrhea include medication side effects and food allergies or intolerances.

◆ **Gastroesophageal reflux disease (GERD):** GERD can be acute or chronic, caused by the reflux of stomach acid into the esophagus from a variety of causes. Complications may occur if GERD occurs chronically and is not treated; these include inflammation of the esophagus and cellular changes of the esophageal cells, known as Barrett esophagus, which can cause cancer. Treatment of GERD is like that of PUD and is aimed at reducing gastric acidity and GERD symptoms. Nonpharmacologic interventions focus on lifestyle changes, which include small frequent meals, sleeping with the head of the bed elevated, avoiding foods that worsen symptoms, sitting upright for 2 hours after eating, and avoidance of eating prior to bedtime.

◆ **Peptic ulcer disease (PUD):** PUD refers to erosion and ulceration of the gastric mucosa, most commonly the stomach or duodenum. Normal protective factors that help prevent erosion include adequate blood supply to the gastric mucosa, bicarbonate (a base to decrease gastric acidity), prostaglandins, and the production of mucus to protect the gastric lining. The most common cause of PUD is *Helicobacter pylori* (*H. pylori*), a gram-negative bacterium that increases gastric acidity. The second most common cause of PUD is the chronic use of nonsteroidal anti-inflammatory drugs (NSAIDs). Alternatively, when one or several of the protective mechanisms fail, PUD can occur. Treatment depends on the cause and may include acid reducers such as proton pump inhibitors ("-zoles") or histamine-2 receptor blockers ("-dines") and triple antibiotic therapy, if *H. pylori* is the cause. Smoking increases the risk of recurrence. If possible, clients should avoid high-dose, long-term NSAID use.

CLINICAL PEARLS: GASTROINTESTINAL DISORDERS

Nausea and Vomiting

Assessment/Signs and Symptoms
Nausea is a sign of potential vomiting and a subjective symptom that may include a feeling of an unsettled stomach, with increased salivation. If vomiting occurs, it is important to assess the client for potential dehydration and acid–base and electrolyte imbalances and document it as a form of output.

Diagnostics
Determining the underlying cause of the nausea and subsequent vomiting is the priority in management. Characteristics of the emesis can aid in diagnosis because it may indicate the rate of gastric emptying. Color may help in diagnosing the cause as well. Bright red emesis indicates bleeding, which may be caused by gastric ulcers, esophageal variceal rupture, or other disorders in which bleeding is possible. If the emesis is dark, "coffee ground" in appearance, it may indicate

Table 8-1

Normal Serum Electrolyte Levels

Potassium	3.5–5 mEq/L (3.5–5 mmol/L)
Sodium	135–145 mEq/L (135–145 mmol/L)
Chloride	96–106 mEq/L (96–106 mmol/L)
Calcium	8.6–10.2 mg/dL (2.15–2.55 mmol/L)
Magnesium	1.5–2.5 mEq/L (0.75–1.25 mmol/L)
Phosphorous	2.4–4.4 mg/dL (0.78–1.42 mmol/L)
Serum osmolality	275–295 mOsm/kg (275–295 mmol/kg)
Blood urea nitrogen	6–20 mg/dL (2.14–7.14 mmol/L)
Creatinine	0.2–1 mg/dL (15.25–76.25 µmol/L)

partially digested blood originating lower in the gastrointestinal tract. Timing of nausea is also important to note.

Pertinent Laboratory Values

If persistent vomiting occurs, serum electrolyte levels, serum osmolality, serum creatinine, and arterial pH and bicarbonate levels must be monitored (see Tables 8-1 and 8-2).

Constipation

Assessment/Signs and Symptoms

Infrequent, hard bowel movements with associated straining to pass stool are characteristic of constipation. Elimination frequency varies on an individual basis, so a baseline status should be obtained. The client may also have abdominal bloating, cramping, or discomfort as stool accumulates in the colon. Underlying causes of constipation include a diet that is low in fiber; dehydration; pregnancy; and side effects of medications, most commonly opioids.

Diagnostics

Constipation is usually diagnosed based on history and physical examination. An abdominal x-ray may be used to identify the presence of stool in the large intestine.

Pertinent Laboratory Values

For constipation associated with poor intake of fluids, laboratory values may indicate dehydration, although this is not common (see Tables 8-1 and 8-2).

Table 8-2

Normal Arterial Acid–Base Levels

Arterial pH	7.35–7.45 (7.35–7.45)
Arterial oxygen (Pao$_2$)	80–100 mm Hg (10.64–13.3 kPa)
Arterial carbon dioxide (Paco$_2$)	35–45 mm Hg (4.66–5.99 kPa)
Serum bicarbonate (HCO$_3$)	22–26 mEq/L (22–26 mmol/L)

Diarrhea

Assessment/Signs and Symptoms

Diarrhea involves frequent, watery, and loose stools that may occur with urgency. The client may have abdominal cramping immediately before an episode of diarrhea. Dehydration as well as electrolyte and acid–base imbalances are possible complications associated with long-standing diarrhea. Fever may indicate a bacterial infection that may require antibiotic therapy. The client's abdomen may be tender and/or distended. The perineum should be assessed for skin breakdown. Intake and output and daily weights should be recorded. Diarrhea should be documented as a form of liquid output (measured or approximated) for monitoring of fluid volume status.

Diagnostics

Diagnosis is again based on history and physical examination. Production of loose stool more than three times per day is diagnostic of diarrhea. If a bacterial infection or *C. difficile* is suspected, a stool culture may be obtained. Offending agents or medications should be stopped immediately. Treatment of diarrhea depends on the causative factor.

Pertinent Laboratory Values

Serum electrolyte levels, serum osmolality, serum creatinine, and arterial pH and bicarbonate levels must be monitored (see Tables 8-1 and 8-2).

Gastroesophageal Reflux Disease

Assessment/Signs and Symptoms

Clients frequently report the sensation of heartburn that is worse after eating. Regurgitation of stomach contents may also occur. Less often, GERD can cause a dry cough and can exacerbate asthma symptoms.

Diagnostics

Diagnosing GERD is usually based on the client's symptoms. If the client does not respond to treatment, an endoscopy may be performed to evaluate the gastric mucosa and assess for the presence of erosion, inflammation, or PUD.

Peptic Ulcer Disease

Assessment/Signs and Symptoms

Clinical manifestations of PUD depend upon the ulcer location. Most commonly, ulcers occur in the stomach (gastric) or the first portion of the small intestine, the duodenum. Both types of ulcers have a high chance of reoccurring. Gastric ulcers cause pain ~1 to 2 hours after eating, and food may increase or decrease pain. Duodenal ulcers cause pain 2 to 5 hours after eating, and pain is decreased with ingestion of food. The pain is described as "burning" and occurs in the epigastric area. Clients may have no symptoms of ulcers, especially those caused by NSAIDs. Major complications of PUD include hemorrhage and perforation of the ulcer, which are both medical emergencies.

Diagnostics

The best way to diagnose PUD is via endoscopy. During this procedure, the gastric cells are biopsied to test for *H. pylori*. Other less invasive ways to screen for *H. pylori* include a serum blood test, urea breath test, or stool culture. To assess for bleeding of the ulcer, a complete blood count (CBC) with hemoglobin and hematocrit measurements should be obtained.

Pertinent Laboratory Values

Low hemoglobin, hematocrit, and red blood cell count on the CBC may indicate bleeding of the peptic ulcer. If the bleeding is slow and chronic, the client may develop iron-deficiency anemia. The client would present with low red blood cell indices. Low mean corpuscular volume and the mean corpuscular hemoglobin represent a microcytic, hypochromic anemia consistent with chronic blood loss and low iron levels.

MEDICATION OVERVIEW

Total or Central Parenteral Nutrition

For clients who are unable to use the gastrointestinal tract for nutrition, complete nutrition is available to be delivered parenterally either through a peripheral (peripheral parenteral nutrition or PPN) or central intravenous line (total parenteral nutrition or TPN). TPN is customized to provide the nutritional requirements of each individual and is always delivered through a central venous line or a peripherally inserted central catheter. In the event of gastrointestinal disorders, TPN is a potential option to continue to provide calories, fat, protein, vitamins, and electrolytes while the gastrointestinal disorder is treated. TPN is considered a medication that requires verification by two registered nurses prior to administration. It is infused through specialized intravenous tubing with a filter. A fat emulsion may be infused simultaneously as a piggyback on the TPN. Both PPN and TPN are hypertonic solutions. Due to the risk of bacterial colonization of the intravenous (IV) tubing because of the high amounts of dextrose, the IV tubing is changed every 24 hours. Intake and output, daily weights, and laboratory values are monitored daily to evaluate parenteral nutrition effectiveness. Elevated or decreased blood glucose levels may occur while a client is receiving parenteral nutrition. Due to the high dextrose content, blood sugars should be monitored every 4 to 6 hours. The client may require insulin while on parenteral nutrition, even if the client does not have diabetes mellitus. Insulin can be added to the PPN or TPN solution if needed. Once approved to transition to oral intake, a clear liquid diet is ordered and advanced as the client tolerates.

Nausea and Vomiting

There are a variety of medications available to treat nausea and vomiting. See Table 8-3 for treatment options and information.

Constipation

Laxatives used for constipation are named by class and grouped by the time it takes for the laxative to exert an effect (see Table 8-4).

Table 8-5 discusses the classes of medications used to treat constipation.

Table 8-3

Drugs Used in the Treatment of Nausea and Vomiting

Class	Prototype	Mechanism of Action	Major Side and Adverse Effects	Critical Information	Indications
Serotonin antagonist	Ondansetron	Blocks serotonin receptors in the brain that are involved in activating vomiting	Most common side effects: headache and constipation Most serious adverse effect: prolongation of QT interval, which can cause fatal dysrhythmias	Safe in pregnancy, although data are emerging about increased risk of cleft lip and palate Do not give to clients with a long QT interval	Nausea from various sources
Dopamine antagonist	Promethazine	Block dopamine receptors in the brain	Common side effects: anticholinergic (dry mouth, blurred vision, urinary retention, and constipation) as well as sedation and decreased blood pressure Possible severe respiratory depression Local tissue injury when administered parenterally	Must not be given to children younger than 2 years of age Extravasation can occur if given IV. A large-bore IV catheter must be used and checked for patency prior to administration of medication	Nausea
Substance P/neurokinin 1 antagonists	Aprepitant	Block neurokinin 1 receptors in the brain	Fatigue, dizziness, diarrhea	Best when combined with another class of antiemetic Many potential drug interactions	Nausea from chemotherapy
Cannabinoids	Dronabinol	Exact mechanism of action unknown	Tachycardia and hypotension can also occur Potential for abuse related to effects similar to smoking marijuana	Must not be given to clients with psychiatric disorders	

IV, intravenous(ly).

Table 8-4

Classification of Laxatives Based on Time to Expected Effect

Laxative Group	Time to Expected Effect
I	2–6 hr
II	6–12 hr
II	1–3 days

Table 8-5

Drugs Used to Treat Constipation

Class	Prototype	Mechanism of Action	Major Side and Adverse Effects	Critical Information	Indications
Bulk-forming	Psyllium	Acts like dietary fiber; causes stool to swell and increase ease of passage Group III	Minimal side effects Esophageal obstruction if compound does not pass through the esophagus and swells there	Must be taken with a full glass of water	Constipation
Osmotic	Polyethylene glycol	Pulls water into the colon to soften stool via osmosis Group II—works in 6–12 hours	Water loss, signs of dehydration Nausea, flatulence	Increase fluid intake to prevent dehydration	Diverticulosis, IBS, dietary fiber supplement
Stimulant	Bisacodyl	Increase motility of colon to move stool forward Increase water in the intestine to soften stool Group II if given orally Group I if given rectally—works in 15–60 minutes	Burning sensation of rectum if given rectally Risk of dehydration	Large potential for abuse of this laxative	Constipation, bowel cleansing before colonoscopy
Surfactant	Docusate sodium	Increase amount of water in stool to ease passage Group III	Well tolerated	Administer with full glass of water Use caution with clients with heart failure, because sodium component may increase water retention and exacerbate heart failure symptoms	Constipation, relief of opioid-induced constipation, increased peristalsis

IBS, inflammatory bowel syndrome.

Diarrhea

Diarrhea is a symptom that is most commonly treated with opioid-containing medications. See Table 8-6 for the overview of the treatment options.

> **BLACK BOX WARNING:** Loperamide can cause torsades de points and sudden cardiac death in high doses and is contraindicated in clients younger than 2 years of age.

> **SAFETY ALERT!** Be aware of signs and symptoms of dehydration, such as dry mucous membranes; sunken eyes; hypotension; tachycardia; and weak, thready pulses. Remember that daily weights are the best indicator of fluid volume status.

GERD and PUD

A variety of medications are used in the management of GERD and PUD, outlined in Table 8-7.

> **BLACK BOX WARNING:** Misoprostol can cause abortion, premature birth, and/or birth defects and should be avoided in women of child-bearing age unless they can comply with contraception to prevent pregnancy.

Table 8-6

Drugs Used to Treat Diarrhea

Class	Prototype	Mechanism of Action	Major Side and Adverse Effects	Critical Information	Indications
Opioids	Diphenoxylate/atropine (controlled substance) Loperamide (available over the counter)	Bind to opioid receptors to decrease GI motility	Common side effects of diphenoxylate: nausea and abdominal pain High doses of diphenoxylate can cause respiratory and CNS depression Common side effects of loperamide constipation and nausea Serious adverse effects: Stevens-Johnson syndrome and toxic megacolon	Diphenoxylate has a potential for abuse–it is combined with atropine to discourage abuse	Noninfectious diarrhea

CNS, central nervous system; GI, gastrointestinal.

Table 8-7

Drugs Used to Treat GERD and PUD

Class	Prototype	Mechanism of Action	Major Side and Adverse Effects	Critical Information	Indications
PPIs	Omeprazole	Irreversible inhibition of the proton pump, which decrease production of gastric acid	Headache, nausea, and diarrhea are the most common side effects	Most effective acid reducers available	PUD
			Pneumonia may occur due to an increase in gastric acidity, especially in those prone to aspiration	Monitor for signs and symptoms of pneumonia (productive cough, fever, weakness)	GERD
			Hypersecretion of gastric acid if the medication is discontinued abruptly	PPIs interact with clopidogrel, decreases its effectiveness. For clients on both medications, they should be taken 12 hours apart.	
			Hypomagnesemia		
			Decreased calcium absorption by the bones, causes osteoporosis and fractures (long-term risk)	If *Clostridium difficile* is suspected, the medication must be stopped immediately	
			Clostridium difficile		
H2RAs	Ranitidine	Antagonist of histamine type 2, which is responsible for the formation of gastric acid production	Well-tolerated medication	More potent and better tolerated than older H2RAs (e.g., cimetidine)	PUD
			Pneumonia due to increased gastric pH	Does not affect histamine type 1, which is responsible for allergic reactions	GERD
Mucosal protectants	Sucralfate	Sticky gel that coats ulcers to allow for healing	Not systemically absorbed, so very few side effects	Administer all other medications 2 hours before or after sucralfate, because the coating it produces interferes with medication absorption	Hypersecretory disorders
			Constipation is the most common side effect		
Prostaglandin analog	Misoprostol	Acts to replace prostaglandins lost by NSAID use to increase secretion of mucous and bicarbonate and decreasing gastric acid secretion	Side effects include diarrhea, abdominal pain, and abnormal vaginal bleeding in women	Pregnancy is an absolute contraindication for use	Prevention of NSAID-induced ulcers
				It must be confirmed that women of child-bearing age are not pregnant before this medication can be prescribed	

(continued)

Table 8-7

Drugs Used to Treat GERD and PUD (continued)

Class	Prototype	Mechanism of Action	Major Side and Adverse Effects	Critical Information	Indications
Antibiotics (see Chapter 6 for overview of antibiotics)	Clarithromycin (macrolide)				PUD caused by H. Pylori
	Amoxicillin (penicillin)				
	Tetracycline				
	Metronidazole (nitroimidazole)				
Antacids	Three different formulations used for PUD and GERD:	Neutralize gastric acid to decrease destruction of the gastric mucosa	Magnesium: diarrhea, hypermagnesemia if renal insufficiency or failure is present	Alters stomach pH; administer all other medications 2 hours before or after antacids	GERD
	Magnesium (magnesium hydroxide)		Aluminum: constipation	Need to be taken 7 times per day to treat PUD, which makes compliance difficult	PUD
	Aluminum (aluminum hydroxide)		Calcium: constipation and flatulence	Magnesium antacids cannot be given to clients with renal dysfunction, as they may lead to potentially fatal hypermagnesemia	
	Calcium (calcium carbonate)			Magnesium can also be used as an osmotic laxative (milk of magnesia)	
				Aluminum antacids are usually used to counteract diarrhea from magnesium antacids	
				If dose exceeds recommended amount, calcium antacids can lead to metabolic alkalosis	

GERD, gastroesophageal reflux disease; H2RA, histamine-2 receptor blocker; NSAID, nonsteroidal anti-inflammatory drug; PPI, proton pump inhibitor; PUD, peptic ulcer disease.

Practice Questions and Rationales

1. A client reports to the nurse that bowel movements only occur every 4 days and requests a laxative. What is the **best** response by the nurse?
   1. "We will need to obtain an x-ray of your abdomen to see what is going on."
   2. "Have you needed a laxative in the past for this problem?"
   3. "I will contact your provider to request a laxative for you immediately."
   4. "Please describe your most recent bowel movement for me."

2. During intravenous infusion of promethazine, a client reports burning at the intravenous insertion site. What is the correct action by the nurse?
   1. Discontinue the infusion.
   2. Slow down the rate of infusion.
   3. Apply a warm compress to the site.
   4. Assess the area for redness or swelling.

3. A postoperative client is on telemetry and reports nausea. The rhythm strip on the telemetry device shows the following rhythm.

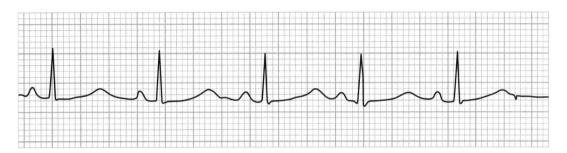

   Which medication, if ordered by the prescriber, would require the nurse to intervene?
   1. Dexamethasone
   2. Promethazine
   3. Ondansetron
   4. Lorazepam

4. A pregnant client experiencing morning sickness does not want to take medications to treat her nausea. What nonpharmacologic alternatives would the nurse suggest to help reduce the client's nausea? Select all that apply.
   1. Increase dietary fat.
   2. Avoid known triggers of nausea.
   3. Eat a small snack immediately after waking.
   4. Engage in perinatal massages regularly.
   5. Drink 8 to 10 glasses of water daily.

5. A client with a past medical history of opioid abuse has several episodes of noninfectious diarrhea. The nurse is about to administer the prescribed loperamide when the client states "I do not want to take that, it will make me high." What is the **best** response by the nurse?

     1. "I understand your concern, but it is important to decrease your diarrhea."
     2. "Have you used this medication to make you high before?"
     3. "I will contact the prescriber and request diphenoxylate instead."
     4. "Even though it contains an opioid, it will not make you high."

6. A client arrives to the emergency department reporting more than six episodes of diarrhea per day for the last 5 days. The nurse assesses the client for what signs or symptoms associated with frequent diarrhea?

     1. Serum osmolality 260 mOsm/L (260 mmol/L)
     2. Urine output 60 mL/hr
     3. Bicarbonate 30 mEq/dL (30 mmol/L)
     4. Muscle cramps
     5. Flattened T waves on electrocardiogram

7. A client with peptic ulcer disease has been taking omeprazole for the past 10 years and is concerned about long-term effects of the medication. Which are potential long-term effects the nurse should discuss with the client? Select all that apply.

     1. Hyperkalemia
     2. Osteopenia
     3. Hypomagnesemia
     4. Stomach cancer
     5. Renal insufficiency

8. Which laboratory value for a client who has recently been prescribed misoprostol for peptic ulcer disease would require **immediate** action by the nurse?

     1. Serum sodium 133 mEq/dL (133 mmol/L)
     2. Hemoglobin 10.2 mg/dL (102 g/L)
     3. Arterial pH 7.46 (7.46)
     4. Human chorionic gonadotropin 30 mIU/mL (30 IU/L)

9. A client has been diagnosed with peptic ulcer disease caused by *Helicobacter pylori*. Which instruction will the nurse provide to the client with regard to the medication regimen for this diagnosis?

     1. "You will need to limit intake of all medications containing acetaminophen."
     2. "You may need to take two or three different antibiotics to properly treat this disease."
     3. "The *Helicobacter pylori* in your stomach will be treated with high doses of antifungal medications."
     4. "The best way to treat this disease is through alterations in your diet to increase the acidity of your stomach."

10. A client with symptomatic gastroesophageal reflux disease (GERD) has requested the medication regimen be switched from ranitidine to sucralfate. Which response by the nurse is appropriate?

    1. "Sucralfate is not as strong as ranitidine, so you should continue your current regimen."
    2. "You should use both of these medications to provide maximum symptom relief."
    3. "Sucralfate will not improve your symptoms unless you have an ulcer."
    4. "There are many side effects of sucralfate, it is not recommended for you to switch medications."

11. A client with peptic ulcer disease taking pantoprazole develops a fever and white blood cell count of 13,500/μL (13.5 × 10⁹/L). What is the **priority** nursing action?

    1. Obtain a urine specimen for culture and sensitivity.
    2. Palpate for tactile fremitus.
    3. Check a complete set of vital signs.
    4. Palpate the abdomen for distention or masses.

12. A client with diabetes and peptic ulcer disease has been prescribed clarithromycin for the treatment of *Helicobacter pylori*. Which statement made by the client indicates teaching by the nurse was effective?

    1. "If I develop a rash, I should limit my sun exposure."
    2. "I will stop this medication immediately if I have an episode of diarrhea."
    3. "A change in the taste of food may indicate a serious reaction to the medication."
    4. "If I develop hearing loss while taking this medication, it is reversible."

13. A client with severe constipation has developed abdominal pain, distention, nausea, and inability to pass stool. Which medication will the nurse request to provide the **best** relief for the client?

    1. Docusate sodium
    2. Ondansetron
    3. Bisacodyl suppository
    4. Ranitidine

14. Which assessment findings would alert the nurse to potential adverse effects for a client receiving total parenteral nutrition (TPN) containing insulin? Select all that apply.

    1. Absent bowel sounds
    2. Absolute neutrophil count 9,000/μL (9 × 10⁹/L)
    3. Blood glucose 50 mg/dL (2.77 mmol/L)
    4. Mean arterial pressure (MAP) 50 mm Hg
    5. 2+ peripheral pulses

15. A pediatric client weighing 38 lb is prescribed promethazine 0.1 mg/kg every 6 hours. Calculate the total daily dose. Round your answer to the nearest tenth.

    _____ mg/day

9

CANCER MEDICATIONS

BRIEF OVERVIEW OF CANCER

Cancer is not a single disease but rather a term that is used to describe over 100 diseases that can affect almost any tissue or organ within the body. Cancer represents abnormalities in the normal balance of cellular processes controlling programmed cell death (apoptosis), repair, metabolism, reproduction, and proliferation. These abnormalities lead to the behavioral characteristics of cancerous cells such as uncontrolled growth and reproduction, evading the body's normal immune defenses, the ability to invade surrounding tissues, and spread to distant sites (metastasis).

CLINICAL PEARLS

◆ The signs and symptoms of cancer vary with each type of cancer.
◆ The National Cancer Institute (NCI) encourages individuals to seek medical evaluation for the following signs and symptoms that persist for more than 2 weeks:
  ● Unexplained weight gain or loss
  ● Pain
  ● Skin changes including those involving warts, moles, or sores that do not heal
  ● Changes in bowel or bladder habits
  ● Persistent cough, hoarseness, or sore throat
  ● Unusual bleeding or discharge including blood in urine, stools, or from the vagina
  ● A thickening or lump in the breast or other part of the body
  ● Change in size or shape of the breast or nipple
  ● Continued indigestion, changes in appetite, or trouble swallowing
  ● Unexplained night sweats
  ● Persistently feeling week or very tired
◆ The diagnostic evaluation of all forms of malignancy begins with history and physical examination and includes clinical and pathologic examinations. Clinical staging is accomplished through diagnostic imaging procedures, such as computed tomography (CT), magnetic resonance imaging (MRI), and ultrasound to assess tumor size, location, involvement of adjacent structures or lymph nodes, and metastasis to other parts of the body. Diagnostic imaging procedures to identify metastasis are dependent on the clinical examination, presence of symptoms, and other assessment parameters that might indicate organ or bone involvement.
◆ Pathologic assessment of tumor tissue identifies cancer cell type and growth characteristics, and microscopic evidence of spread to lymph nodes, surrounding, or distant tissues. Tissue is also tested to identify genetic, biochemical, or molecular biomarkers that provide information about prognosis, cancer cell behavior, and potential treatment options.

- Additional diagnostic procedures (i.e., blood cell counts, electrolyte levels, or pulmonary function tests) are performed to assess the effects of cancer on normal body functions.
- According to the American Cancer Society (ACS), the two most common types of cancer affecting both males and females are lung and colorectal cancer.
- In women, breast cancer is the most common type of cancer; in men, prostate cancer is the most common form of cancer.

Lung Cancer

Overview

- Lung cancer, the leading cause of cancer death for both genders, accounts for 25% of all cancer-related deaths.
- Most clients present with advanced or metastatic lung cancer, in part, because signs and symptoms do not develop early in the disease. With recent implementation of lung cancer screening for individuals at high risk, it is anticipated over time that lung cancer will be diagnosed at an earlier stage.
- Tobacco smoking is the leading risk factor for lung cancer. The risk is proportional to the number of cigarettes smoked per day and the number of years of tobacco use. Individuals with a 20- to 30-pack-year history (a pack year is defined as 20 cigarettes smoked daily for 1 year) are considered at high risk for developing lung cancer. Secondhand exposure for nonsmokers is also a risk factor.
- Other risk factors include occupational or environmental exposure to general air pollution, asbestos, radon, and metals such as arsenic, nickel, and chromium.

Signs and Symptoms

- Clinical manifestations include cough, hemoptysis, dyspnea, shortness of breath, and dysphagia.
- Clients may develop a variety of symptoms associated with advanced disease such as pain, or headache, weight loss, anorexia, fatigue, and neurologic symptoms.
- Clients with lung cancer are at risk for disorders, referred to as paraneoplastic syndromes, that stem from the metabolic effects of lung cancer on body tissues. Examples of these disorders include electrolyte and endocrine abnormalities such as elevated calcium levels, syndrome of inappropriate antidiuretic hormone (SIADH), and Cushing syndrome.

Diagnostics

- Clinical staging of lung cancer includes chest x-ray and CT scan of the chest, abdomen, and pelvis to identify the primary tumor and metastasis.
- MRI of the brain is performed for clients who have neurologic symptoms; radionucleotide bone scan is done for clients with bone pain or an elevated serum alkaline phosphatase level.
- The least invasive method for tissue for biopsy is chosen based on the location of the tumor or enlarged lymph nodes. Biopsy is performed through bronchoscopy, radiologic image-guided percutaneous access, mediastinoscopy, or excision performed during the surgical intervention. Aspiration of pleural effusion may allow identification of cancer cells.

Colorectal Cancer

Overview

- Colorectal cancer is the fourth most frequently diagnosed cancer and the second leading cause of cancer death in the United States.
- Risk factors associated with colorectal cancer include inherited genetic abnormalities, family history of colorectal cancer, personal history of inflammatory bowel disease, tobacco smoking, alcohol intake, diets lacking in fruits and vegetables, consumption of red and processed meats, low levels of physical activity, metabolic syndrome, diabetes mellitus, obesity/high body mass index (BMI), and colonic polyps.

Signs and Symptoms

- There may be no signs or symptoms in early stages of colorectal cancer. As the disease progresses, clients may experience rectal bleeding or blood in stools (melena), changes in bowel habits, cramping abdominal pain and distension, a palpable abdominal mass, weakness, fatigue, unintended weight loss, enlarged lymph nodes, and/or anemia.

Diagnostic Indicators

- Diagnostic evaluation and staging of colorectal cancer include colonoscopy and CT scan of the chest, abdomen, and pelvis.

Pertinent Laboratory Values

- Complete blood cell count (CBC), serum chemistry, and carcinoembryonic antigen (CEA) measurement may be obtained to help arrive at a diagnosis.

Breast Cancer

Overview

- In women, breast cancer is the leading cause of cancer and the second most common cause of cancer-related death. Breast cancer is 100 times more common in women than in men (Siegel et al., 2018).
- While the overall incidence of breast cancer is slightly higher in white women, African American women are diagnosed at a younger age, with higher rates of regional or advanced disease, and have a higher mortality rate than do white women.
- Risk factors associated with breast cancer include inherited genetic abnormalities, family history of breast cancer in a first-degree relative; age (especially greater than 55 years or older); early menarche; nulliparity; first full-term pregnancy after age 30; no history of breast-feeding; late age of menopause; use of hormone replacement therapy, oral contraceptives, or both; high-fat diet; obesity; high amount of alcohol use; smoking tobacco; and prior thoracic radiation therapy.
- Risk assessment is performed prior to treatment planning to identify which clients are most likely to respond to treatment, have aggressive disease, or develop metastasis regardless of treatment. Factors considered in the risk assessment include close blood relative with history of breast, ovarian, metastatic prostate, or pancreatic cancer; age of onset of breast cancer for client or close blood relative; and client or close blood relative with certain known inherited genetic mutations or cancer syndromes.

Signs and Symptoms

◆ A new lump or mass, swelling of all or part of a breast or axilla, skin irritation or dimpling (sometimes looking like an orange peel), breast or nipple pain, nipple retraction (turning inward), redness, scaling, or thickening of the nipple or breast skin and nipple discharge (other than breast milk).

◆ Most breast cancers are identified through a screening mammogram rather than through self-breast examinations.

Diagnostic Indicators

◆ Diagnostic evaluation and staging of breast cancer begin with a bilateral diagnostic mammogram. If additional imaging is needed to clarify the findings, ultrasound and/or MRI are used.

◆ When feasible, the preferred method of tissue biopsy is a percutaneous core breast biopsy where multiple core tissue samples are obtained. Most often, a stereotactic core biopsy is performed; the procedure uses radiologic imaging from mammography, MRI, or ultrasound to more accurately locate the target biopsy location. Excisional biopsy is performed when the core biopsy provides indeterminate results or if rare cancer cell types are suspected. Fine needle aspiration (FNA) using a very thin, hollow needle may be used to sample a small amount of fluid and very small pieces of tissue from the tumor. This type of biopsy is not routinely used because it does not provide adequate tissue sample for full analysis.

◆ Sentinel lymph node biopsy to identify spread to the initial lymph nodes into which a tumor drains is most often the preferred procedure to confirm lymph node involvement.

  ● The cancer stage reflects the genetic, biochemical, and molecular analysis of cancer cells; tumor size; presence of local tissue invasion; spread to lymph nodes; and/or metastasis to distant sites.

  ● The cancer stage is used to determine the need for combined treatments (called multimodality therapy) involving surgery and/or radiation and/or chemotherapy.

Prostate Cancer

Overview

◆ Except for skin cancer, prostate cancer is the most common cancer in men in the United States. It is anticipated that one in nine men will develop prostate cancer during their lifetime.

◆ African American men or those with a close relative diagnosed with prostate cancer before the age of 65 appear to be at higher risk than white men for the development of prostate cancer. These individuals are encouraged to discuss prostate cancer screening with their physicians beginning at age 45.

◆ Increasing age is the most well-documented risk factor linked to prostate cancer. In addition to African American ancestry, other risk factors include a familial predisposition in 5% to 10% of cases, inherited genetic mutations, and smoking tobacco.

◆ Risk assessment is performed prior to treatment planning to identify which clients are most likely to respond to treatment, have aggressive disease, or develop metastasis regardless of treatment. Factors considered in the risk assessment include the prostate-specific antigen (PSA) level, the size of the tumor palpated by digital rectal examination (DRE), and Gleason score (aggressiveness of the cancer cells in the biopsy specimen).

Signs and Symptoms

◆ Early stages of prostate cancer may have no signs or symptoms. As the cancer advances, signs and symptoms include weak or interrupted urine flow; difficulty starting or stopping urine flow; urinary frequency, especially at night; hematuria and/or dysuria. Pelvic, spine, and rib pain are often associated with metastasis to bone.

Diagnostic Indicators

◆ Diagnostic evaluation and staging of prostate cancer include physical examination, DRE, PSA level, and prostate biopsy.

◆ Endorectal or prostate ultrasound, CT, and MRI (with or without rectal coil) are used by some physicians to assist with diagnostic evaluation and clinical staging.

Pertinent Laboratory Values

Prostate-specific antigen: The serum values vary based on ethnicity and age. Levels over 4 ng/mL (4 µg/L) warrant prostate biopsy.

CHEMOTHERAPY

◆ Defined as a systemic treatment for cancer that uses drugs to stop the growth of cancer cells, either by killing the cells or by stopping them from reproducing.

◆ Chemotherapy may be classified by mechanism of action in relation to the cell cycle (a multistage process of reproduction).

- Drugs that exert their maximal effect during specific phases of the cell cycle are termed cell cycle–specific agents. Actively proliferating cancer cells progressing through the cell cycle are most sensitive to the effects of chemotherapy.
- Drugs that act independently of cell cycle phases are termed cell cycle nonspecific agents.

◆ Chemotherapy drugs may also be categorized into chemical groups, each with differing mechanisms of action. These include the alkylating agents, nitrosoureas, antimetabolites, antitumor antibiotics, topoisomerase inhibitors, plant alkaloids (also referred to as mitotic inhibitors), and hormonal and miscellaneous agents. The classification, mechanism of action, cell cycle specificity, and common side effects of selected types of chemotherapy are included in Table 9-1.

General Approaches to Use of Chemotherapy in Cancer Treatment

◆ Chemotherapy is administered in repeated doses over time to maximize the number of cancer cells that are destroyed and/or prevented from reproducing.

◆ Two or more chemotherapy agents from different categories, called combination chemotherapy, are used together to leverage varying mechanisms of action, maximize cancer cell

| Table 9-1 |

Chemotherapy Classification

Class	Prototype	Mechanism of Action	Cell Cycle Specificity	Major Side and Adverse Effects	Indications
Alkylating Agents					
Nitrogen mustards	Melphalan, mechlorethamine, cyclophosphamide, ifosfamide, bendamustine	Damages DNA resulting in impaired cell functioning and reproduction processes; leads to cell death	Cell cycle nonspecific	Bone marrow suppression, nausea, vomiting, alopecia, secondary malignancy	Melphalan: Recurrent epithelial ovarian cancer Cyclophosphamide: Breast cancer Bendamustine: Non-Hodgkin lymphoma
Platinum-based antineoplastic ("platins")	Cisplatin, carboplatin, and oxaliplatin			Delayed hypersensitivity; Nausea, vomiting, renal, neuro and ototoxicity; bone marrow suppression, cold-induced peripheral, perioral, and/or pharyngolaryngeal dysesthesia, (oxaliplatin)	Carboplatin: Epithelial ovarian and lung cancer Oxaliplatin: Colorectal cancer Cisplatin: Lung cancer
Nitrosoureas (cross the blood–brain barrier)	Carmustine, lomustine, and streptozocin			Pulmonary and hepatic impairment; prolonged bone marrow suppression	Carmustine and lomustine: Brain tumor Streptozocin: Neuroendocrine adrenal and islet cell cancer
Hydrazine and triazine agents	Procarbazine, dacarbazine, and temozolomide			Bone marrow suppression, nausea, vomiting, secondary malignancy; monoamine oxidase inhibitor properties (procarbazine)	Temozolomide and procarbazine: Bain cancer Dacarbazine: Advanced malignant melanoma
Alkane sulfonate agent	Busulfan			Seizures with high doses	Busulfan: Prior to stem cell transplant for leukemia

(continued)

Table 9-1

Chemotherapy Classification (continued)

Class	Prototype	Mechanism of Action	Cell Cycle Specificity	Major Side and Adverse Effects	Indications
Antimetabolite Agents					
Pyrimidine antagonists	Cytosine arabino-side, 5-fluorouracil, capecitabine, cytarabine, fludarabine, azacytidine, decitabine, gemcitabine	Interferes with the biosynthesis of metabolites necessary for RNA and DNA synthesis; inhibits DNA replication and repair	Cell cycle—S phase specific	Nausea, vomiting, diarrhea, hand–foot syndrome (capecitabine), hepatotoxicity (6-thioguanine)	Cytosine arabinoside: Acute myeloid leukemia 5-Fluorouracil and capecitabine: Colorectal cancer Gemcitabine: Large cell lymphoma
Folate antagonists	Methotrexate, peme-trexed, and pralatrexate			Bone marrow suppression, mucositis; renal impairment, urine crystal formation, dermatitis, tumor lysis syndrome, arachnoiditis, and encephalopathy (methotrexate)	Pemetrexed: Lung cancer Methotrexate: Acute lymphoblastic leukemia
Microtubule Agents					
Plant alkaloids	Vinblastine, vincris-tine, vinorelbine, and vindesine	Arrest metaphase by inhibiting mitotic tubular formation (spindle); inhibit DNA and protein synthesis	Cell cycle G2 and M phase specific	Myelosuppression—especially neutropenia, peripheral and autonomic neuropathy (bloating, constipation, ileus), fever, pulmonary, and liver toxicity	Vincristine: Brain cancer Vinblastine: Testicular cancer Vinorelbine: Lung cancer
Taxanes	Paclitaxel and docetaxel			Hypersensitivity, myelosuppression, neurotoxicity	Paclitaxel and docetaxel: Epithelial ovarian cancer
Epothilones	Ixabepilone			Prolonged myelosuppression	Ixabepilone: metastatic breast cancer

Topoisomerase Inhibitor Agents

	Camptothecins: Irinotecan and topotecan (crosses blood–brain barrier); etoposide, teniposide	Cell cycle nonspecific	Induce breaks in the DNA strand and interferes with reproduction	Myelosuppression, diarrhea (irinotecan); smokers may require lower doses; topotecan: lower doses needed with history of renal failure; etoposide and teniposide associated with increased risks of secondary acute myeloid leukemia; stomatitis	Etoposide: Non-Hodgkin lymphoma and testicular cancer Topotecan: Ovarian cancer
Anthracyclines (also classified as antitumor antibiotics)	Epirubicin, daunorubicin, doxorubicin, and idarubicin	Cell cycle nonspecific	Interfere with DNA synthesis by binding DNA; prevent RNA synthesis	Bone marrow suppression; anorexia, nausea, and vomiting; alopecia; cardiac toxicity (daunorubicin, doxorubicin), red urine (doxorubicin, idarubicin, epirubicin)	Idarubicin and daunorubicin: acute myeloid leukemia Doxorubicin: Breast cancer

Glucocorticoid Agents

Corticosteroids	Prednisone, hydrocortisone, methylprednisolone, and dexamethasone	N/A	Induces apoptosis; when given in pharmacologic doses, growth of tumors is inhibited in certain types of cancers	Weight gain, osteoporosis, hyperglycemia, and mood effects	Dexamethasone: Multiple myeloma Prednisone: Non-Hodgkin lymphoma

Hormonal Agents

Antiestrogens	Tamoxifen and toremifene	N/A	Blocks estrogen-binding site in cancer cells and prevents tumor growth in cancers dependent on estrogen	Tamoxifen: Increased incidence of endometrial cancer and thromboembolic events	Tamoxifen and toremifene: Breast cancer
Estrogen antagonist	Fulvestrant	N/A	Blocks estrogen-binding site in cancer cells and prevents tumor growth in cancers dependent on estrogen	Injection site pain, nausea, bone pain, headache, fatigue, arthralgias	Fulvestrant: Breast cancer

(continued)

Table 9-1

Chemotherapy Classification (continued)

Class	Prototype	Mechanism of Action	Cell Cycle Specificity	Major Side and Adverse Effects	Indications
Aromatase inhibitor	Anastrozole, exemestane, letrozole	Decrease circulating estrogen levels thereby preventing tumor growth in cancers dependent on estrogen	N/A	Hot flashes, musculoskeletal pain, vaginal dryness, and headache; increased incidence of bone fractures and osteoporosis	Anastrozole, exemestane, and letrozole: Breast cancer
Estrogens	Chlorotrianisene, diethylstilbestrol, estramustine	Makes estrogen receptors less sensitive to estrogen; decreases estrogen levels	N/A	Increased risk of thrombosis, including fatal and nonfatal myocardial infarction, male gynecomastia and impotence, nausea, diarrhea	Diethylstilbestrol and estramustine: Prostate cancer
Progestins	Megestrol medroxyprogesterone (use is limited)	Makes estrogen receptors less sensitive to estrogen; decreases estrogen levels	N/A	Weight gain most common side effect; less frequently hypertension, congestive heart failure, thrombophlebitis, and pulmonary embolism	Megestrol: Advanced breast cancer
Gonadotropin-releasing hormone antagonist	Degarelix	Cause a decrease in testosterone in men to stop prostate cancer growth	N/A	Injection site reactions (e.g, pain, erythema, swelling, or induration), hot flashes, increased weight, fatigue, and increases in serum levels of transaminases and GGT	Degarelix: Prostate cancer
Luteinizing hormone-releasing hormone analogue	Leuprolide, goserelin acetate	Cause a decrease in androgen levels in men to stop prostate cancer growth and estrogen levels in women interfering with breast cancer growth	N/A	Temporary transient increase in androgen level; implant site reaction and soreness, hot flashes, sweating, tiredness, headache, nausea, diarrhea, constipation, stomach pain, acne, gynecomastia	Leuprolide, and goserelin acetate: Prostate cancer
Nonsteroidal antiandrogens	Bicalutamide, flutamide, nilutamide	Binds to the androgen receptors and prevents tumor growth	N/A	Gynecomastia, sexual dysfunction, vasomotor symptoms, liver enzyme abnormalities, osteoporosis, and gastrointestinal symptoms	Bicalutamide, flutamide, and nilutamide: Prostate cancer

Miscellaneous Agents

	Agent	Mechanism		Adverse effects	Indication
	L-Asparaginase, bleomycin, procarbazine, tretinoin	L-Asparaginase depletes an amino acid needed for leukemia cell survival	N/A	Anaphylaxis, hypersensitivity: Thrombosis, pancreatitis, glucose intolerance, liver toxicity, coagulopathy, pulmonary fibrosis (bleomycin)	L-Asparaginase: Acute lymphoblastic leukemia Bleomycin: Testicular cancer Tretinoin: Acute promyelocytic leukemia
Miotic inhibitor	Amsacrine	Binds with DNA to prevent reproduction	N/A	Myelosuppression, mucositis, perirectal abscess	Amsacrine: Acute myeloid leukemia
	Arsenic trioxide	Not completely understood	N/A	Differentiation syndrome, (can be fatal if not treated) Symptoms may include fever, dyspnea, acute respiratory distress, pulmonary infiltrates, pleural or pericardial effusions, weight gain or peripheral edema, hypotension, and renal, hepatic, or multiorgan dysfunction. Electrocardiographic abnormalities	Arsenic trioxide: Acute myeloid leukemia

GGT, gamma-glutamyltransferase.

destruction, offer potential synergistic effects, prevent development of drug-resistant cancer cells, and minimize overlapping toxicities.

- Single-agent chemotherapy, as an initial treatment for limited or advanced cancer, is avoided because over time cancer cells develop resistance to a single drug.
- Single-agent chemotherapy is used for clients with advanced cancer who have experienced disease progression following the use of combination chemotherapy.
◆ Treatment choices are based on the type of cancer as well as the cancer stage.
  - In addition to the type of cancer and stage, the choice of chemotherapy and other treatment options are based on the following: age, functional abilities, past medical history, comorbidities, organ function, and other medications prescribed for the client.
◆ Chemotherapy dosing is most often calculated based on body surface area that reflects height and weight.
◆ Routes of chemotherapy administration are presented in Table 9-2.

Chemotherapy-Related Toxicities (Adverse Effects)

◆ Both cancer and normal cells are subject to the effects of chemotherapy. In normal cells, the effects of chemotherapy result in toxicities or adverse effects, which are defined as unfavorable or unintended signs, symptoms, or diseases associated with the use of a medical treatment or procedure.
◆ The incidence and magnitude of toxicities are influenced by the mode of administration, dose, and treatment schedule. Clients who have are frail, have a poor performance status, and/or have comorbid illnesses, tend to be more susceptible to adverse effects associated with chemotherapy and other cancer treatments.
◆ Although other medications used to treat cancer, such as targeted therapy and immunotherapy, often have unique side effect profiles, some of the toxicities overlap with those associated with chemotherapy.
◆ Almost all body systems or organs are subject to chemotherapy-related toxicity and include gastrointestinal (GI), hematopoietic, integumentary, neurologic, genitourinary, reproductive, pulmonary, cardiovascular, endocrine, and electrolyte balance.
◆ The NCI Common Toxicity Criteria for Adverse Events (CTCAE v5.0) is a descriptive terminology grading system developed to provide consistent and standardized toxicity assessment criteria for clients receiving cancer treatments such as chemotherapy.
  - Although specific parameters according to organ or system categories apply to the grading criteria, the general approach to toxicity grading is as follows: grade 1 (mild), grade 2 (moderate), grade 3 (severe), grade 4 (life threatening), and grade 5 (death occurring during treatment).
  - The CTCAE is used to determine the need for changes in the chemotherapy treatment plan such as dosing modifications.
  - The CTCAE is used in clinical trials to report toxicities that may be associated with investigational drugs.

Gastrointestinal Adverse Effects: Chemotherapy-Induced Nausea and Vomiting

◆ Chemotherapy-induced nausea and vomiting (CINV) is a result of complex central and peripheral nervous system communication pathways involving neurotransmitters such as neurokinins (NKs), serotonin ($5-HT_3$), cannabinoid, and dopamine (D2)

Table 9-2

Routes of Chemotherapy Administration

Route	Rationale	Considerations	Nursing Care
Oral	Allows home administration	Adherence and safety issues	Assess client ability to follow oral regimen, manage toxicities, and maintain drug safely at home
	Facilitates independence	Clients seen less often by providers	Assess and address barriers that may interfere with adherence and toxicity management
	Less disruptive or invasive	Financial barriers may interfere with adherence	Client teaching regarding drug regimen, toxicity management, and drug storage safety
			Monitor adherence and toxicities in between provider visits
Intravenous	Systemic distribution and absorption	Repeated IV placement may be difficult and painful	Assess veins prior to initiation of therapy; discuss long-term venous access with care team as warranted
	Necessary for drugs that can cause tissue damage with extravasation	Drugs can lead to venous sclerosing	Obtain chemotherapy certification and adhere to ASCO/ONS guidelines for chemotherapy administration
		Extravasation of irritant and vesicant drugs can cause mild to severe tissue damage necessitating skin grafts	Monitor intravenous site for extravasation: pain, redness, edema, discoloration
			Monitor for catheter-related infection
Subcutaneous	Allows home administration depending of the drug	Absorption may be less reliable	Monitor for infection, thrombocytopenia, clotting dysfunction, or evidence of bleeding, bruising, or hematoma
	Less invasive	Difficult in very thin clients or those with cachexia	
Intramuscular	Less time intensive than traditional intravenous route	Absorption may be less reliable	Monitor for infection, thrombocytopenia, clotting dysfunction, or evidence of bleeding, bruising, or hematoma
		Difficult clients with muscle wasting or those with cachexia	

(continued)

Table 9-2

Routes of Chemotherapy Administration (continued)

Route	Rationale	Considerations	Nursing Care
Intrathecal	Allows direct access to cerebral spinal fluid	Access necessitates client endure lumbar puncture or placement of ventricular reservoir or implanted pump device	Monitor client for evidence of infection
Intraventricular		Special training and skills required for drug administration	Monitor client for signs of elevated intracranial pressure (headache, nausea/vomiting, seizures, change in mental status)
			Monitor reservoir or pump for occlusion or malfunction
Intravesical	Administration of chemotherapy directly into the bladder through a Foley catheter allows direct contact with bladder wall and area of resected tumor	Chemotherapy administration may occur in the postanesthesia care setting immediately after surgical resection of the bladder tumor or in the physician's office ambulatory setting	Follow institutional policy and procedure for use of closed system to prevent client and others' exposure to hazardous drugs
		Clients may be sent home with indwelling Foley catheter for 1–2 days until postoperative visit	Clients are assisted to turn frequently to promote maximum bladder wall exposure to chemotherapy
			Several chemotherapy agents have been used for intravesical therapy. Although side effects may vary according to the chemical properties of the agent, clients are monitored for symptoms of cystitis, pain hematuria, dysuria, and urgency. In clients with traumatic catheterization, bladder irritation, or use of vesicant chemotherapy, there may be a greater incidence of cystitis and pain
			Some agents used may be absorbed into the circulation through the bladder wall. Therefore, clients are monitored for systemic toxicities associated with specific chemotherapy drugs. Provide clients education about care of indwelling Foley catheter and drainage bag/urine disposal using safe handling precautions; signs and symptoms of urinary infection and bleeding, and pain management

Intrapleural	Pleurodesis: Injection of sclerosing agent, which may or may not be chemotherapy, into pleural space to cause inflammatory reaction so that the parietal and visceral layers of the pleura adhere to each other; goal to eliminate space for reaccumulation of pleural effusion (Lenker, Mayer, & Bernard, 2015)	Requires placement of pleural catheter to drain effusion prior to intrapleural administration of chemotherapy sclerosing agent
		Catheters are placed into the pleural space via thoracoscopic video-assisted surgical procedures or tunneled into place as an outpatient procedure with imaging guidance
		Clients with tunneled pleural catheters are managed in the home and require teaching regarding catheter care and drainage of pleural fluid
		Monitor clients for signs and symptoms of catheter-elated infection
		Clients are monitored for effusion reaccumulation including dyspnea and shortness of breath
Intraperitoneal	Allows abdominal structures to be in direct contact with chemotherapy agents	The procedure is very complicated, associated with multiple potential complications. Best outcomes are experienced by multidisciplinary collaboration, specially trained physicians and centers with high volumes of clients undergoing this procedure. Careful assessment for eligible clients is critical. Clinical trials continue to explore best approaches to client selection and treatment procedures
	Hyperthermic intraperitoneal chemotherapy (HIPEC) following surgical removal of cancer that has spread to peritoneal surfaces, while the client is still in the operating room, a heated solution of chemotherapy is infused into the abdominal cavity. After a limited period, the solution is drained and the needed procedures to close the abdomen are completed. Used to treat a select group of clients with cancers that metastasized to the abdominal region such as mesothelioma, colorectal, and ovarian cancer	Nursing care for chemotherapy administration is guided by policy and procedure for temperature of chemotherapy solution, chemotherapy instillation, amount of time drug remains in abdomen (dwell time), and drainage
		Requires frequent turning of the client to facilitate maximum exposure of abdominal surfaces to chemotherapy
		Postoperatively assess client for pain, abdominal distention, nausea, vomiting, ileus, bowel perforation, wound integrity, peritoneal infection, fluid and electrolyte, and renal and cardiopulmonary status
		Postoperative care includes maintenance of the nasogastric tube, venous thromboembolism prophylaxis, administrations of antiemetics, hydration, electrolytes, and analgesics

(continued)

Table 9-2

Routes of Chemotherapy Administration (continued)

Route	Rationale	Considerations	Nursing Care
Intra-arterial	Chemotherapy delivered through arterial circulation directly to the tumor Decreased systemic side effects depending on doses	Most frequent approach is via infusion pump implanted in abdomen for treatment of hepatic metastasis commonly related to gastrointestinal cancers Clinical trials are exploring percutaneous arterial catheter placement guided through radiographic procedures such as arteriography. Treatment for liver tumors may combine chemotherapy and/or an agent that cuts off artery supplying blood flow to tumor tissue in order to cause tumor necrosis and tumor cell death (referred to as chemoembolization therapy)	In order to fill the pump reservoir with chemotherapy, the pump access is performed by specially trained nurses or physicians with noncoring needle Following insertion of pump, clients are instructed to report fever and swelling at the insertion site; avoid contact sports, use of heat over pump, spending time in a sauna or hot tub, scuba diving; and importance of maintaining appointment schedule For hepatic arterial chemoembolization monitor for intra-abdominal bleeding, nausea, vomiting, anorexia, pain, fever, edema, liver impairment, ascites, encephalopathy, renal dysfunction, infection, diarrhea Monitor prothrombin time and activated partial thromboplastin time Monitor for thrombus or embolism

ASCO/ONS, American Society of Clinical Oncology/Oncology Nursing Society.

SAFETY ALERT! Vesicant drugs are those that can cause severe tissue damage if they leak out of the vein into surrounding tissues (referred to as extravasation) during intravenous administration. Nurses or other state-defined health care providers must receive specialized education and training and demonstrate chemotherapy administration competencies to be certified and permitted to administer chemotherapy (Neuss et al., 2017). Many components of the medical and nursing interventions to manage extravasation of vesicants are dependent on the chemical characteristics of the specific chemotherapy agent.

Table 9-3

Chemotherapy Agents Listed in Terms of Risk of Associated Nausea and Vomiting

High Risk (>90% Incidence)	Moderate Risk (30%–90% Incidence)	Low Risk (10%–30% Incidence)	Minimal Risk (<10% Risk)
Cisplatin	Carboplatin	Paclitaxel	Bevacizumab
Mechlorethamine	Ifosfamide	Docetaxel	Bleomycin
Streptozotocin	Doxorubicin ($\leq$60 mg/m^2)	Mitoxantrone	Busulfan
Cyclophosphamide	Irinotecan	Pemetrexed	Fludarabine
(>1,500 mg/m^2)	Etoposide	Methotrexate	Nivolumab
Doxorubicin (>60 mg/m^2)	Oxaliplatin	Gemcitabine	Pembrolizumab
Ifosfamide (>2 g/m^2)	Temozolomide	Cytarabine ($\leq$100 mg/m^2)	Rituximab
Dacarbazine	Cytarabine (>1 g/m^2)	5-Fluorouracil	Trastuzumab
		Cetuximab	Vinblastine
			Vincristine

Chemotherapy agents may be rated according to the risk of causing nausea and vomiting (Table 9-3).

◆ Classification of CINV:
  ● Acute CINV occurs in the first 24 hours after chemotherapy.
  ● Delayed CINV occurs 24 hours to 7 days with a maximal intensity 48 to 72 hours following treatment.
  ● Anticipatory CINV, a conditioned response, occurs prior to administration of chemotherapy. It is triggered by sights, sounds, or odors associated with the period just prior to treatment and is seen in clients with a history of poorly controlled CINV.
  ● Breakthrough CINV occurs despite prophylactic measures.
  ● Refractory CINV is not responsive to standard treatment approaches.
◆ Additional factors may contribute to CINV such as concurrent symptoms (i.e., pain), comorbidities, the effects of the cancer, constipation, and other medications.
◆ The experience of CINV may affect appetite, nutrition status, fluid and electrolyte balance, wound healing, functional abilities, utilization of health care resources, quality of life, psychological status, and willingness to continue potentially useful or curative anticancer treatment.

Anorexia is common in clients receiving some types of chemotherapy and may be potentiated by CINV, cancer cell metabolites, alterations in taste, the effects of other cancer treatments, as well as physical and psychosocial distress.

Assessment of CINV

◆ Assess for factors contributing to anorexia, nausea, and vomiting.
◆ Monitor patterns of CINV and responsiveness to treatment.
◆ Monitor for Mallory-Weiss tear (esophageal tear due to vomiting).

◆ Monitor for signs and symptoms of inadequate fluid and nutritional intake and fluid and electrolyte losses such as fatigue, lethargy, postural dizziness, poor skin turgor, dry skin and mucus membranes, increased thirst, oliguria, and muscle cramps.

Diagnostic Indicators

- ◆ Elevated Hgb/Hct
- ◆ Elevated BUN/creatinine
- ◆ Electrolyte imbalance
- ◆ Tachycardia
- ◆ Hypotension, orthostatic hypotension
- ◆ Tachypnea
- ◆ Decreased urine output, concentrated urine
- ◆ Decreased jugular venous pressure
- ◆ Weight loss

Antiemetic Medications

- ◆ The key principles of CINV medication management that are based on national guidelines include the following:
  - Prophylactic antiemetic therapy is initiated prior to chemotherapy when the chemotherapy has greater than 10% risk of emesis and is continued long enough to cover the duration of emetic risk.
  - When combination chemotherapy regimens are used, choice of antiemetic is based on the chemotherapy agent with the highest risk of CINV.
- ◆ Management of CINV involves combinations of antiemetic medications or single drugs that inhibit the peripheral and central pathways and neurotransmitters involved in the physiology of nausea and vomiting. Table 9-4 provides examples of antiemetic regimens recommended by national guidelines.
- ◆ Other medications and nonpharmacologic strategies are used to prevent and manage CINV.

Mucositis

- ◆ An inflammatory process, associated with certain chemotherapy agents, involving the membranes of the oral cavity, the GI tract, and occasionally the vaginal mucosa.
- ◆ Depending on the drug, the process usually begins 5 to 14 days after chemotherapy administration and usually abates within approximately 2 to 4 weeks after the last dose of chemotherapy.
- ◆ Diarrhea, the most common symptom of GI tract mucositis, may become severe leading to malabsorption, bleeding, fluid and electrolyte imbalance, rectal excoriation, and secondary infection.
- ◆ Mucositis involving the tissues of the mouth, also referred to as stomatitis, ranges from mild tissue redness to severe and painful ulcerations, bleeding, and secondary infection.
  - Oral mucositis occurs in 40% to 80% of clients depending on the chemotherapy regimen; close to 100% of clients treated with high-dose chemotherapy used for hematopoietic stem cell transplantation (HSCT).
  - The incidence and severity of oral tissue involvement is greater in clients with head and neck cancers receiving both radiotherapy and chemotherapy.
  - Severe oral mucositis may impact swallowing, fluid and nutritional intake, speech, and quality of life.

Table 9-4

Examples of Antiemetic Regimens

High Risk of CINV With IV Chemotherapy: Address Acute and Delayed CINV

Drug Target	Day 1	Days 2, 3, 4	Clinical Pearls
Neurokinin	Aprepitant 125 mg po × 1	Aprepitant 80 mg po daily on days 2, 3 (if aprepitant used on day 1) **AND** Dexamethasone 8 mg po/IV on days 2, 3, 4	Neurokinin is used to prevent CINV not for management of symptoms
(NK antagonist)	Fosaprepitant 150 mg IV × 1		
(choose one)	Netupitant/palonosetron 0.05 mg po × 1		
Serotonin	Ondansetron 16–24 mg po × 1		Serotonin agents may cause headache and constipation: nurses provide clients with education regarding management of constipation
(5-HT3 antagonist)	Granisetron 0.01 mg/kg IV × 1		
(choose one)	Palonosetron 0.25 mg IV × 1		
Steroid	Dexamethasone 12 mg po/IV 1		Steroids may cause dyspepsia and hyperglycemia especially in clients with diabetes: clients may require acid blocking therapy and additional monitoring and management of hyperglycemia

Moderate Risk of CINV with IV chemotherapy: Address Acute and Delayed CINV

Drug Target	Day 1	Days 2, 3	Clinical Pearls
NK antagonist	Palonosetron 0.25 mg IV × 1	Olanzapine 10 mg po on days 2, 3	As above
Steroid	Dexamethasone 12 mg po/IV 1		As above
Blocks neurokinin, serotonin, and dopamine neurotransmitters	Olanzapine 10 mg po once		Olanzapine associated with mild short-term sedation: consider safety when using in clients at risk for falls or orthostatic hypotension. May cause extrapyramidal symptoms when used with other dopamine blockers such as prochlorperazine, haloperidol, and promethazine

CINV, Chemotherapy-induced nausea and vomiting; NK, neurokinin.

◆ Advanced oral and GI mucositis can affect coping abilities, adherence to ongoing treatment, frequency of health care visits, hospitalizations, and health care costs. Debilitating symptoms and sequelae of severe mucositis may necessitate changes in chemotherapy dosing, treatment delays, and/or premature treatment termination.

Assessment

◆ Assess risk factors and comorbidities that may contribute to oral mucositis: tobacco use, alcohol use, poor oral hygiene, dental disease, diminished self-care capabilities, previous radiation therapy involving the head and neck, impaired salivary gland function.

◆ Assess risk factors that contribute to both oral and GI mucositis: advanced age, concurrent medications known to dry mucous membranes, myelosuppression, previous chemotherapy known to cause mucositis, diminished renal function, impaired nutritional status, and chronic disease affecting the GI mucosa.

◆ Visual inspection of the oropharyngeal mucosa is performed to assess for areas of redness, ulcerations, white patches, or other evidence of infection.

◆ Clients are assessed for changes in oral tissue sensation, burning and pain, decreased tolerance to temperature extremes of food, sore throat, ability to maintain oral fluid and nutritional intake, speech, and swallowing status.

◆ Clients with bone marrow suppression are monitored for evidence of systemic infection because in clients with mucositis the oral cavity is one of the most commonly documented sources of sepsis.

◆ Clients are monitored for signs and symptoms of GI mucositis including diarrhea, rectal and vaginal tissue pain, redness, excoriation, bleeding, and evidence of infection. In clients with limited mobility and self-care capabilities, there is an increased risk of rectal and perineal infection–associated diarrhea-related tissue excoriation.

Diagnostic Indicators

◆ Dehydration and electrolyte imbalance (see diagnostic indicators as previously presented in discussion of diagnostic indicators for nausea and vomiting) may develop in clients unable to maintain sufficient fluid and nutrition intake.

◆ Secondary viral, bacterial, or fungal infections evidenced by organisms identified in culture and sensitivity results.

Hematologic Adverse Effects

The hematologic adverse effects of chemotherapy result in decreased bone marrow production of blood cells; this is referred to as myelosuppression.

Assessment

◆ Myelosuppression is characterized by decreased levels of white blood cells (WBCs) (leukopenia), neutrophils (neutropenia), hemoglobin and hematocrit levels (anemia), and platelets (thrombocytopenia).

◆ Decreased WBCs and neutrophils are associated with an increased risk of infection.
  ● Other factors contributing to infection risk are assessed such as skin wounds, intravenous, bladder or other catheters, invasive procedures, other medications, immobility, diarrhea, nutritional impairments, and the effects of advanced cancer on organ and vessel integrity.
  ● Monitor for signs and symptoms of infection such as chills and fever greater than 100.5°F (38.5°C); and signs of inflammation in common sites of infection such as sinuses, periodontium, pharynx, lungs, skin including intravenous catheter and invasive drainage catheters, perianal/perineal area, and bladder. Fever and redness may be the only signs of infection when WBCs are very low.

◆ Monitor for evidence of anemia including pallor, shortness of breath, dyspnea on exertion, fatigue, light-headedness, syncope, and chest pain.

◆ Monitor for signs and symptoms of thrombocytopenia including bruising, hematoma, petechiae, purpura, vaginal spotting, hematuria, melena, hematemesis and epistaxis, and bleeding gums.
  ● Severe or life-compromising bleeding due to thrombocytopenia is evidenced by hemodynamic shock including hypotension, tachycardia, pallor, diaphoresis, diminished mental status, shortness of breath or difficulty breathing, and chest pain.

Table 9-5

Diagnostic Indicators of Myelosuppression

	Diagnostic Indicators
Leukopenia	WBC < 3,500 cells/μL (3.5 x 10⁹/L)
Neutropenia	Neutrophils < 1,500/μL (1.5 x 10⁹/L)
Anemia (2018q)	Hemoglobin <13.5 g/dL (8.38 mmol/L) (males) <12.0 g/dL (7.45 mmol/L) (females)
	Hematocrit <38.8% (0.39 proportion of 1.0) (male) <34.9% (0.35 proportion of 1.0) (female)
	Tachycardia: Pulse greater than 100 beats/min
	Tachypnea: Respirations greater than 20 breaths/min
Thrombocytopenia	Platelets < 150,000/μL (150 x 10⁹/L)
	Positive fecal occult blood test

Diagnostic Indicators
◆ Indicators of myelosuppression are described in Table 9-5.

SAFETY ALERT! Chemotherapy agents with the potential to cause severe myelosuppression are labeled by the FDA with a black box warning that severe myelosuppression may occur and result in serious infection, septic shock, requirement for transfusions, hospitalization, and death. Nurses assess the client's complete blood cell and neutrophil values prior to administration of agents associated with myelosuppression. Nurses notify the prescribing physician regarding laboratory values that indicate evidence of neutropenia, anemia, and/or thrombocytopenia to obtain medication orders for dose modifications or need to omit chemotherapy administration. Client teaching is provided by nurses regarding signs and symptoms of infection, bleeding, and anemia. Nurses also instruct clients about energy conservation, prevention of infection, and bleeding.

Chemotherapy Handling
◆ In general, chemotherapy agents are considered hazardous drugs because of well-documented evidence of carcinogenicity, teratogenicity, genotoxicity, and health care worker adverse effects (skin rashes, nausea, hair loss, abdominal pain, nasal sores, allergic reactions, cancer, miscarriage, and delayed time to conception).

SAFETY ALERT! To prevent occupational exposure to hazardous drugs, nurses administering chemotherapy or handling blood and body fluids of clients receiving chemotherapy adhere to guidelines and use personal protective equipment (PPE) as strongly endorsed by several government entities and professional organizations including the Oncology Nursing Society (ONS), the Occupational Safety and Health Administration (OSHA), The National Institute for Occupational Safety and Health (NIOSH), and the US Pharmacopeia.

MEDICATION OVERVIEW: NOVEL MEDICATIONS USED IN CANCER TREATMENT: TARGETED AND IMMUNE-BASED AGENTS

Although chemotherapy has been the primary pharmaceutical approach for cancer treatment, recent advances in understanding the immune system, the genetic basis of cancer and mechanisms of cellular biology, novel classes of medications have been added to the strategies for treating cancer. Targeted therapies use drugs to identify and block the activity of biomolecules involved in the growth, reproduction and spread of specific types of cancer cells. Immune-based medications leverage the cells of the immune system to kill cancer cells or deliver lethal substances directly to cancer cells so that they are destroyed or prevented from reproducing. These novel classes of medications to treat cancer are often less toxic to normal cells than chemotherapy. However, both targeted therapies and immunotherapies have side effects that are monitored by physicians, nurses, and other health care providers. The majority of current and future clinical trials will focus on novel medications used alone or in combination with each other and/or chemotherapy agents.

CANCER-RELATED PAIN

- ◆ Cancer clients experience both acute and chronic pain related to the underlying cancer, diagnostic procedures, cancer treatments, and preexisting comorbidities unrelated to cancer.
- ◆ The experience of cancer pain is influenced by prior pain experiences and physical, psychosocial, cultural, and spiritual factors.

Assessment

- ◆ A comprehensive pain assessment, recommended to be performed routinely throughout the continuum of cancer, includes the following:
  - ● Pain characteristics: Location(s), type and quality of pain, onset, duration, course, intensity, and referral/radiation patterns. The characteristics of pain are important because pain syndromes (somatic, visceral, and neuropathic) often have different treatment algorithms.
  - ● Pain intensity rating is identified by clients using a pain intensity scale such as a numeric scale where zero represents no pain and ten represents the "worse pain that you can imagine." Based on this numeric scale, pain intensity can be categorized as mild (1 to 3), moderate (4 to 6), and severe (7 to 10).
  - ● Factors that exacerbate or relieve pain including effectiveness and limitations of the current pain management strategies; presence of breakthrough or refractory pain.
  - ● Effect of pain on activity, mobility, sleep, psychological distress, usual roles, spiritual well-being.
  - ● Previous pain experiences including successful or ineffective interventions.
  - ● Client's perception of what the pain signifies; cultural influences and beliefs regarding pain management.
  - ● Client goals for pain management and level of pain that is tolerable.

Diagnostic Indicators

◆ Acute pain is characterized by rapid onset but is usually a short duration ranging from weeks to months. Clients display signs and symptoms of distress including crying, wincing, grimacing, diaphoresis, tachycardia, hypertension, and pallor. It is associated with diagnostic procedures, surgery, chemotherapy, radiation, and some oncologic emergencies.

◆ Chronic pain lasts for greater than 3 months and is associated with significant physical, psychosocial, and social ramifications. Clients generally do not display the same signs and symptoms commonly observed with acute pain. Chronic pain is associated with advanced cancer and in some individuals, the long-term effects of cancer treatments.

Medications: Pain Management

◆ The most widely cited algorithm for pharmaceutical pain management is the WHO analgesic ladder (1986) that suggests a stepwise approach, based on the severity of pain, from lower strength nonopioid analgesics to strong opioids.

  ● Step 1 includes use of nonopioid analgesics (i.e., acetaminophen or nonsteroidal anti-inflammatory drugs) with or without adjuvant medications (i.e., antidepressants or anticonvulsants).

  ● Step 2 includes use of low-potency opioids (i.e., codeine) with or without adjuvant medications.

  ● Step 3 includes use of high-potency opioids (i.e., morphine or oxycodone) with or without adjuvant medications.

  ● Although not included in the original version of the WHO analgesic ladder, Miguel (2000) has suggested a 4th step including integrative therapies, analgesic interventions (i.e., nerve blocks, epidural injections, and spinal stimulators). See Figure 9-1 for the WHO analgesic ladder.

  ● Examples of Medications Used to Manage Cancer-Related Pain can be found in Table 9-6.

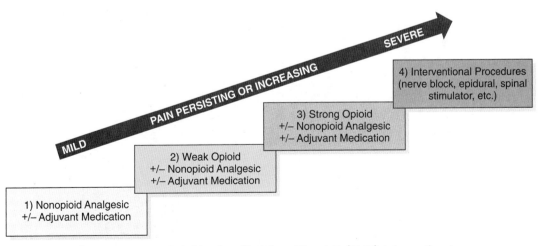

■ **Figure 9-1** Analgesic ladder. (Modified from Miguel, R. (2000). Interventional Treatment of Cancer Pain: The Fourth Step in the World Health Organization Analgesic Ladder? *Cancer Control*, 7(2), 149–156. doi:10.1177/107327480000700205.)

Table 9-6

Examples of Medications Used to Manage Cancer-Related Pain

Drug Classification	Common Side Effects	Nursing Implications	Indications
Opioids			
Low potency: Codeine, tramadol, hydrocodone High potency: Morphine, oxycodone, fentanyl, hydromorphone, methadone	Nausea, constipation, sedation that may decrease over time, urinary retention, myoclonus, pruritus, delirium, and respiratory depression	Assess for side effects on ongoing basis Provide measures to prevent constipation with the initiation of opioid therapy Monitor for respiratory depression Client teaching regarding safety measures for sedative and respiratory effects Use with caution in clients with renal impairment: Monitor renal function tests Methadone pharmacokinetics may be altered with agents used to treat infections and corticosteroids	Low-potency opioids: Mild to moderate pain High-potency opioids: Moderate to severe pain
Nonsteroidal anti-inflammatory drugs: Ibuprofen, naproxen, celecoxib, sulindac, and indomethacin	Gastric and duodenal ulceration, bleeding, renal impairment, increased risk of myocardial infarction, and cerebrovascular accident	Assess for gastric or duodenal irritation or bleeding Monitor Hgb/Hct, renal function Avoid in clients receiving anticoagulants or steroids	Mild to moderate pain Bone metastasis, fever, tissue inflammation
Tricyclic antidepressants: Amitriptyline, nortriptyline, duloxetine, venlafaxine	Constipation, dry mouth, sedation, agitation, tachycardia, cardiac conduction abnormalities	Provide measures to prevent constipation Client teaching regarding safety measures for sedation	Mild to moderate pain Neuropathic pain such as chemotherapy-induced neuropathy, postherpetic neuralgia, tumors infiltrating nerves
Anticonvulsants: Gabapentin, pregabalin, and lamotrigine	Sedation, bone marrow suppression, nausea	Client teaching regarding safety measures for sedation and dizziness Monitor complete blood count May require trial and error with several agents	Mild to moderate pain Neuropathic pain such as chemotherapy-induced neuropathy, postherpetic neuralgia, tumors infiltrating nerves

Medication	Side Effects	Nursing Considerations	Indication
Corticosteroids: Dexamethasone and methylprednisolone	Dyspepsia and hyperglycemia especially in clients with diabetes	Monitor for hyperglycemia Monitor GI symptoms; clients may require acid-blocking therapy	Mild to moderate pain Neuropathic pain, lymphedema, increased intracranial pressure
Acetaminophen	Liver impairment, may have increased risk with alcohol consumption	Client teaching regarding dosing limitations	Mild to moderate pain
Benzodiazepines: Alprazolam, clonazepam, and lorazepam	Sedation, dizziness, impaired motor coordination, delirium, respiratory depression	Client teaching regarding safety measures for sedative, motor, and respiratory effects Use with caution in clients receiving medications with sedative and respiratory depression effects	Anxiety Associated with pain, procedures, or muscle spasm
Topical anesthetics: Lidocaine (patch or cream), capsaicin cream	Rash where medication is applied	Monitor for skin rash Instruct client to avoid having cream touch other body parts (i.e., eyes); apply covering to area where cream is applied	Mild to moderate pain Peripheral neuropathies related to chemotherapy, postherpetic neuralgia, tumors infiltrating nerves
Opioids			
Low potency: Codeine, tramadol, and hydrocodone	Nausea, constipation, sedation that may decrease over time, urinary retention, myoclonus, pruritus, delirium, and respiratory depression	Assess for side effects on ongoing basis Provide measures to prevent constipation with the initiation of opioid therapy Monitor for respiratory depression Client teaching regarding safety measures for sedative and respiratory effects Use with caution in clients with renal impairment: Monitor renal function tests Methadone pharmacokinetics may be altered with agents used to treat infections and corticosteroids	Low-potency opioids: Mild to moderate pain
High potency: Morphine, oxycodone, fentanyl, hydromorphone, and methadone			High-potency opioids: Moderate to severe pain

(continued)

Table 9-6

Examples of Medications Used to Manage Cancer-Related Pain (continued)

Drug Classification	Common Side Effects	Nursing Implications	Indications
Nonsteroidal anti-inflammatory drugs: Ibuprofen, naproxen, celecoxib, sulindac, indomethacin	Gastric and duodenal ulceration, bleeding, renal impairment, increased risk of myocardial infarction, and cerebrovascular accident	Assess for gastric or duodenal irritation or bleeding Monitor Hgb/Hct, renal function Avoid in clients receiving anticoagulants or steroids	Mild to moderate pain Bone metastasis, fever, tissue inflammation
Tricyclic antidepressants: Amitriptyline, nortriptyline, duloxetine, venlafaxine	Constipation, dry mouth, sedation, agitation, tachycardia, cardiac conduction abnormalities	Provide measures to prevent constipation Client teaching regarding safety measures for sedation	Mild to moderate pain Neuropathic pain such as chemotherapy-induced neuropathy, postherpetic neuralgia, tumors infiltrating nerves
Anticonvulsants: Gabapentin, pregabalin, and lamotrigine	Sedation, bone marrow suppression, dizziness, nausea	Client teaching regarding safety measures for sedation and dizziness Monitor complete blood count May require trial and error with several agents	Mild to moderate pain Neuropathic pain such as chemotherapy-induced neuropathy, postherpetic neuralgia, tumors infiltrating nerves
Corticosteroids: Dexamethasone, methylprednisolone	Dyspepsia and hyperglycemia especially in clients with diabetes	Monitor for hyperglycemia Monitor GI symptoms; clients may require acid-blocking therapy	Mild to moderate pain Neuropathic pain, lymphedema, increased intracranial pressure
Acetaminophen	Liver impairment may have increased risk with alcohol consumption	Client teaching regarding dosing limitations	Mild to moderate pain

Medication	Side Effects	Nursing Considerations	Use
Benzodiazepines: Alprazolam, clonazepam, lorazepam	Sedation, dizziness, impaired motor coordination, delirium, respiratory depression	Client teaching regarding safety measures for sedative, motor, and respiratory effects Use with caution in clients receiving medications with sedative and respiratory depression effects	Anxiety Associated with pain, procedures, or muscle spasm
Topical anesthetics: Lidocaine (patch or cream), capsaicin cream	Rash where medication is applied	Monitor for skin rash Instruct client to avoid having cream touch other body parts (i.e., eyes); apply covering to area where cream is applied	Mild to moderate pain Peripheral neuropathies related to chemotherapy, postherpetic neuralgia, tumors infiltrating nerves

GI, gastrointestinal; Hgb/Hct, hemoglobin/hematocrit.

◆ For clients with continuous or frequent episodes of pain, where as-needed (PRN) dosing is not sufficient to manage pain, around the clock dosing or a long-acting opioid preparation is necessary.

◆ In addition to around the clock or long-acting opioid agents, breakthrough pain is managed with PRN doses of short-acting opioid preparations. The breakthrough dose should be 10% to 20% of the 24-hour long-acting dose.

◆ Both the long-acting and breakthrough medication doses are titrated upward over time to achieve and maintain adequate pain control.

◆ When higher doses of analgesics are required, drug preparations combining an opioid with other medications (i.e., oxycodone and acetaminophen) should be avoided in order to avoid toxicities associated with the nonopioid component.

◆ Routes of pain medications administration include oral (preferred), intravenous, intramuscular, subcutaneous, transdermal, topical, buccal, nasal, and rectal.

◆ Physical tolerance develops over time in all clients receiving opioids such that they will require increased doses to maintain the same amount of pain control. This is not addiction.

◆ Physical dependence develops over time in all clients receiving opioids. Abrupt cessation of opioids will result in withdrawal syndrome. This is not addiction.

◆ Addiction is psychological dependence, drug craving, and compulsive use of the drug without the need for analgesic effect and despite potential toxicities associated with uncontrolled drug use.

Practice Questions and Rationales

1. A nurse is reviewing the past medical history of a client who has been admitted for breast cancer. Which factor in the client's history is associated with breast cancer?

    1. Current age of 31 years
    2. Bearing two children to full term before 25 years
    3. Breast-feeding two children
    4. Oral contraceptive use

2. A client with cancer overhears the interdisciplinary team discussion about cell cycle–specific and nonspecific chemotherapy agents. The client asks the nurse for a further explanation of the difference. Which statement explains how cell cycle–specific and cell cycle nonspecific chemotherapy agents differ?

    1. Cell cycle nonspecific agents exert effect during specific phases of the cell cycle.
    2. Cell cycle–specific agents act independently of the cell cycle phases.
    3. Both cell cycle–specific agents and nonspecific agents are used in cancer treatment.
    4. Chemotherapy agents are used when surgical intervention is not possible or unavailable.

3. A nurse is teaching a client about the toxicities of chemotherapy. Which statement by the nurse is included in the teaching plan?

    1. "At times, you may experience palpitations and dizziness."
    2. "Monitoring your food and fluid intake is important."
    3. "Appling lotion daily to your dry skin after baths and showers will nourish your skin."
    4. "If you start to get headaches, make sure you call your primary care physician for treatment."

4. A nurse is preparing to administer chemotherapy to a client with cancer. Which agent is **most** likely to cause chemotherapy-induced nausea and vomiting?

    1. Cisplatin
    2. Docetaxel
    3. Bleomycin
    4. Methotrexate

5. A nurse is caring for client who is receiving cisplatin. Which laboratory value is **most** concerning to the nurse?

    1. Potassium level of 4.9 mEq/L (4.9 mmol/L)
    2. Sodium level of 160 mEq/L (160 mmol/L)
    3. Magnesium level of 2 mEq/L (1 mmol/L)
    4. Calcium level of 9.2 mg/dL (2.3 mmol/L)

6. A nurse is caring for a client who is receiving chemotherapy for lung cancer. During the morning assessment, the nurse assess the client's oral cavity. Which documented assessment requires the nurse to call the prescriber?

    1. "The client denies numbness or tingling to tongue."

    2. "The client is concerned about soreness with swallowing."

    3. "The client ate 70% of meal with 200 mL of fluids."

    4. "The client communicates with appropriate tone and speech as on admission."

7. A nurse is caring for a client that has been admitted for myelosuppression secondary to breast cancer treatment. Which diagnostic indicator does the nurse expect to observe in the client's electronic health record?

    1. Elevated white blood (cell) count (WBC)

    2. Decreased neutrophils

    3. Increased hemoglobin

    4. Low potassium level

8. A nurse is caring for a client who has been prescribed ondansetron prior to administration of etoposide. What statement should the nurse include prior to administering the ondansetron?

    1. "This will increase your neutrophil count."

    2. "The medication will improve your appetite."

    3. "It will assist in preventing nausea and vomiting."

    4. "The medication is known to improve the sodium level."

9. Which statement by the client receiving ondansetron for chemotherapy-induced nausea and vomiting warrants additional instruction?

    1. "I will add fluids and fiber in my diet."

    2. "Headache is common with this medication."

    3. "This medication should decrease my nausea."

    4. "I may feel depressed when taking this."

10. A nurse is caring for a client who is receiving acetaminophen and an antidepressant for pain control. Which step of the World Health Organization pain scale is this considered?

    1. Step 1

    2. Step 2

    3. Step 3

    4. Step 4

11. A nurse is caring for a client with cancer. After review of the medication administration record, the nurse determines that the client has asked for increasing doses of an analgesic for the past 5 days. Which does the nurse suspect is occurring with the client?

    1. Physical tolerance

    2. Withdrawal syndrome

    3. Drug craving

    4. Drug toxicity

12. A nurse is reviewing the medication administration record of a client with cancer. The client reports weight gain and an increase in their blood glucose since the last visit. Which medication does the nurses suspect is the cause of the client's issues?

    1.   Prednisone

    2.   Toremifene

    3.   Irinotecan

    4.   Cisplatin

13. A nurse is reviewing the laboratory values of a client receiving chemotherapy. The client reports frequent nosebleeds and abnormal bruising. Which laboratory value does the nurse suspect is related to the client's issues?

    1.   Hemoglobin of 15 g/dL (150 g/L)

    2.   Hematocrit of 36% (0.36 proportion of 1.0)

    3.   Neutrophil of 3,000/µL (3 x 10^9/L)

    4.   Platelets of 125,000/µL (125 x 10^9/L)

14. A nurse from another area of the hospital is shadowing on the bone marrow transplant and chemotherapy nursing division. Which statement by the shadow nurse is appropriate regarding the clients and medications used in this area?

    1.   "I need to make sure that all the clients here are well cared for."

    2.   "I noticed that there are special procedures for administering the drugs here."

    3.   "PPE is used during routine morning care to the clients."

    4.   "Many of the clients have supportive and engaged families."

15. A client who has been in the hospital for an extended stay to receive chemotherapy is planning for discharge. For which signs and symptoms does the nurse teach the client to seek medical evaluation? Select all that apply.

    1.   Unexplained weight loss

    2.   A persistent cough

    3.   Difficulty swallowing

    4.   Dry patches on the skin of the feet

    5.   White spots on the tongue

10

PERIPHERAL NERVOUS SYSTEM MEDICATIONS

BRIEF OVERVIEW OF THE PERIPHERAL NERVOUS SYSTEM

The peripheral nervous system consists of the parts of the nervous system outside the brain and spinal cord. It includes the peripheral nerves, neuromuscular junctions, cranial nerves, and spinal nerves. The peripheral nervous system is divided into the somatic nervous system and the autonomic nervous system with the somatic nervous system responsible for voluntary control, whereas the autonomic nervous system is "self-regulating," affecting the functions of such things as the heart rate and digestive system. The autonomic nervous system is further broken up into the parasympathetic and sympathetic nervous systems. Simply stated, the parasympathetic system is responsible for slowing down body functions while the sympathetic system increases body functions (Fig. 10-1).

Autonomic Nervous System Responses

The sympathetic nervous system, which is activated during a "fight-or-flight" response, uses neurotransmitters such as norepinephrine and epinephrine; heart rate is increased, and blood flow is shunted to the muscles, while noncritical functions, like digestion, are slowed. The parasympathetic nervous system primarily uses the neurotransmitter acetylcholine and performs the "housekeeping functions" of the body, also known as the "rest and digest" functions: regulation of heart rate, salivation, digestion, and elimination functions. Medications affecting the autonomic nervous system are separated into two groups based on the neurotransmitter they involve, cholinergic (acetylcholine) or adrenergic (norepinephrine or epinephrine), and function by either stimulating or blocking the receptors for each neurotransmitter (see Table 10-1).

Sympathetic Nervous System/Adrenergic Receptors

The adrenergic receptors are composed of two types: alpha and beta. The alpha receptors (α_1 and α_2) respond to both of the major sympathetic nervous system neurotransmitters, epinephrine and norepinephrine, and epinephrine also activates both of the beta receptors (β_1 and β_2). However, only β_1 receptors respond to norepinephrine (not β_2). Each receptor has distinct actions and effects and are used to treat a variety of medical issues (Table 10-2).

CLINICAL PEARLS—PERIPHERAL NERVOUS SYSTEM

★ **STUDY TIPS** – The somatic nervous system is responsible for voluntary muscles, whereas the autonomic nervous system is responsible for involuntary responses that regulate physiologic functions.

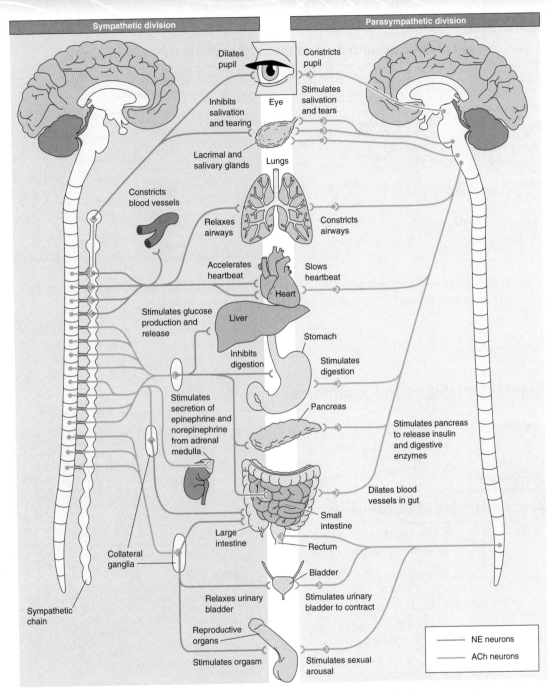

Figure 10-1 Schema explaining how parasympathetic and sympathetic nervous systems regulate functioning organs. (Modified from Bear MF, Connors BW, and Parasido, MA. *Neuroscience - Exploring the Brain*, 2nd ed. Philadelphia: Lippincott Williams & Wilkins. 2001.)

A Comparison of the Sympathetic and Parasympathetic Nervous Systems

	Sympathetic (SNS)	Parasympathetic (PNS)
Major neurotransmitter involved	Norepinephrine, epinephrine	Acetylcholine
Receptor types	α_1, α_2, β_1, β_2	Nicotinic and muscarinic
Pupils	Dilates	Constricts
Salivary glands	Inhibits	Stimulates
Heart rate	Increases	Decreases
Bronchi	Dilates	Constricts
Digestion	Inhibits	Stimulates
Intestinal motility	Inhibits	Stimulates
Bladder	Relaxes	Contracts

★ **STUDY TIPS** – Remembering the beta-adrenergic receptors can be easily done: β_1 has its largest effects on the heart, and β_2 has its largest effects on the lungs.

- β_1 = 1 heart
- β_2 = 2 lungs

Assessment/Signs and Symptoms

- Clients' past medical history as well as their current symptoms should be assessed.
- Signs and symptoms will vary depending on the condition and which medication is being used.

Table 10-2

Basic Description of Adrenergic Receptors

Receptor	Action and Uses	Effects
α_1	Smooth muscle contraction	Vasoconstriction
	Pupil dilation for eye examination	Pupil dilation
	Uses • Nasal congestion • Hypotension	Decreased secretions Decreased GI motility
α_2	Smooth muscle contraction	Decreased norepinephrine release
	Uses • Hypertension	Decreased insulin release
β_1	Heart muscle contraction	Increased heart rate
	Uses • Cardiac arrest • Heart failure • Shock	Increased cardiac output Increased stroke volume Increased contractility Increased renin release
β_2	Smooth muscle relaxation	Bronchial relaxation
	Uses • Asthma • Premature labor	Uterine relaxation Vasodilation of skeletal muscle

Diagnostics

◆ Blood tests and/or cultures may be indicated for certain conditions or to evaluate the client's health status.

MEDICATION OVERVIEW

There are a variety of medications that affect the peripheral nervous system and are generally characterized into two groups: the cholinergic medications and the adrenergic medications (Table 10-3). The cholinergic medications act on receptors that are activated by acetylcholine, and the adrenergic medications act on receptors that are activated by epinephrine or norepinephrine. In either group, the medications exert their actions by stimulating or blocking the receptors of the peripheral nervous system.

★ **STUDY TIPS** – Committing the normal responses of the most popular receptors: muscarinic, nicotinic, α_1, α_2, β_1, and β_2 can help to easily identify the actions of the medications that interact with them. For example, by understanding the effects of muscarinic activation, it is easy to predict what muscarinic agonists will do (mimic the effects) and what muscarinic antagonists will do (block the effect).

Table 10-3

Peripheral Nervous System Medications

Class	Prototype	Mechanism of Action	Major Side and Adverse Effects	Critical Information	Indications
Cholinergic Medications					
Muscarinic agonist	Bethanechol	Reversibly binds to muscarinic cholinergic receptors, thereby affecting the heart (bradycardia), exocrine glands (increasing sweating and salivation), smooth muscle (bronchial constriction, increased motility of GI system, vasodilation, and increased bladder emptying), and eyes (miosis and near vision accommodation)	Side effects relatively rare Hypotension (related to vasodilation) and bradycardia Excessive salivation, abdominal cramping and diarrhea Bronchoconstriction	Also known as parasympathomimetic drugs Contraindicated for use in hypotensive clients and clients with an intestinal obstruction or recent bowel surgery, urinary tract obstruction, or asthma Also contraindicated for clients with hyperthyroidism (may cause dysrhythmias)	Used to treat urinary retention Used off label to treat gastroesophageal reflux
Muscarinic antagonist	Atropine	Block acetylcholine action at the muscarinic receptors resulting in increased heart rate, decreased salivation, relaxation of the bronchi, decreased GI motility, and mydriasis	Dry mouth, blurred vision, photophobia, elevated intraocular pressure, urinary retention, constipation, decreased sweating, and tachycardia	Also known as parasympatholytic medications or anticholinergics Listed on the Beers Criteria, as inappropriate medications for use with the geriatric population At high enough doses, this has the ability to block some nicotinic receptors as well Toxic doses can cause hallucinations and delirium, progressing into coma, respiratory arrest, and death if not treated Although the medications dilate the bronchi, they can also cause the thickening of bronchial secretions, resulting in mucous plugs. It is therefore used with caution in clients who have asthma. Interacts with medications that can cause a muscarinic blockade including antihistamines and tricyclic antidepressants. Concurrent use should be avoided	Can be used to treat bradycardia, as a pre-anesthetic medication, to dilate pupils for an eye exam, diverticulitis, and as an antidote for muscarinic agonist poisoning

Adrenergic Medications

Category	Drug	Action	Side Effects	Nursing Considerations	Uses
Adrenergic agonists	Epinephrine	Can activate all four receptor subtypes (α_1, α_2, β_1, and β_2) and produce a wide variety of effects α_1: vasoconstriction β_1: increase cardiac workload β_2: bronchial dilation	Hypertensive crisis, cerebral hemorrhage, cardiac dysrhythmias, angina, hyperglycemia, and tremors	Cannot be given orally, must be given topically or parenterally (subcutaneously, intramuscularly or intravenously) Clients receiving the medication via IV route must be on continuous cardiac monitoring related to increased risk of hypertension Contraindicated for use in hyperthyroid clients related to elevated risk of dysrhythmias	Used to delay absorption of local anesthesia, and elevate blood pressure (α_1) Used to treat AV heart block, and used to treat clients in cardiac arrest (β_1) Used to treat anaphylactic shock (α_1, α_2, β_1, and β_2)
α_1-Adrenergic agonist	Phenylephrine	Reduce nasal congestion by activating α_1-adrenergic receptors in the nasal blood vessels causing vasoconstriction. When α_1-adrenergic receptors are activated on blood vessels, vasoconstriction will occur	Rebound congestion, central nervous system excitation, vasoconstriction	Can be coadministered intravenously with local anesthetics to delay absorption Rebound congestion can be minimized by limiting the use of topical application to 3–5 days Caution should be taken for oral or IV use with clients with previous cardiac disorder due to vasoconstriction	Can be given intranasally to treat nasal congestion Can be given parenterally to treat hypotension Can be given via an ophthalmic preparation to dilate pupils
α-Adrenergic antagonists	Prazosin	Blocks the α_1 adrenergic receptors causing dilation in the blood vessels and relaxation of bladder and prostate	Orthostatic hypotension, reflex tachycardia, and nasal congestion	"First-dose effect": severe postural hypotension resulting in loss of consciousness with first dose. A small dose is given at bedtime for first dose and titrated up slowly thereafter to help prevent this from occurring. Geriatric clients are particularly at risk for these effects This class of medication is listed on the Beers Criteria, as inappropriate medications for use with the geriatric population due to risk of orthostatic hypotension	Used to treat hypertension Off label, used to treat benign prostatic hyperplasia

(continued)

Table 10-3

Peripheral Nervous System Medications *(continued)*

Class	Prototype	Mechanism of Action	Major Side and Adverse Effects	Critical Information	Indications
β_2-Adrenergic agonists	Albuterol	Activates primarily β_2 receptors resulting in a bronchodilation In large doses, the selectivity for β_2 receptors is lost and both β_1 and β_2 receptors are activated	Tachycardia, angina, seizures	Cardiac arrest and/or death may occur with an overdose of short acting β_2-adrenergic agonists	Used to treat asthma and COPD
β-Adrenergic antagonists	Propranolol (nonselective)	Blocks both β_1 and β_2 receptors (nonselective) resulting in decreased heart rate, decreased ventricular contraction, and decreased conduction through the AV node	Related to β_1: bradycardia, reduced cardiac output, AV heart block, rebound cardiac excitation Related to β_2: bronchoconstriction and inhibition of glycogenolysis	Significant first-pass effect with metabolization (<30% of drug reaches circulation) Can exacerbate heart failure and should be used cautiously by clients with increased risk for heart conditions Can mask symptoms of hypoglycemia; used with caution for clients with or at risk for developing diabetes Other contraindications: AV heart block, bradycardia, and asthma Client's blood pressure and pulse should always be assessed prior to taking medication Clients should be taught to change positions slowly Metoprolol (β_1 selective) can be used safely for clients with asthma as it does not block β_2 receptors at therapeutic doses (selectivity is lost at high doses)	Used to treat angina, hypertension, cardiac dysrhythmias, and migraines Also used as part of treatment plan after a myocardial infarction

AV, atrioventricular; GI, gastrointestinal; IV, intravenous.

Practice Questions and Rationales

1. A client with a history of urinary retention presents to the emergency department with symptoms of excessive salivation, blurred vision, diarrhea, and abdominal cramping. Upon examination, the client's blood pressure is 92/54 mm Hg. The nurse recognizes that these symptoms are consistent with which situation?

    1. Anticholinergic poisoning.
    2. First-dose effect.
    3. Muscarinic poisoning.
    4. Anaphylactic shock.

2. Which client would be an appropriate candidate for treatment using a muscarinic agonist?

    1. A client with urinary retention following a total knee replacement
    2. A client with urinary retention related to a mass in the urinary tract
    3. A client with postoperative urinary retention and a past medical history of asthma
    4. A client with urinary retention newly diagnosed with an atonic bladder currently being treated for hyperthyroidism

3. A new nurse graduate is discussing the use of epinephrine with the nurse manager. Which statement by the new nurse graduate demonstrates an understanding of the medication?

    1. "When epinephrine is taken orally, it should be separated from other medications and food by at least 1 hour."
    2. "Epinephrine given subcutaneously will absorb faster than if given intramuscularly."
    3. "Epinephrine given intravenously requires continuous cardiac monitoring related to an increased risk of arrhythmias and hypertension."
    4. "Epinephrine should be used cautiously in clients with diabetes due to the risk of hypoglycemia."

4. The anticholinergic medication atropine would be contraindicated in a client with which concurrent diagnosis?

    1. Hypotension
    2. Constipation
    3. Asthma
    4. Glaucoma

5. A client is taking albuterol, to treat asthma. The client presents for a follow-up appointment and asks why their hands sometimes shake when taking the medication. Which response by the nurse is correct?

    1. "When $beta_2$ receptors are activated, they cause the contraction of smooth muscle, resulting in tremors."
    2. "The activation of $beta_2$ receptors in the skeletal muscles causes an increase in the contraction of muscles, resulting in tremors."
    3. "$Beta_2$ receptor activation can cause hypoglycemia, resulting in tremors."
    4. "The activation of $beta_2$ receptors may result in constriction of the blood vessels, causing tremors."

6. A nurse is taking care of a client who is currently prescribed propranolol to treat hypertension. The client mentions to the nurse a history of asthma but always forgets to include

it on the past medical history because it has not required treatment for several years. The nurse checks the client's medical chart and sees that asthma is not listed in the past medical history. What is the **priority** action of the nurse?

1. Ensure that the provider is aware that asthma is not listed in the client's past medical history and question the prescribed propranolol.
2. Add asthma to the client's past medical history in the chart and ensure that the pulse oximetry is monitored every shift.
3. Ensure the provider is aware that the client's past medical includes a diagnosis of asthma and anticipate an order for a nebulizer treatment.
4. Include the conversation in the nursing shift note; however, since the client has not had recent asthma flares, it is not necessary to alert the provider.

7. The client is given a new prescription of prazosin and asks about the medication. Which information should the nurse provide the client?

1. Take this medication 1 hour before eating or 2 hours after.
2. Prazosin may result in sexual dysfunction.
3. Clients should be monitored closely for risk of bradycardia.
4. The first dose of this medication should be small and given before going to bed.

8. Which statement is accurate regarding the nurse's understanding of alpha blockade?

1. "Alpha antagonist medications lower blood pressure by the dilation of the arterioles, directly reducing arterial pressure."
2. "Alpha blockade results in contraction of the smooth muscle, helping to treat conditions such as benign prostatic hyperplasia."
3. "Alpha antagonist medications can help to treat nasal congestion by constriction of the blood vessels in the nasal cavity."
4. "Alpha blockade may result in bradycardia by triggering the baroreceptor reflex."

9. A client begins taking a beta-adrenergic antagonist medication after experiencing a myocardial infarction. Which assessment finding would alert the nurse that the client is experiencing an adverse effect of the medication? Select all that apply.

1. Bradycardia
2. Swelling of extremities
3. Shortness of breath
4. Bronchodilation
5. Hyperglycemia

10. A client with a diagnosis of hypertension and a past medical history of asthma is prescribed a beta$_1$-selective adrenergic antagonist. Which statement is accurate regarding the client's understanding of the medication selection?

1. "By taking a beta$_1$-selective adrenergic antagonist medication, it ensures that I will never experience bronchoconstriction as an adverse effect."
2. "I am prescribed a beta$_1$-selective adrenergic antagonist medication because a nonselective beta-adrenergic blocker may affect my asthma."
3. "Since I am taking a beta$_1$-selective adrenergic antagonist instead of a nonselective beta-adrenergic antagonist, I can expect that a lower dose of medication will be used."
4. "I need to be aware of the increased risk of developing diabetes while taking beta$_1$-selective adrenergic antagonists."

11

CENTRAL NERVOUS SYSTEM MEDICATIONS

BRIEF OVERVIEW OF CHRONIC NEUROLOGIC DISORDERS AND THEIR MEDICATIONS

The neurologic system is a network of complex structures, which include neurons and specialized cells, that carry electrical and chemical signals between the brain and the body's various organs and tissues. The neurologic system is responsible for coordinating information humans receive (sensory) from their external environment and generating responses to that information (motor). The neurologic system controls the entire body and communication among its organs.

The neurologic system is divided into two main parts: the central nervous system (CNS) and the peripheral nervous system (PNS). The CNS is composed of the brain and spinal cord. The PNS is composed of structures outside the CNS and helps connect the CNS to the rest of the body. Cranial and spinal nerves make up the PNS, along with their nerve branches and ganglia. The PNS can further be divided into the somatic and autonomic nervous systems (ANS). The somatic system contains pathways that regulate *voluntary* motor control, while the ANS controls automatic or *involuntary* functions of the body. The neurologic system also contains various neurotransmitters and receptors. Medications used to treat neurologic disorders will enhance, suppress, or mimic the activity of neurotransmitters at their receptor sites. Specific neurologic disorders include the following:

- *Alzheimer disease (AD)*: This is the most common type of dementia in the United States. There are two classes of drugs available to treat AD: acetylcholinesterase inhibitors and N-methyl-D-aspartate (NMDA) receptor antagonists. Both of these classes of medication work on neurotransmitters that are believed to have a role in the pathology of AD.
- *Parkinson disease (PD)*: PD is a chronic, neurodegenerative disorder that is characterized by motor and nonmotor symptoms. Neurons that produce dopamine undergo a degenerative destruction that causes decreased production of this neurotransmitter. Medications used to treat the symptoms of PD work by increasing the level of dopamine in the brain or work as agonists. In addition, some PD meds work on brain enzymes that break down dopamine. Anticholinergics are also used to treat tremor associated with PD, although they have fallen out of favor due to associated side effects in this drug class. Amantadine is also used in PD to primarily treat dyskinesias associated with long-term levodopa therapy.
- *Multiple sclerosis (MS)*: MS is a chronic, neurodegenerative, autoimmune disease of the CNS. Antibodies are produced, which destroy myelin in the brain and spinal cord. Medications used to treat MS are designed to stop the autoimmune destruction of myelin. Medication classes include drugs that modify the disease course, treat exacerbations, and manage the multiple symptoms of MS.
- *Epilepsy (seizure disorder)*: Epilepsy is a chronic CNS disease that affects individuals across the life span and causes recurrent seizure episodes. Seizures are characterized by an acute

involuntary and transient alteration in behavior, motor activity, sensory functioning, consciousness, or autonomic activity accompanied by abnormal electrical discharges in the brain. The development of a seizure involves many nervous system components including neurons, ion channels, neurotransmitters, receptors, and inhibitory and excitatory synapses. The antiepileptic drugs (AEDs) alter chemical activity to stop excitatory processes, which terminate or prevent seizure activity. The AEDs are organized by their main mechanism of action.

CLINICAL PEARLS: CHRONIC NEUROLOGIC DISORDERS

Alzheimer Disease

Assessment/Signs and Symptoms

◆ AD is a clinical diagnosis characterized by initial episodic memory impairment, executive dysfunction, and visuospatial impairment. As AD progresses, language deficits and behavioral disturbance occur.

◆ Symptoms are insidious, and may interfere with work-related activities or usual daily activities.

◆ There are five main stages of AD: initial, early, middle, late, and end stage.

◆ Although certain drugs help improve functioning and may delay disease progression for a period of time, they do not halt the degenerative process.

Diagnostics

There is no specific diagnostic test for AD; the diagnosis rests on a complete health history, physical examination, and ruling out other reversible causes of cognitive impairment. Symptoms must not be attributable to delirium or major psychiatric disorder.

Parkinson Disease

Assessment/Signs and Symptoms

◆ The cardinal motor features of PD are resting tremor, bradykinesia, and muscular rigidity.

◆ There are several nonmotor symptoms that affect individuals with PD. These include autonomic dysfunction, neuropsychiatric diagnoses, fatigue, sleep disturbance, cognitive impairment, and sexual dysfunction.

Diagnostics

◆ There is no specific diagnostic test for PD.

◆ Diagnosis is based on a complete history and physical examination

Multiple Sclerosis

Assessment/Signs and Symptoms

◆ MS is a chronic demyelinating, neurodegenerative, and autoimmune disease of the CNS that has a wide variety of clinical manifestations.

◆ Symptoms are dependent on the location of damaged myelin.

◆ Clinical manifestations may include visual disturbances (diplopia, decreased visual acuity, blurred vision), sensory changes, motor weakness, fatigue, imbalance, spasticity, coordination, impaired gait, intention tremors, bladder and/or bowel difficulties, sexual dysfunction, vertigo, pain, depression, emotional lability, and cognitive impairment.

Diagnostics

◆ There is no conclusive diagnostic test for MS. Diagnosis rests largely on clinical characteristics, brain and spinal imaging studies, and laboratory evaluation.
◆ Blood work and/or lumbar puncture may be needed to aid in diagnosis.
◆ Diagnostic criteria necessitates the documentation of two or more episodes of symptoms and two or more signs that indicate pathology (demyelination) in anatomically different regions of the CNS.

Epilepsy ("Seizure Disorder")

Assessment/Signs and Symptoms

◆ Main classification: Focal (also termed partial) and generalized
◆ *Focal/partial*: Epileptogenic focus is limited to one side of the brain; three categories of focal/partial seizure are as follows:
  ● *Simple partial*: No change in loss of consciousness (LOC); may have motor, sensory, autonomic symptoms or a combination of all three; individuals with simple partial seizures may experience a "sensory march" where a numbness or tingling spreads to different parts of a limb or the body; may have auditory, olfactory, or visual manifestations; symptoms dependent on brain region affected.
  ● *Complex partial*: Various combination of cognitive, affective, and psychomotor symptoms may have LOC or alteration of consciousness; individuals affected commonly have automatisms; postictal state can follow.
  ● *Partial with secondary generalization*: Seizure starts as simple partial and progresses to bilateral hemispheres in the brain; symptoms similar to primary generalized.
◆ *Generalized*: Epileptogenic focus occurs in bilateral brain hemispheres and involves the thalamus and reticular activating system (RAS), which results in positive LOC. Categories include absence (petite mal), atypical absence, myoclonic, atonic (drop attack), or tonic–clonic (grand mal).
  ● *Absence (petite mal)*: Typically occur in children, and affected individuals may exhibit poor academic performance; brief episodes, which last seconds; person unaware of surrounding environment.
  ● *Atypical absence*: Presence of accompanying myoclonic jerks or automatisms (repetitive movements, lip smacking).
  ● *Myoclonic*: Brief and involve single or multiple "jerks" of one of more muscle groups.
  ● *Atonic (drop attack)*: Acute and abrupt loss of muscle tone; falls and injuries are commonly sustained; may have myoclonic movements.
  ● *Tonic–clonic*: "Grand mal"; acute LOC followed by tonic phase (muscle rigidity), which lasts ~10 to 15 seconds; individual may open mouth and eyes, and there is lower extremity extension with upper extremity adduction; after tonic phase, the person will have clonic activity, which consists of rhythmic, involuntary muscle contractions lasting 1 to 2 minutes; tongue biting, urinary or bowel incontinence may occur during event; diaphoresis, tachycardia, and apnea may occur during clonic phase; postictal phase follows.

Diagnostics

◆ Electroencephalograms (EEGs) can help to identify seizure type.

◆ Neurologic exams will also assist in the diagnosis of epilepsy.

◆ During the assessment phase, other tests such as MRIs, blood tests, etc., may be ordered to rule out other diagnoses.

MEDICATION OVERVIEW

Alzheimer Disease

Drugs used to treat AD do not cure the disease, and clients and families need ongoing education regarding expectations of treatment (Table 11-1). Two classes of medications are used: the cholinesterase inhibitors and the NMDA receptor antagonists. Cholinesterase inhibitors provide modest

Table 11-1

Drugs Used to Treat Alzheimer Disease

Class	Generic Name(s)	Mechanism of Action	Major Side and Adverse Effects	Critical Information	Indications
Cholinesterase inhibitors	Donepezil (PO)	Increases the concentration of acetylcholine at synapses	*Donepezil*: nausea, diarrhea, vivid dreams/nightmares	*Donepezil*: administer in AM to reduce nightmares/sleep disturbance	Mild to moderate AD
	Galantamine (PO)		*Galantamine*: nausea, vomiting, diarrhea, anorexia, weight loss	*Galantamine*: avoid in ESRD and severe hepatic impairment	
	Rivastigmine (PO or transdermal patch)		*Rivastigmine*: oral formulation: nausea, vomiting, anorexia, headaches	*Rivastigmine*: transdermal dose should be lower in mild to moderate hepatic impairment; avoid in severe hepatic impairment	
			Transdermal formulation: skin irritation	*Cholinesterase inhibitors are contraindicated in clients with baseline bradycardia and known cardiac conduction system disease*	
N-methyl-D-aspartate (NMDA) receptor antagonist	Memantine (PO)	Blocks the effects of excessive levels of glutamate	Dizziness	*May* increase agitation and delusions in some clients with AD	Moderate to severe AD

AD, Alzheimer disease; ESRD, end-stage renal disease.

symptomatic treatment for cognition and overall global functioning in AD. NMDA receptor antagonists may provide modest benefit for moderate to severe AD and may have some neuroprotective properties

Parkinson Disease

The medication treatment plan for PD aims to increase the level of dopamine in the CNS either by utilizing dopamine precursors (levodopa), dopamine receptor agonists, or monoamine oxidase inhibitors. The best available medication to treat motor symptoms in PD is carbidopa–levodopa ("L-dopa"); however, dopamine may be preferred for certain clients. Other medications such as amantadine and anticholinergics may be used to help treat some of the symptoms associated with PD. The medications for PD should be taken on a strict administration schedule to minimize symptoms, improve mobility, reduce the risk of adverse events such as falls, and improve "on" time and quality of life. See Table 11-2 for further information.

SAFETY ALERT! Abrupt cessation of L-dopa and dopamine agonists can result in parkinsonism–hyperpyrexia syndrome. Medications should always be slowly weaned. This syndrome resembles neuroleptic malignant syndrome and requires urgent recognition. Clinical signs and symptoms include significant hyperthermia, severe muscle rigidity, mental status changes, and autonomic system instability.

SAFETY ALERT! Avoid dopamine-blocking agents in clients with PD. These include all antipsychotics with the exception of clozapine and quetiapine. Also, certain antiemetics should not be used in this population as they have dopamine-blocking properties. Specific antiemetics are metoclopramide, prochlorperazine, promethazine, and chlorpromazine. Clients with PD who receive these medications can have a sudden worsening of their PD symptoms.

Multiple Sclerosis

The medications used in MS can be broken down into three main categories: disease-modifying agents (immunomodulators and immunosuppressants), agents to manage acute exacerbations (glucocorticoids, covered in the respiratory chapter), and symptom management agents. The disease-modifying agents can help to decrease the frequency and severity of relapses as well as maintain the quality of life. Medications used to manage the acute exacerbations (glucocorticoids) should be used short term, and their frequent use (more than three times a year and/or for more than 3 weeks at a time) is discouraged due to the long-term side effects of glucocorticoids such as osteoporosis. Lastly, the symptom management agents are used to treat things such as bladder dysfunction, bowel dysfunction, fatigue, depression, pain, and tremors (list is nonexclusive). These medications are not covered in this section as many are discussed within their respective chapter, and they are client specific but are an important part of the treatment plan for clients with MS. See Table 11-3 for further information on the disease-modifying agents used to treat MS.

Table 11-2

Drugs Used to Treat Parkinson Disease

Class	Generic Name(s)	Mechanism of Action	Major Side and Adverse Effects	Critical Information	Indications
Levodopa (L-dopa)	Carbidopa–levodopa (PO)	Carbidopa is given with L-dopa (a dopamine precursor) to prevent the breakdown of L-dopa in the gastrointestinal tract (before it crosses the blood–brain barrier) and to reduce nausea, vomiting, and orthostatic hypotension associated with L-dopa alone	Nausea, dizziness, somnolence, and headache *Older adults* are more prone to orthostatic hypotension, confusion, hallucinations, delusions, agitation, and psychosis	Most effective drug to treat PD symptoms Long-term use of L-dopa associated with motor fluctuations, "on–off" phenomenon, abnormal movements (dyskinesias, cramping, dystonia)	Symptomatic management of bradykinesia, rigidity, and tremors. May be given at any stage but often in younger clients, dopamine agonists are used first due to L-dopa's association with wearing off and dyskinesias with long-term use
Dopamine agonists	Pramipexole (PO) Ropinirole (PO) Rotigotine (transdermal patch)	Synthetic agents that directly stimulate dopamine receptors	Nausea, vomiting, sleepiness, orthostatic hypotension, confusion, hallucinations, peripheral edema Rotigotine: skin reactions and above adverse effects	Use of these drugs can lead to impulse control disorders, and clients need ongoing assessment to identify problematic obsessive or compulsive behaviors	May be preferred initial agents in PD for younger clients as no association with long-term motor fluctuations or emergence of abnormal movements
Dystonias	Amantadine	Mechanism of action unknown in the treatment of PD	Side effects: dizziness, headache, insomnia, and nausea Adverse effects: CHF, dysrhythmias, and psychosis	Contraindicated for use in breastfeeding women and in clients with renal failure	To treat dyskinesias that occur as a result of long-term levodopa therapy
Anticholinergics	Benztropine	Antagonizes acetylcholine and histamine receptors	Side effects: urinary retention, nausea, headache, blurred vision Adverse effect: psychosis	These agents must be used with caution especially in older adults, due to their adverse effects (cognitive impairment, confusion, and hallucinations) Trihexyphenidyl and Benztropine may still be used in individuals < 70 yr of age to treat tremor Contraindicated in clients with glaucoma or obstructive uropathy	To treat tremor, rigidity, or drooling

PD, Parkinson disease.

Table 11-3

Drugs Used to Treat Multiple Sclerosis

Class	Generic Name(s)	Mechanism of Action	Major Side and Adverse Effects	Critical Information	Indications
Immunomodulators	Interferon beta-1b; interferon beta-1a (SC or IM)	Suppresses immune response through various mechanisms	Injection site reactions including necrosis, flu-like symptoms, depression, leukopenia, anemia, asymptomatic liver dysfunction	SC or IM injection depending on specific agent; dosing varies	Relapsing–remitting MS (RRMS)
		Disease-modifying agent		Periodic monitoring of CBC, LFTs, and TSH	
			Less common: suicidal ideation, hepatotoxicity	LFTs should be monitored monthly for first 6 mo	
				Clients can premedicate prior to each injection with acetaminophen or ibuprofen to decrease flu-like symptoms	
Immunomodulator	Glatiramer acetate (SC)	Suppresses immune response	Injection site reactions; transient systemic postreaction symptoms (flushing, chest pain, dyspnea, palpitations, anxiety)	SC injection	RRMS
				No necessary lab monitoring	
Immunomodulator	Dimethyl fumarate (PO)	Suppresses the immune response; may be neuroprotective	Flushing, diarrhea, nausea, abdominal pain; lymphocytopenia; elevated liver enzymes	Give medication with food	RRMS
				Obtain CBC and LFTs prior to drug initiation; 6 mo after and yearly thereafter	
Immunomodulator	Teriflunomide (PO)	Suppresses the immune response	Diarrhea, nausea, hair thinning, elevated liver enzymes, PN	Contraindicated in pregnancy and in women trying to conceive	RRMS
				Monitor LFTs prior to and after treatment initiation; monitor for S&S of PN	

(continued)

Table 11-3

Drugs Used to Treat Multiple Sclerosis (continued)

Class	Generic Name(s)	Mechanism of Action	Major Side and Adverse Effects	Critical Information	Indications
Immunomodulator	Fingolimod (PO)	Suppresses the immune response by mobilizing lymphocytes in the lymph nodes	More common: headache, influenza, diarrhea, back pain, elevated liver enzymes, cough Less common: increased infection risk, atrioventricular block, possible increased risk of basal cell carcinoma, macular edema	Contraindications: MI (in last 6 mo), unstable angina, stroke, TIA, prolonged QT interval Clients need BP and EKG monitoring for first 6 hr after drug initiation Clients need CBC, LFTs, ophthalmologic exam, varicella serology checked prior to initiation	RRMS
Immunomodulator	Natalizumab (IV infusion monthly)	Suppresses the immune response	Headache, flushing, nausea, dizziness, fatigue, allergic reactions, anxiety, infections	Increased risk of progressive multifocal leukoencephalopathy Obtain anti-JC virus (John Cunningham virus) antibodies prior to initiation and then at 1 yr	RRMS

BP, blood pressure; CBC, complete blood count; EKG, electrocardiographic; LFT, liver function test; PN, peripheral neuropathy; RRMS, relapsing–remitting multiple sclerosis; TIA, transient ischemic attack; TSH, thyroid-stimulating hormone.

> **BLACK BOX WARNING FOR TERIFLUNOMIDE:**
> ◆ Contraindicated in clients with severe hepatic impairment.
> ◆ Avoid using in conjunction with other hepatotoxic drugs.
> ◆ Contraindicated in pregnancy and in women of birth age who are not utilizing reliable contraception; exclude pregnancy prior to drug initiation and counsel women to avoid becoming pregnant while on drug.

> **BLACK BOX WARNING FOR NATALIZUMAB:**
> ◆ Increases the risk of progressive multifocal leukoencephalopathy (PML), which may lead to severe disability or death.
> ◆ Risk for PML increases with the therapy duration, use of prior immunosuppressant drugs, and presence of anti-JC virus antibodies.

Epilepsy

Medications used to treat seizures are called AEDs. There are first-, second-, and third-generation AEDs available and are additionally classified as either narrow or broad spectrum based on the types of seizures they have the ability to treat. Older agents, first generation, have a wider range of adverse effects and increased association with toxic events. As mentioned earlier AEDs can be categorized as either narrow or broad spectrum. Narrow-spectrum AEDs mainly target focal and absence seizures, whereas broad-spectrum AEDs are used for generalized and focal seizures.

Table 11-4 on the next page summarizes some of the most commonly used AEDs.

> **SAFETY CONSIDERATIONS:** *There is an FDA class warning on all AED drugs regarding the possible increased risk of suicidal ideation while on these medications.*

> **BLACK BOX WARNING FOR PHENYTOIN SODIUM INTRAVENOUS SOLUTION:**
> ◆ IV rate administration for phenytoin sodium should not exceed 50 mg/min in adults and 1 to 3 mg/kg/min or 50 mg/min in pediatric clients due to risk of severe hypotension and cardiac arrhythmias.

> **BLACK BOX WARNING FOR CARBAMAZEPINE:**
> ◆ Monitor for life-threatening dermatologic reactions including Stevens-Johnson syndrome and toxic epidermal necrolysis.
> ◆ Aplastic anemia and agranulocytosis have been reported. Obtain a complete blood count with differential prior to initiation and periodically during therapy.

Table 11-4

Drugs Used to Treat Epilepsy

Class	Generic Name(s)	Mechanism of Action	Major Side and Adverse Effects	Critical Information	Indications
Narrow spectrum; first generation	Phenytoin sodium (PO or IV)	Blocks sodium channels	Blood dyscrasias, gingival hyperplasia, ataxia, confusion, dizziness, drowsiness, hepatotoxicity, rash, IV site reactions, decreased bone mineral density Ongoing CBC, LFTs, phenytoin serum levels (narrow therapeutic range) Monitor signs and symptoms of toxicity	Avoid IV use in clients with PMH: SB, second- and third-degree blocks Give slowly via IV with inline filter; IV requires continuous telemetry monitoring Therapeutic range: 10–20 mcg/mL	Generalized and complex partial seizures; status epilepticus (IV)
Narrow spectrum; first generation	Phenobarbital (PO)	Improves the effect of GABA in the CNS to cause neuronal hyperpolarization	CNS depression, respiratory depression (IV use); anemia, depression, hepatic impairment Caution in renal impairment and hyperthyroidism Monitor CBC, CMP, TSH during therapy	May cause cognitive impairment and gait instability especially in older adults	Generalized and complex partial seizures; status epilepticus (IV)
Narrow spectrum; first generation	Carbamazepine (PO)	Binds to sodium channels to inhibit the generation of rapid action potentials in the CNS	GI upset, weight gain, blurred vision, CNS depression, bone marrow suppression, hyponatremia, hepatotoxicity Monitor serum sodium levels, LFTs, CBC, and serum phenobarbital levels	Monitor for renal toxicity Monitor for skin reactions and rash Older adults more likely to develop hyponatremia	Generalized and partial seizures
Narrow spectrum; first generation	Oxcarbazepine (PO)	Binds to sodium channels to inhibit the generation of rapid action potentials in the CNS	GI upset, weight gain, blurred vision, CNS depression, bone marrow suppression, hyponatremia, hepatotoxicity Monitor serum sodium levels, LFTs, and CBC	Monitor for renal toxicity Older adults more likely to develop hyponatremia	Generalized and partial seizures

Classification	Drug	Mechanism of action	Adverse effects / Monitoring	Warnings / Considerations	Indications
Narrow spectrum; second generation	Lacosamide (PO)	Enhances slow inactivation of sodium channels	CNS depression, dizziness, nausea, tremor	Check EKG in individuals with cardiac conduction disorders prior to drug initiation	Partial-onset seizures
Broad spectrum; second generation	Valproic acid (PO)	Increases availability of GABA, an inhibitory neurotransmitter	CNS depression, blood dyscrasias, hepatotoxicity, alopecia, tremor Monitor CBC, LFTs prior to and during therapy	Avoid in clients with hepatic disease; may cause liver failure Monitor serum levels and signs and symptoms of toxicity Monitor for increased ammonia levels	Generalized, partial, partial complex, and absence seizures
Broad spectrum; second generation	Lamotrigine (PO)	Inhibits release of glutamate, an excitatory amino acid; inactivates voltage-dependent sodium channels	Nausea, rash, insomnia, drowsiness, rash Monitor renal function, CBC, LFTs, serum levels for adherence	Stephens-Johnson syndrome rare but caution clients	All seizure type; monotherapy or adjunctive
Broad spectrum; second generation	Levetiracetam (PO)	Inhibits presynaptic calcium channels and may also modulate GABA activity	Fatigue, mood changes, drowsiness, weakness	Monitor effects on mood	Partial, myoclonic, generalized seizures
Broad spectrum; second generation	Topiramate (PO)	Blocks voltage-dependent sodium channels; enhances GABA activity	Paresthesias, anorexia, nausea, cognitive changes May decrease sodium bicarbonate Monitor BMP prior to and during therapy	Contraindicated in pregnancy and in women trying to get pregnant Increases risk of renal calculi, metabolic acidosis	Monotherapy or adjunctive in generalized or partial seizures
Broad spectrum; second generation	Zonisamide (PO)	Blocks voltage-dependent sodium and T-type calcium channels	Drowsiness, anorexia, nausea Monitor BMP prior to and during therapy	Avoid in those with sulfonamide allergy Increases risk of nephrolithiasis, metabolic acidosis	Monotherapy or adjunctive in generalized or partial seizures

BMP, basic metabolic panel; CBC, complete blood count; CMP, comprehensive metabolic panel; CNS, central nervous system; EKG, electrocardiogram; GABA, gamma-aminobutyric acid; LFT, liver function test; TSH, thyroid-stimulating hormone.

BLACK BOX WARNING FOR VALPROIC ACID:

◆ Hepatotoxicity has been reported.
◆ Use is contraindicated in clients with known mitochondrial disorders caused by mitochondrial DNA polymerase gamma (POLG) mutations or if mitochondrial disease is suspected in children younger than 2 years old.
◆ Valproic acid is teratogenic, and its use should be avoided in women of childbearing age unless its use is critical to manage a medical condition.
◆ Use has been associated with life-threatening pancreatitis.

BLACK BOX WARNING FOR LAMOTRIGINE:

◆ Monitor for life-threatening dermatologic reactions including Stevens-Johnson syndrome and toxic epidermal necrolysis.

Practice Questions and Rationales

1. A nurse is caring for a client with challenges in memory recall. The client is being treated with a *N*-methyl-ᴅ-aspartate (NMDA) receptor antagonist medication. Which disease is part of the client's history?
   1. Alzheimer disease
   2. Parkinson disease
   3. Multiple sclerosis
   4. Seizure disorder

2. A nurse is caring for a client diagnosed with Parkinson disease (PD). The client is prescribed levodopa. Which are expected assessments of a client with PD? Select all that apply.
   1. Tremors to hands at rest
   2. Confusion of person, place, and time
   3. Postural rigidity
   4. Sexual dysfunction
   5. Motor weakness
   6. Altered level of consciousness

3. A nurse is caring for a client diagnosed with a seizure disorder. Which laboratory value would the nurse assess prior to administration of phenytoin?
   1. Sodium level
   2. Potassium level
   3. White blood cell count
   4. Hemoglobin and hematocrit

4. A client is diagnosed with complex partial seizures and is prescribed phenobarbital. After 1 hour, the nurse assesses the client. Which assessment finding requires immediate action?
   1. Heart rate of 69 beats/min
   2. Respiratory rate of 8 breaths/min
   3. Blood pressure of 130/78 mm Hg
   4. Pain rating of 2 on a scale of 1 to 10, with 10 as the highest rating

5. Which other antiepileptic medications, besides phenobarbital, are used for generalized and partial seizures and work on the sodium channels? Select all that apply.
   1. Carbamazepine
   2. Oxcarbazepine
   3. Lacosamide
   4. Valproic acid
   5. Phenobarbital

6. A nurse is caring for a client diagnosed with partial seizures and prescribed zonisamide. Which statement is included in teaching the client about the medication?

    1. "The medication enhances GABA activity making you more alert and focused."

    2. "This medication works on the sodium and calcium channels of the brain, causing drowsiness."

    3. "This medication depresses the CNS activity producing irritability and insomnia."

    4. "The medication is responsible for the release of glutamate, an excitatory amino acid, causing nausea and insomnia."

7. A nurse is receiving report about a client who was recently admitted to the nursing unit with multiple sclerosis. Which are expected clinical manifestations? Select all that apply.

    1. Motor impairment

    2. Difficulty walking

    3. Feelings of sadness

    4. Difficulty sleeping

    5. Double vision

8. A nurse is preparing to administer interferon beta-1b to the client with multiple sclerosis. Which nursing intervention is performed prior to the administration of the medication?

    1. Perform a depression survey.

    2. Complete a full set of vital signs.

    3. Assess laboratory values such as complete blood count and liver function tests.

    4. Administer acetaminophen or ibuprofen as prescribed.

9. A nurse is caring for a client diagnosed with Parkinson disease (PD). Prior to the administration of a scheduled dose of carbidopa–levodopa, the nurse observes the client having an increase in tremors and rigidity. The nurse plans to call the prescriber. Which statement might the nurse make to the prescriber?

    1. "The client's medication is not working and needs a larger dose."

    2. "The client's family is agitating the client and not allowing for rest."

    3. "The client's mood suggesting toxicity and suggest discontinuing the medication and adding pramipexole."

    4. "The client's dose is wearing off before the next dose and needs to be administered more frequently."

10. A nurse is caring for a client admitted to the nursing unit with pneumonia and a history of late stage Alzheimer disease. The nurse is assessing the client, when a family member tells the nurse that the family is not happy with the effects of memantine. The family member reports no change in the client's memory. Which statement by the nurse is therapeutic to the client's family member?

    1. "Not all drugs work the same on all Alzheimer patients."

    2. "We should have a family meeting to discuss the medications."

    3. "Medications for Alzheimer's do not slow the progression of the disease."

    4. "Let's write down your thoughts and we can address them with the prescriber in the morning."

11. A nurse is caring for a child who is being discharged from the acute care unit after diagnosis and treatment of a seizure disorder. The mother is assisting her child after discharge and is involved in his care. Which statement by the mother warrants additional instruction regarding the medications for the seizure disorder?

    1. "I should allow my child to take rests throughout the day."
    2. "If necessary, I will allow extra time for morning care."
    3. "I am prepared to assist with meals and doctor appointments."
    4. "I will not worry if my child talks about hurting himself."

12. A nurse is teaching a young woman about a new medication, topiramate. Which statement is included in the instruction?

    1. "If you are allergic to sulfa drugs, you should not take this medication."
    2. "Take this medication in the morning and with a full glass of water."
    3. "The medication should not be taken if you plan to get pregnant."
    4. "Prior to taking this medication, take your blood pressure."

13. A nurse is reviewing a client's electroencephalogram (EEG) report. Which chronic neurologic disorder in the client's history has a diagnostic test of EEGs?

    1. Epilepsy
    2. Multiple sclerosis (MS)
    3. Alzheimer disease (AD)
    4. Parkinson disease (PD)

14. A nurse is caring for a client with Parkinson disease (PD). The client asks how the disease causes motor dysfunction. Which is the nurse's correct response?

    1. "The medications affect the cholinergic receptors."
    2. "It is caused by a destruction of dopamine neurotransmitter."
    3. "Serotonin, a neurotransmitter is overproduced by the brain."
    4. "The cause is related to the autoimmune destruction of myelin."

15. A nurse is caring for a client with a history of multiple sclerosis (MS). The client asks the nurse why so many medications are prescribed. Which statements explain why many medications are used in the treatment of MS? Select all that apply.

    1. "The medications manage acute exacerbations."
    2. "The medications aid in diagnosis of the disease."
    3. "The medications modify the disease."
    4. "The medications are used to assist with symptom management."
    5. "The medications are used to slow the progression of the disease process."

12

PSYCHOTHERAPEUTIC MEDICATIONS

BRIEF OVERVIEW OF PSYCHIATRIC DISORDERS

◆ **Major depressive disorder:** Major depressive disorder is characterized by single or recurrent episodes of unipolar (nonbipolar) depression resulting in significant changes in functioning (typically social, occupational, and/or self-care). This condition significantly increases the risk of suicidal thoughts and behaviors. It is one of the leading causes of disability in the United States. Treatment is aimed at restoring optimal daily functioning and may include psychopharmacology, counseling therapy, and/or electroconvulsive therapy (ECT).

◆ **Bipolar disorder:** Bipolar disorder is a mood disorder characterized by recurrent exacerbations of depression and mania that typically emerges in late adolescence or early adulthood. Periods of illness (depression or mania) alternate with periods of normal functioning. The manic phase is characterized by bizarre, hyperactive, paranoid, and/or psychotic behavior. Treatment is aimed at restoring optimal daily functioning and may include psychopharmacology, community services, counseling therapy, and/or ECT.

◆ **Schizophrenia:** Schizophrenia is a thought disorder characterized by alterations in thinking, behavior, emotions, and perceptions of reality. This condition likely results from a combination of genetic, neurobiologic, and nongenetic factors. The typical onset is teens to early 20s. Treatment is aimed at restoring optimal daily functioning and may include psychopharmacology, community services, counseling therapy, and/or behavioral therapy.

◆ **Generalized anxiety disorder:** Generalized anxiety disorder is characterized by excessive worry and anxiety more than 50% of the time, for at least 3 months. Anxiety is often (but not always) related to domains of life, such as family, health, finances, school, or work. If untreated, it may lead to a panic disorder. Treatment is multifaceted and may include psychopharmacology, counseling therapy, and behavioral therapy.

CLINICAL PEARLS—PSYCHIATRIC DISORDERS

Major Depressive Disorder

Assessment/Signs and Symptoms

◆ Common signs and symptoms of major depressive disorder include anergia, anhedonia, anxiety, restlessness, reduced or increased appetite, weight loss or weight gain, change in bowel habits, insomnia or hypersomnia, and change in sexual functioning.

◆ In addition, somatic complaints, blunted affect, poor grooming and hygiene, isolative behavior, psychomotor retardation or agitation, slowed speech, and delayed response may also be seen.

Diagnostics

◆ Diagnosis is by psychiatric assessment, including history and physical examination as well as laboratory results to exclude physiologic causes of symptoms, including serum thyroid and vitamin D levels and/or pregnancy test.

◆ Several depression screening tools are available: Hamilton Depression Scale, Beck Depression Inventory, Geriatric Depression Scale, Zung Self-Rating Depression Scale.

Bipolar Disorder

Assessment/Signs and Symptoms

◆ Bipolar mania is characterized by abnormally elevated mood (euphoria), expansive thoughts, agitation, irritability, intolerance of feedback/criticism, grandiosity, poor judgment, poor boundaries, poor impulse control, emotional lability, insomnia, inattention to activities of daily living, and excessive amounts of energy. Delusions and hallucinations are possible.

◆ Bipolar depression is also characterized by the symptoms present in major depressive disorder.

Diagnostics

◆ Diagnosis is by psychiatric assessment, including history and physical examination.

◆ A laboratory workup should be done to exclude physiologic causes of symptoms, including serum thyroid levels and urine screening for substance use.

Schizophrenia

Assessment/Signs and Symptoms

◆ Positive symptoms (manifestations of things that are normally not present):
  ● Hallucinations (visual, auditory, olfactory, tactile, or gustatory)
  ● Delusions (persecution, grandeur, somatic delusions, jealousy, thought broadcasting, thought insertion, religiosity, thought withdrawal, delusions of control)
◆ Negative symptoms (absence of things that are normally present):
  ● Affect (blunted, flat)
  ● Alogia (poverty of speech, poverty of thought)
  ● Anergia (lack of energy)
  ● Avolition (lack of motivation)
◆ Cognitive and affective symptoms: Disordered thinking, indecisiveness, problem-solving impairment, poor concentration, impaired memory, hopeless, suicidal ideation

Diagnostics

◆ Psychotic thinking or behavior present for at least 6 months. There is significant impairment in several areas of functioning, including school, work, self-care, and interpersonal relationships.

◆ Diagnosis is by psychiatric assessment, including history and physical examination.

◆ A laboratory workup should be done to exclude physiologic causes of symptoms, including serum white blood cell count to rule out infection and urine screening for urinary tract infection and/or substance-induced psychosis.

Generalized Anxiety Disorder

Assessment/Signs and Symptoms

◆ Common signs and symptoms include the following:
  ● Mild anxiety: Restlessness, irritability, increased motivation
  ● Moderate anxiety: Increased heart rate, discomfort, muscular tension, perspiration, restlessness, rapid speech
  ● Severe anxiety: Dizziness, diarrhea, headache, feelings of dread, insomnia, nausea, hyperventilation, trembling, tachycardia, urinary frequency, focusing on self
  ● Panic anxiety: Delusions, hallucinations, sweating, dilated pupils, palpitations, feelings of impending doom, insomnia, trembling, aggressive behavior, withdrawal into self/mutism

Diagnostics

◆ Characterized by excessive anxiety or worry for more than 3 months, and at least one of the following behaviors:
  ● Avoidance of activities or events that may have a potentially negative outcome
  ● Excessive time and energy spent preparing for events that may have a negative outcome
  ● Procrastination in decision-making or in behavior due to worry
  ● Seeking repeated reassurances from others due to worry

MEDICATION OVERVIEW

Major Depressive Disorder

Medications along with psychotherapy or counseling are the primary treatment of major depressive disorder. Antidepressants seek to balance the neurotransmitters in the brain responsible for the regulation of emotions, stress, sleep, appetite, and sexuality. The choice of which medication to use is generally made by the provider based on the client's severity of symptoms, presence of comorbidities, and any other factors that may be contributing to current state of the disorder. See Table 12-1 for more information about these medications.

> **BLACK BOX WARNING:** All antidepressants carry a black box warning for an increased risk of suicide in children, adolescents, and young adults. Risks versus benefits should be weighed prior to prescribing these medications to these populations. Clients taking these medications should be closely observed by their families and caregivers, and close communication with the providers for behavior changes or suicidal ideation should be done.

SAFETY ALERT! MAOIs interact with many medications and can result in serious harm. Clients should be educated not to take any medications, including over-the-counter medications and herbal remedies, unless they have been discussed with their provider.

Bipolar Disorder

Bipolar disorder is most effectively treated when a combination of medication and psychotherapy is used. It is a lifelong illness, and treatment should be focused in helping clients to balance themselves out, minimizing the extreme mood swings that can occur with the disorder. Mood stabilizers, atypical antipsychotics, and antidepressants are the cornerstones of medication management for bipolar disorder. See Table 12-2 for further information.

SAFETY ALERT! Lithium toxicity can result in serious complications for the client. Close monitoring and routine lithium monitoring of clients taking lithium is essential. Normal range of lithium is 0.6 to 1.2 mEq/L. Clients with mild lithium toxicity (1.5 to 2.0 mEq/L) may experience blurred vision, tinnitus, gastrointestinal upset (nausea, vomiting, diarrhea), and ataxia. Clients with severe lithium toxicity (>3.5 mEq/L) may experience impaired consciousness, nystagmus, seizures, coma, oliguria/anuria, and myocardial infarction. Clients with moderate lithium toxicity (2.0 to 3.5 mEq/L) may experience excessive urine output, tremors, confusion, irritability, and psychomotor retardation.

Schizophrenia

Schizophrenia is a complex, lifelong illness and as such, treatment is highly individualized based on the presentation of symptoms and response to treatment. The goals of management are to treat the symptoms present, prevent a relapse from occurring, and maintain quality of life. Psychotherapy along with pharmacologic management is a crucial aspect as this is a chronic disorder.

Treatment of schizophrenia is separated into two categories: the acute phase and maintenance therapy. During the acute phase, treatment is focused on returning the client to normal functioning levels and close titration of medications must be done to stabilize the client. Once the client is back to baseline, maintenance therapy is the focus of treatment, with the goal of preventing relapse. In most cases, second-generation antipsychotics are the first-line treatment for schizophrenia; however, first-generation antipsychotics may be used as well (see Table 12-3 for more information).

Generalized Anxiety Disorder

Medications used to treat generalized anxiety disorder (GAD) are often given in conjunction with the client receiving psychotherapy. Antidepressants, SSRIs in particular, are the most frequently used medications to treat GAD (SSRIs are covered above in Table 12-1). Other medications such as benzodiazepines and buspirone can be used as well and are discussed below in Table 12-4.

Life Span Considerations: Use benzodiazepines cautiously with elderly clients as they are more susceptible to respiratory depression and paradoxical response.

SAFETY ALERT! The use of benzodiazepines is associated with sleep driving and other complex, sleep-related events. If sleep driving or other like events are reported, discontinuation of the medication should occur to ensure client's safety.

Table 12-1

Drugs Used to Treat Major Depressive Disorder

Class	Prototype	Mechanism of Action	Major Side and Adverse Effects	Critical Information	Indications
Selective serotonin reuptake inhibitors (SSRIs)	Fluoxetine	Blocks the reuptake of serotonin in the synapses, thus enhancing the effects of serotonin	Sexual dysfunction	Report any mental status changes or suicidality, particularly when initiating therapy	Depression
			Serotonin syndrome (potentially lethal; symptoms include fever and confusion)	Stop medication if serotonin syndrome is suspected	Obsessive-compulsive disorder
			CNS stimulation (resulting in insomnia and agitation)	Taper medication when discontinuing	Panic disorders
				Full therapeutic effect may take 6–8 weeks	Bulimia nervosa
			Suicidality (at start of therapy)	Take medication in morning to reduce likelihood of insomnia	Premenstrual dysphoric disorder
					Posttraumatic stress disorder
				Not to be taken concurrently with MAO inhibitors or tricyclic antidepressants	
Atypical antidepressants	Bupropion	Exact mechanism unknown, likely acts by inhibiting uptake of dopamine	Seizures	Contraindicated in clients with seizure disorders	Depression
			Can suppress appetite and cause weight loss	Monitor for seizures	Smoking cessation
				Not to be taken concurrently with MAO inhibitor antidepressants	Seasonal affective disorder
Tricyclic antidepressants	Amitriptyline	Blocks the reuptake of norepinephrine and serotonin in the synapses, thus enhancing their effects	Orthostatic hypotension	Stand slowly to reduce orthostasis Monitor blood pressure and heart rate	Depression
			Anticholinergic effects (dry mouth, blurred vision, urinary retention, constipation)	Treat anticholinergic symptoms	Bipolar depression
			Sedation	Take at bedtime if sedation occurs	Neuropathy
			Toxicity (resulting in dysrhythmias, confusion, seizures, coma, and/or death)	Contraindicated in clients with seizure disorders	Anxiety disorders
				Monitor for seizures	Insomnia
			Seizures	Check baseline electrocardiogram	
				Monitor for signs of toxicity	

Monoamine oxidase inhibitors (MAOIs)	Phenelzine	Blocks MAO in the brain, thus enhancing the effects of norepinephrine, dopamine, and serotonin	CNS stimulation (agitation, anxiety, mania)	Stand slowly to reduce orthostasis Monitor blood pressure and heart rate	Depression Bulimia nervosa
			Orthostatic hypotension	Observe for CNS stimulation	
			Hypertensive crisis (from dietary tyramine)	Observe for hypertensive crisis (headache, nausea, tachycardia, hypertension)	
				Interacts with many medications including antidepressants, meperidine, antihypertensives, digoxin, and antihistamines	
				Avoid/eliminate foods with tyramine (aged cheeses and meats, red wine, avocados, smoked fishes, protein supplements)	

CNS, central nervous system; MAO, monoamine oxidase.

Table 12-2

Drugs Used to Treat Bipolar Disorder

Class	Prototype	Mechanism of Action	Major Side and Adverse Effects	Critical Information	Indications
Mood stabilizer	Lithium	Results in several neurochemical alterations in the brain, notably serotonin receptor blocking	Lithium toxicity (diarrhea, nausea, vomiting, polyuria, muscle weakness, slurred speech, tremors)	Routine lithium level monitoring to ensure therapeutic range and to avoid toxicity (normal range = 0.6–1.2 mEq/L; toxicity can occur at 1.5 mEq/L or higher)	Bipolar disorder
					Alcohol use disorder
			Fine muscle tremors in the hands	Inform provider if hand tremors occur or worsen	Bulimia nervosa
			GI discomfort	Take with food or milk to reduce GI distress	Psychotic disorders
			Increased thirst	Avoid prolonged use of NSAIDs	
			Electrolyte imbalance	Ensure adequate fluid and sodium intake (important to maintain sodium balance and not increase or decrease sodium intake rapidly)	
			Weight gain		
			Renal toxicity	Check baseline kidney and thyroid function, and then check regularly during therapy	
			Hypothyroidism (with long-term treatment)	Use caution when taking diuretics with lithium, as loss of sodium via diuresis can result in retention of lithium, increasing the risk of toxicity	
Mood-stabilizing antiepileptic	Valproic acid	Enhances the inhibitory effects of gamma-aminobutyric acid; inhibits glutamate, thus reducing CNS stimulation	Hepatotoxicity	Contraindicated in clients who are pregnant or have liver disease	Bipolar disorder
			Thrombocytopenia	Routinely monitor liver function tests, platelets, and amylase	
			Teratogenesis		
			Pancreatitis	Report bruising or abdominal pain/discomfort	
			GI discomfort	Routine valproic acid level monitoring to ensure therapeutic range: valproic acid (total) = 50–125 µg/mL	

CNS, central nervous system; GI, gastrointestinal; NSAID, nonsteroidal anti-inflammatory drug.

Table 12-3

Drugs Used to Treat Schizophrenia

Class	Prototype	Mechanism of Action	Major Side and Adverse Effects	Critical Information	Indications
First-generation (typical) antipsychotic	Haloperidol	Inhibits dopamine (D₂), acetylcholine, norepinephrine, and histamine in the brain. D₂ blockade is presumed to inhibit symptoms of psychosis	Acute dystonia (facial and muscular spasms)	Treat positive symptoms of psychosis (hallucinations and delusions)	Psychotic disorders
			Parkinsonism (muscular rigidity, tremors, shuffling, drooling)	Observe for symptoms of dystonia, parkinsonism, akathisia, tardive dyskinesia, and NMS	Schizophrenia spectrum disorders
			Akathisia	Reduce dose or discontinue as needed for side effects	Bipolar disorder
			Tardive dyskinesia (involuntary body movements, lip smacking, slurred speech)	Benztropine and/or anticholinergic medications can be used for symptoms of dystonia and akathisia	
			NMS (fever, labile blood pressure, muscle rigidity, change in level of consciousness)		
			Anticholinergic effects		
			Weight gain and gynecomastia		
			Seizures		
Second-generation (atypical) antipsychotic	Risperidone	Inhibits serotonin, dopamine (D₂), acetylcholine, norepinephrine, and histamine in the brain. D₂ blockade is presumed to inhibit symptoms of psychosis	Agranulocytosis (clozapine only)	Treat positive and negative symptoms of psychosis	Psychotic disorders
			Weight gain	Regular white blood count monitoring is required for clozapine	Schizophrenia spectrum disorders
			Impaired glucose tolerance	Monitor baseline and periodic fasting blood glucose, cholesterol, and weight	Bipolar disorder
			Anticholinergic effects	Encourage healthy diet and exercise	
			Mild EPS (tremors)	Report signs of EPS	
			Orthostasis		
			Hypercholesterolemia		

EPS, extrapyramidal symptoms; NMS, neuroleptic malignant syndrome.

Table 12-4

Drugs Used to Treat Generalized Anxiety Disorder

Class	Prototype	Mechanism of Action	Major Side and Adverse Effects	Critical Information	Indications
Benzodiazepines	Diazepam	Enhances the inhibitory effects of gamma-aminobutyric acid in the CNS	CNS depression (oversedation, decreased respiratory rate, ataxia, light-headedness)	Controlled Substances Act Schedule IV medication class	GAD
				Contraindicated in clients with respiratory depression	Panic disorder
			Anterograde amnesia		Insomnia
			Paradoxical response (excitatory or hyperactivity effect)	Use cautiously with the elderly; this population is more susceptible to respiratory depression and paradoxical response	Seizure disorder
					Alcohol withdrawal
			Acute withdrawal if stopped abruptly (anxiety, insomnia, sweating, tremors)	Monitor respiratory function regularly	Preoperative sedation
				Intended for short-term use due to risk for dependence	
				Avoid alcohol and using heavy equipment when taking	
				Taper medication if use has been long term to minimize withdrawal symptoms	
Atypical/non-barbiturate anxiolytic	Buspirone	Exact mechanism unknown, favorably binds to serotonin and dopamine receptors	Dizziness	Avoid use during breast-feeding	GAD
			Nausea	Contraindicated for use with monoamine oxidase inhibitor antidepressants (may cause hypertensive crisis)	Panic disorder
			Headache		Social anxiety disorder
			Agitation	Full clinical effect may not occur for 3–6 weeks	Obsessive-compulsive disorders
			Light-headedness	Not appropriate for as-needed use; must be taken regularly	Trauma- and stressor-related disorders (PTSDs)
				Avoid grapefruit juice (enhances effect of buspirone)	

Class	Drug	Action	Nursing considerations	Adverse effects	Uses
Beta-blockers	Propranolol	Blocks stimulation of beta1- and beta2-adregnergic receptor sites, thus reducing certain physical manifestations of anxiety (elevated heart rate)	Obtain baseline vital signs	Bradycardia	GAD
			May be used as-needed	Dysrhythmias (A-V node blockade)	PTSD
			Administer with food to increase absorption	Orthostatic hypotension	Alcohol withdrawal
			Assess for skin changes when initiating therapy	Stevens-Johnson syndrome	Aggressive behavior

CNS, central nervous system; GAD, generalized anxiety disorder; PTSD, posttraumatic stress disorder.

Practice Questions and Rationales

1. A nurse is caring for a client who has a new prescription for haloperidol. The nurse knows that client teaching has been successful when the client makes which statement?
   1. "This medication will help improve my desire to be around people."
   2. "This medication will help motivate me to get back to work."
   3. "This medication will help reduce the voices I hear in my head."
   4. "This medication will help me when I have trouble finding words."

2. A client with schizophrenia is starting clozapine therapy. Which information is highest **priority** to include in client teaching?
   1. The client should have periodic fasting glucose levels drawn.
   2. The client should monitor for weight gain and adhere to a healthy diet.
   3. The client should report fine hand tremors to the health care provider.
   4. The client must have regular white blood cell count (WBC) levels drawn.

3. The nurse documents that a client with schizophrenia is experiencing anticholinergic side effects from long-term use of risperidone. Which symptoms has the nurse assessed?
   1. Parkinsonism, dystonia, poverty of speech
   2. Hyperglycemia, hypercholesterolemia
   3. Tachycardia, muscle rigidity, hyperreflexia
   4. Urinary retention, infrequent bowel movements, blurred vision

4. A client who takes lithium, who had a brief seizure in the ambulance, presents to the emergency department with altered consciousness, dysrhythmias, and rapid eye movements. Which serum lithium level would the nurse expect to assess?
   1. 3.6 mEq/L (3.6 mmol/L)
   2. 3.1 mEq/L (3.1 mmol/L)
   3. 2.5 mEq/L (2.5 mmol/L)
   4. 1.7 mEq/L (1.7 mmol/L)

5. A client newly diagnosed with generalized anxiety disorder has been prescribed diazepam and buspirone by an outpatient provider. Which client statement indicates teaching has been effective?
   1. "I will take diazepam and buspirone together for long-term management."
   2. "Buspirone can cause sedation, so I will take it only at night."
   3. "I will take diazepam for a short time until the buspirone takes full effect."
   4. "I can become tolerant of buspirone, so I will take it only when needed."

6. A nurse is caring for a client who has just begun taking diazepam to treat anxiety. The nurse should monitor the client for which side/adverse effect(s) of this medication? Select all that apply.
   1. Light-headedness
   2. Hypertension
   3. Bradypnea
   4. Hearing loss
   5. Anterograde amnesia

7. For which clinical indications would benzodiazepines be prescribed appropriately?
    1. Long-term management of obsessive–compulsive disorder, seizure disorder, and alcohol use disorder
    2. Short-term management of panic disorder, alcohol withdrawal, and preoperative sedation
    3. Short-term management of posttraumatic stress disorder, muscle spasms, and tachycardia
    4. Long-term management of bipolar mania, psoriasis, and insomnia

8. A client with major depressive disorder is prescribed phenelzine by a provider. Which client teaching is the highest **priority?**
    1. Phenelzine's full therapeutic effect may take 6 to 8 weeks.
    2. Phenelzine interacts with many foods and medications.
    3. Phenelzine may cause insomnia and some sexual side effects.
    4. Continue taking phenelzine even after mood improves.

9. A nurse is assuming care of a client diagnosed with depression with suspected serotonin syndrome. Which symptoms would the nurse expect to find upon assessment?
    1. Confusion, sweatiness, labile blood pressure, irritability, tachycardia
    2. Mania, akathisia, panic attacks, cardiac rhythm changes
    3. Nausea, lethargy, orthostasis, headache
    4. Blurred vision, urinary retention, orthostasis, constipation

10. A client diagnosed with major depressive disorder has been prescribed fluoxetine. Which information would the nurse include while providing teaching to the client? Select all that apply.
    1. The medication's full therapeutic effect may take 6 to 8 weeks.
    2. The medication can cause sedation, seizures, and tachycardia.
    3. Taper medication with provider supervision when discontinuing medication.
    4. The medication should be taken as needed during periods of severe depression.
    5. The medication can cause worsening depression and suicidal thoughts.

13

REPRODUCTIVE SYSTEM MEDICATIONS

The reproductive system is a system composed of sex organs that work in an organized manner for the purpose of reproduction. Substances such as fluids, hormones, and pheromones are also important accessories to the reproductive system. This chapter will discuss the female and male reproductive systems, the common conditions and disorders of each system, and their associated pharmacologic and nonpharmacologic treatment recommendations.

BRIEF OVERVIEW OF FEMALE REPRODUCTIVE SYSTEM, ITS CONDITIONS, AND ITS DISORDERS

The external structures of the female reproductive system include the clitoris, labia majora, labia minor, Bartholin glands, the fourchette, and the perineum. The major internal organs of the female reproductive system include the vagina, cervix, uterus, fallopian tubes, and ovaries. The female breast is also a component of female reproduction, especially when lactating.

Female reproductive system disorders consist of abnormalities associated with the menstrual cycle, uterine and/or ovarian function, infections, coagulation disorders, and unknown causes. Pharmacologic management of reproductive disorders, pregnancy prevention, and care of women in labor and during the postpartum period will be discussed in this chapter. Conditions associated with the female reproductive system such as pregnancy and menopause will also be described. Most commonly, the nurse is responsible for collecting a detailed history related to the present concern and obtaining vital sign measurement, with the assessment completed by the health care provider.

Menstrual Cycle Disorders

Disorders of the menstrual cycle involve any deviation from a woman's typical menstrual pattern, which can be either abnormal bleeding or the absence of menses. For any menstrual cycle disorder, a full evaluation by a provider must occur prior to initiation of medications.

- ◆ Abnormal uterine bleeding is bleeding that occurs in the absence of identifiable pelvic pathology, medical condition, or pregnancy. Treatment is with hormones (progestin and/or progestin–estrogen combination).
- ◆ Amenorrhea is a disturbance in the menstrual cycle pattern possibly related to absence of normal ovulation, contributing to irregular stimulation of the uterine lining. Amenorrhea is categorized as primary or secondary absence of menses. Primary amenorrhea is defined as no menses by age 16. Secondary amenorrhea is defined as no menses for longer than 3 months after an established pattern of menses for 1 year. There are a many possible reasons for secondary amenorrhea, including but not limited to: pregnancy or lactation, problems with the hypothalamus, pituitary gland, ovaries, or uterus.

◆ Dysmenorrhea is characterized by painful menses that is classified as primary or secondary. Primary dysmenorrhea can occur anytime without evidence of an underlying diagnosis and is typically related to an increase in prostaglandin production. Secondary dysmenorrhea is painful menses related to an actual medical diagnosis, such as endometriosis, adenomyosis, ovarian cysts, or pelvic inflammatory disease.

Psychiatric Disorders Associated with Hormonal Changes of the Female Reproductive System

◆ Premenstrual syndrome (PMS) and premenstrual dysphoric disorder (PMDD) are a collection of physical and emotional indicators related to the menstrual cycle. The symptoms tend to increase in severity during the latter half of the cycle, known as the luteal phase, and resolve with the start of the menstrual flow. PMDD is the severe form of PMS. Treatment is based on the severity of symptoms. For mild-to-moderate symptoms, nonpharmacologic options may include avoidance of alcohol, salt, caffeine, nicotine, simple carbohydrates, and simple sugars and increased intake of complex carbohydrates and protein. More severe symptoms are treated with a combination of nonpharmacologic and pharmacologic methods.

◆ Postpartum depression (PPD) is depression that occurs within 6 months of birth. Common causes of PPD include rapid changes in hormone levels, history of depression, fatigue, lack of social support, social stressors, or emotional factors relating to pregnancy/birth/health status of the infant.

Vaginal Infections

Infections in the vagina may be caused by yeast, bacteria, and/or products that alter the vaginal pH. Treatment depends on the underlying cause. Client education should be directed toward eradication of the underlying cause and prevention of future infections, if possible.

◆ Bacterial vaginosis is a vaginal infection found more commonly in sexually active females. It is considered a sexually associated infection related to an overgrowth of bacteria, causing a rise in vaginal pH.

◆ Candidiasis (yeast) is a fungal infection where vaginal pH is normal.

◆ Group B streptococcus (GBS) is a bacterial infection that can be passed to a fetus during labor and birth. The mother is screened for GBS around 36 weeks of pregnancy.

There are additional infections of the reproductive system associated with sexual activity (vaginal, anal, and/or oral) with an infected person. For all infections, the nurse will obtain a thorough history and review of systems. The provider will complete the physical assessment and obtain necessary diagnostic tests. Screening can occur for those at high risk (multiple partners, incarcerated individuals, geographical areas where sexually transmitted infections [STIs] are prevalent), clients who request screening, and screening as indicated in pregnancy and in the Centers for Disease Control and Prevention (CDC) screening guidelines, summarized in Table 13-1. Treatment varies depending on the infectious agent (refer to Table 13-2). Several STIs can result in systemic complications if left untreated. The various STIs, their symptoms, and treatment regimens are discussed below.

◆ Chlamydia is a bacterial infection caused by *Chlamydia trachomatis* and is the most commonly reported STI in women in the United States. Chlamydia can affect both males and females. Symptoms in women include pelvic pain, pain and/or bleeding with intercourse, and vaginal discharge. Treatment requires antibiotics.

Table 13-1

Screening Guidelines for Sexually Transmitted Infections According to the Centers for Disease Control and Prevention

Infection	Guidelines
Chlamydia/gonorrhea	Sexually active and <25
Genital herpes	At client request
Syphilis	First prenatal visit of pregnancy
Trichomonas	If high risk

◆ Gonorrhea is a bacterial infection caused by the organism *Neisseria gonorrhoeae* that can infect both males and females. Gonorrhea most often affects the urethra, rectum, or throat. In females, gonorrhea can also infect the cervix. Symptoms are similar to chlamydia, and treatment is with antibiotics.

◆ Genital herpes is a viral infection caused by the herpes simplex virus. Herpes simplex virus-1 typically causes cold sores, and genital herpes is most commonly caused by an infection with the herpes simplex virus-2. However, both types can be found orally and genitally. Treatment consists of antiviral agents.

◆ Human papillomavirus (HPV) is the most common sexually transmitted infection. HPV on the cervix is not visible to the naked eye, and the higher risk strains are associated with cancers, including those of the cervix, vagina, and vulva. Low-risk HPV strains present with genital warts in the rectal and vaginal areas.

◆ Pelvic inflammatory disease (PID) is an infection of a woman's reproductive organs. It is a complication often caused by some STIs such as chlamydia and gonorrhea. Symptoms include fever, pelvic pain, and painful intercourse. Treatment consists of identification of the underlying cause, antibiotics, treatment of the sexual partner, and temporary abstinence.

◆ Syphilis is a bacterial infection caused by *Treponema pallidum*. It can have very serious and systemic complications when left untreated. Primary syphilis includes a painless ulcer. Secondary syphilis presents as a rash, weight loss, and lymphadenopathy. Tertiary syphilis is systemic infection that affects the nervous system and heart when syphilis is left untreated. Tertiary syphilis can be fatal. Latent syphilis occurs when the infection lies dormant and no symptoms are present, but the infection can still be transmitted. Treatment of syphilis consists of an antibiotic regimen.

◆ Trichomonas is a very common STI, frequently called "trich." It is caused by infection with a protozoan parasite called *Trichomonas vaginalis*. Symptoms include foul-smelling discharge, painful urination, vaginal itching, and burning. Treatment requires antibiotics.

Mastitis

Mastitis is inflammation of the breast tissue, which may cause a bacterial infection. It is diagnosed ≥24 or more postpartum in a woman with a temperature over 100.4°F (38°C) and associated breast pain, swelling, warmth, and redness. It occurs most commonly in breast-feeding women. Treatment consists of antibiotics, nonsteroidal anti-inflammatory drugs (NSAIDs), warm compresses to the affected breast, and frequent lactation. If untreated or treatment is subtherapeutic, mastitis can lead to a breast abscess.

Table 13-2

Medications for Sexually Transmitted Infections

Class	Prototype Medication	Mechanism of Action	Major Side Effects and Adverse Effects	Critical Information	Indications
Macrolide (see Table 6-1)	Azithromycin	Inhibits protein synthesis (bactericidal)	Angioedema Anaphylaxis Cholestatic jaundice Pancreatitis	Caution in elderly Caution in renal impairment	Chlamydia infection
Cephalosporin (see Table 6-1)	Ceftriaxone	Inhibits cell wall peptide synthesis (bactericidal)	Anaphylaxis Bronchospasm Stevens-Johnson syndrome		Gonorrhea
Penicillin (see Table 6-1)	Penicillin G	Inhibits cell wall synthesis (bactericidal)	Anaphylaxis Hypersensitivity to drug Superinfection Clostridium difficile Nausea Vomiting Diarrhea Pruritus Fever Rash	Anaphylactic reaction to beta-lactams	Syphilis

(continued)

Table 13-2

Medications for Sexually Transmitted Infections *(continued)*

Class	Prototype Medication	Mechanism of Action	Major Side Effects and Adverse Effects	Critical Information	Indications
Vaccine	Human papillomavirus-9-valent vaccine	Induces antibody formation	Hypersensitivity	Hypersensitivity to yeast	Immunization for the prevention of several strains of the human papillomavirus
			Anaphylaxis	Caution if acute illness or immunocompromised	
			Injection site reaction—pain, swelling, redness	Prevention against the most common cancer causing types: 6, 11, 16, 18, 31, 33, 45, 52, and 58	
			Headache		
			Fever	Given in either 2 or 3 doses depending on age at vaccine administration	
			Nausea		
			Fatigue	Will not cure any strain that the client has already contracted	
			Cough		
Bactericidal	Metronidazole (see Table 6-1)	Reduces metabolite formed by anaerobes	Seizures	Pregnancy first trimester	Trichomoniasis
		Disrupts DNA	Aseptic meningitis	Avoid alcohol use during antibiotic course and 24 hr after last dose	
			Optic neuropathy		
			Hypersensitivity	Avoid disulfuram use within 14 days	
			Nausea		
			Vomiting		
			Epigastric discomfort		
			Rash		
			Headache		
			Metallic taste		
Topical acid	Trichloroacetic acid topical	Cauterizes abnormal tissue	Burns, severe	Hypersensitivity	Warts/condyloma

Menopause

Menopause is defined as the cessation of menstruation for 1 year. Treatment is directed at symptom management.

Pregnancy Prevention

Pharmacologic (hormonal) methods of contraception include oral contraceptives, etonogestrel implants, injectable medroxyprogesterone acetate, intrauterine devices, vaginal rings, and transdermal patches. These medications are also approved for the treatment of many reproductive disorders. Nonpharmacologic methods to prevent pregnancy include abstinence, barrier contraceptives (condoms), and natural family planning methods. Pregnancy prevention can be accomplished by interfering with the reproductive process at any step from gametogenesis to implantation of a fertilized ovum. The various types of hormonal contraceptives are as follows:

- ◆ Combined oral contraceptives: Hormonal contraception that contains estrogen and progestin that act by suppressing ovulation, thickening cervical mucus, and causing atrophy to endometrial lining creating an inhospitable environment for implantation.
- ◆ Progestin-only oral contraceptives: Hormonal contraception that contains only progestin that acts similarly to combined oral contraceptives but is less effective in suppressing ovulation.
- ◆ Emergency oral contraception: Pill taken after unprotected or forced intercourse to interfere with implantation.
- ◆ Transdermal contraceptive patch: A transdermal patch that delivers continuous estrogen and progestin through the skin and absorbed into the tissue.
- ◆ Injectable progestins: Medroxyprogesterone in an injection given every 11 to 13 weeks, which offers continuous release of medication to prevent pregnancy.
- ◆ Contraceptive vaginal ring: A ring inserted into the vagina that contains estrogen and progestin delivered continuously.
- ◆ Implantable progestin: A minor surgical procedure to implant a single progestin-containing rod into the subdermal tissue of the inner/upper aspect of the arm that delivers continuous medication for up to 3 years.
- ◆ Intrauterine device (IUD): A chemically active T-shaped device inserted into the uterus that delivers progestin continuously. The time frame for use of an IUD varies by type.

Labor and Birth

Labor and birth represent the time period during which the baby and placenta are delivered and up to 1 to 2 hours following birth. Medications can be used for a variety of labor and birth situations, described below.

- ◆ Labor induction: The stimulation of uterine contractions during pregnancy before labor begins on its own to achieve a vaginal birth. Labor can be induced by stimulating uterine contractions and/or cervical ripening. A nonpharmacologic option available to induce labor is an amniotomy.
- ◆ Preterm labor: Labor that occurs before the 37th week of pregnancy with contraction of the uterus that leads to dilation and effacement of the cervix. Preterm labor is categorized as a high-risk pregnancy. Treatment focuses on stopping labor (using tocolytics), if possible, and/or promoting lung maturation in the fetus (such as with betamethasone acetate) to prepare for birth.

◆ Preinduction cervical ripening: The softening of the cervix that typically begins prior to the onset of labor contractions and is necessary for cervical dilation and the passage of the fetus. This can be accomplished with medications if necessary.

◆ Preeclampsia: An elevation of blood pressure with or without proteinuria after 20 weeks' gestation with a return to normal blood pressure levels after birth. Treatment focuses on blood pressure management, magnesium supplementation to prevent eclampsia and seizure activity, and bed rest.

◆ Eclampsia: Hypertension with tonic–clonic seizure activity in a pregnant woman without another identifiable cause. Treatment focuses on seizure prophylaxis with magnesium sulfate and birth of the fetus, if necessary.

◆ Magnesium toxicity: An electrolyte disturbance in which there is a high level of magnesium in the blood that can occur following the treatment of preeclampsia with magnesium sulfate. Calcium gluconate is the treatment of choice for magnesium toxicity.

◆ Postpartum hemorrhage: Excessive (>500 to 1,000 mL) bleeding within 24 hours after birth. Causes of postpartum hemorrhage can include loss of tone in the uterine muscles, a bleeding disorder, the placenta failing to come out completely, and lacerations of the cervix or vagina. The client is at risk for anemia (normocytic/normochromic) and alterations in hemodynamic stability (low blood pressure, elevated heart rate). The nurse must evaluate the client for these conditions if a large volume of blood is lost.

CLINICAL PEARLS: FEMALE REPRODUCTIVE DISORDERS

Menstrual Cycle Disorders

Abnormal Uterine Bleeding

◆ Assessment/Signs and Symptoms: Bleeding or spotting between periods, after menopause, after intercourse, or heavy bleeding during menses, menses lasting longer than 9 days, or menstrual cycle longer than 38 days or shorter than 24 days.

◆ Diagnostics:
  ● Menstrual cycle history, physical examination, and serum hormone levels.
  ● The nurse should evaluate the baseline and trend hemoglobin and hematocrit levels and assess for signs and symptoms of anemia (fatigue, shortness of breath with exertion, easy bruising, palpitations).
  ● Ultrasound or endometrial biopsy may be performed.

Amenorrhea

◆ Assessment/Signs and Symptoms: Based on underlying cause in addition to the absence of menses. Assess dietary and exercise patterns, excessive androgen symptoms, nipple discharge, and obtain a sexual history.

◆ Diagnostics: Laboratory values of human chorionic gonadotropin (HCG), luteinizing hormone (LH), follicle-stimulating hormone (FSH), thyroid-stimulating hormone (TSH) and prolactin. Pelvic ultrasound and laboratory testing may be performed, if indicated.

Dysmenorrhea

◆ Assessment/Signs and Symptoms: Client report of pain during menstruation

◆ Diagnostics: Client-produced menstrual calendar with symptoms, pelvic examination, ultrasound, and, in some cases, laparoscopic surgery

Endometriosis

- Endometriosis is an example of secondary dysmenorrhea.
- Assessment/Signs and Symptoms: Chronic pain with menses and pain with intercourse, bowel movements, and/or urination.
- Diagnostics: Often diagnosed by symptom profile, physical and pelvic examination, and potential laparoscopic surgery.
- The treatment of endometriosis is hormonal contraception.

Psychiatric Disorders Associated with Hormonal Changes of the Female Reproductive System

PMS/PMDD

- Assessment/Signs and Symptoms: Physical symptoms include headache, hot flashes, abdominal bloating, sleep disturbance, and breast tenderness. Emotional symptoms include depression, anger, anxiety, irritability, or social withdrawal.
- Diagnostics:
  - PMS: A pattern of symptoms associated with the menstrual cycle must be established, which includes symptoms that occur 5 days before the start of menses for at least three consecutive menstrual cycles and end within 4 days of the start of menses with disruption of normal activities of daily living.
  - PMDD: five symptoms total, with the additional criteria including the following:
    - At least one of the following: mood swings, irritability, depressed mood, or anxiety
    - At least one of the following: limited interest in usual activity, poor concentration, decreased energy, changes in appetite, insomnia or hypersomnia, or a sense of being overwhelmed, and/or a physical symptom, as described above

PPD

- Assessment/Signs and Symptoms: Characterized by persistent feelings of sadness and intense mood swings that can occur up to 1 year after having a baby.
- Diagnostics: Based on a thorough history and physical examination. The nurse should evaluate for possible suicidal or homicidal ideations to ensure safety.

Vaginal Infections

Bacterial Vaginosis

- Assessment/Signs and Symptoms: White/yellow, odorous discharge and vaginal burning
- Diagnostics: Based on a sample of vaginal discharge, microscopy, whiff test, vaginal pH, and physical examination

Candidiasis

- Assessment/Signs and Symptoms: Extreme vaginal and vulva itching, erythema, and curdy white discharge that may also cause dysuria
- Diagnostics: Same as for bacterial vaginosis

GBS

- ◆ Assessment/Signs and Symptoms: Usually asymptomatic
- ◆ Diagnostics: Sample of vaginal discharge

Mastitis

- ◆ Assessment/Signs and Symptoms: In addition to fever, mastitis also causes flu-like symptoms and erythema of the infected breast.
- ◆ Diagnostics: Based on history and physical examination. An elevation in white blood cell count may be noted but is not required for diagnosis.

Menopause

- ◆ Assessment/Signs and Symptoms: In addition to the absence of the menstrual cycle, it is often linked to symptoms like hot flashes, mood swings, bone loss, night sweats, and vaginal dryness.
- ◆ Diagnostics: Based on the absence of a period for 1 year or more, an elevated level of FSH and a decreased level of estrogen.

Labor and Birth

Preterm Labor

- ◆ Assessment/Signs and Symptoms: Changes in vaginal discharge (watery/mucous/bloody), pelvic pressure, backache, cramping, rupture of membranes, and/or contractions
- ◆ Diagnostics: Cervical changes on pelvic examination, ultrasound, and fetal fibronectin test

Preeclampsia

- ◆ Assessment/Signs and Symptoms: In addition to elevated blood pressure, signs and symptoms may include edema, weight gain, elevated serum uric acid (≥8 mg/dL or 0.476 mmol/L), and alterations in renal function (elevations in serum blood urea nitrogen and creatinine).
- ◆ Diagnostics:
  - For a diagnosis of preeclampsia, the following must be present (1) systolic blood pressure ≥140 mm Hg or a diastolic blood pressure ≥90 mm Hg in a woman with previously normal blood pressure and (2) new-onset proteinuria (≥0.3 g of protein in 24 hours) or a urinalysis indicating 30 mg/dL (1.785 mmol/L) (1+) of protein.
  - If protein is absent from the urine, and new-onset hypertension is present, a diagnosis of preeclampsia can be made if any of the following are present: thrombocytopenia, renal insufficiency, decreased liver function, pulmonary edema, or visual symptoms.

Eclampsia

- ◆ Assessment/Signs and Symptoms: Preeclampsia symptoms and tonic–clonic seizure activity
- ◆ Diagnostics: Based on the presence of seizures in a preeclamptic pregnant woman

Magnesium Toxicity

◆ Assessment/Signs and Symptoms: Weakness, confusion, decreased respiratory rate, depressed deep tendon reflexes, and cardiac arrest
◆ Diagnostics: Serum levels of magnesium >2.6 mEq/L (1.30 mmol/L) in addition to signs and symptoms

Postpartum Hemorrhage

◆ Assessment/Signs and Symptoms: Uncontrolled bleeding, alterations in vital signs (elevated heart rate, decreased blood pressure).
◆ Diagnostics: Blood loss measuring more than 500 to 1,000 mL within the first 24 hours after birth, decreased red blood cell count, hemoglobin and hematocrit levels. Ultrasound and evaluation of clotting factors may also be included to confirm the diagnosis.

MEDICATION OVERVIEW

Menstrual Cycle Disorders

◆ Treatment of abnormal uterine bleeding consists of progesterone or a monophasic contraceptive (estrogen and progesterone), depending upon the severity of bleeding.
◆ Treatment of amenorrhea may consist of use of a progesterone medication such as prometrium, medroxyprogesterone, or norethindrone acetate to stimulate withdrawal bleed.
◆ Treatment of both primary and secondary dysmenorrhea consists of NSAIDs and/or hormonal contraceptives. If hormonal contraceptives are used, they should be monophasic and on a continuous regimen. A continuous regimen is defined as giving a pill continuously (*discarding the placebo pills*) to cause amenorrhea/anovulation.
◆ Table 13-3 summarizes the medications used to treat abnormal uterine bleeding and amenorrhea.

> **BLACK BOX WARNING:** All estrogen-containing products have the potential for cardiovascular adverse effects, especially in the setting of tobacco use and age>35.

> **BLACK BOX WARNING:** Progestin medications may increase the risk of breast cancer, cardiovascular disease, or dementia.

> **BLACK BOX WARNING:** Medroxyprogesterone acetate may lead to significant bone mineral density loss, increasing the risk of fracture if used for more than 2 years.

Table 13-3

Medications Used to Treat Abnormal Uterine Bleeding and Amenorrhea

Class	Prototype Medication	Mechanism of Action	Major Side and Adverse Effects	Critical Information	Indications
Progestins	Progesterone micronized	Transforms proliferative into secretory endometrium	Thromboembolism Pulmonary embolism Optic neuritis Hypertension Stroke Myocardial infarction Vaginal bleeding Hyperglycemia Photosensitivity Headache Dizziness Breast tenderness Abdominal pain	Do not use if: Allergic to peanuts, undiagnosed vaginal bleeding, liver disease, breast cancer, blood clotting issues, heart attack or stroke, pregnancy	Amenorrhea Secondary amenorrhea Abnormal uterine bleeding

Progestins	Medroxyprogesterone	Inhibits pituitary gonadotropin release; transforms proliferative into secretory endometrium	Thromboembolism Optic neuritis Hypertension Stroke Myocardial infarction Pulmonary embolism Pancreatitis Loss of bone mineral density Headache Dizziness Breast tenderness Abdominal pain	Do not use if: Undiagnosed vaginal bleeding, liver disease, breast cancer, blood clotting issues, heart attack or stroke, or current pregnancy Hazardous drug: use safe handling and disposal precautions	Amenorrhea Secondary amenorrhea Abnormal uterine bleeding
Estrogen–progestin combination	Norethindrone/ethinyl estradiol	Suppresses luteinizing hormone and follicle-stimulating hormone, inhibits ovulation, alters endometrium	Thromboembolism, myocardial infarction, stroke, hypertension, nausea, vomiting, headache	Do not use if pregnant, history of current breast or endometrial cancer, active liver disease, or history of clotting disorders	Abnormal uterine bleeding

Psychiatric Disorders Associated With Hormonal Changes of the Female Reproductive System

◆ PMS/PMDD: Pharmacologic treatment consists of drospirenone-containing contraceptives (e.g., Yaz, Yasmin) and/or vitamin supplementation and selective serotonin reuptake inhibitors (SSRIs).
◆ PPD: Treatment for PPD consists of antidepressants and/or vitamin supplementation and should be in conjunction with cognitive behavioral therapy. Table 13-4 summarizes treatment of PMS, PMDD, and PPD.

Vaginal Infections

The treatment of vaginal infections is dependent upon the causative organism. See Table 13-5 for an overview of medications used to treat vaginal infections that are not sexually transmitted.

◆ Bacterial vaginosis: Oral or vaginal antibiotics
◆ Candidiasis: Oral or vaginal antifungals
◆ GBS: Intravenous antibiotics during labor

Mastitis

This condition is treated with antibiotics, described in Table 13-6.

Menopause

Treatment is based on individual client symptoms, discussed in Table 13-7.

Pregnancy Prevention

This can be achieved through a variety of hormonal contraceptive options, which are outlined in Table 13-8.

Pregnancy

Some medications are recommended during pregnancy for the promotion of fetal growth and development or for the prevention of disease. These are discussed in Table 13-9.

Labor and Birth

Medications can be used for a variety of labor and birth situations. See Table 13-10 for an overview of the medications used in labor and birth.

Table 13-4

Medications Used for Psychiatric Reproductive Disorders

Class	Prototype Medication	Mechanism of Action	Major Side Effects and Adverse Effects	Critical Information	Indications
Vitamin	Pyridoxine (vitamin B6)	Reduction of symptoms of stress, water retention	None reported		PMS/PMDD and postpartum depression
Vitamin	Alpha-tocopherol (vitamin E)	Reduction of symptoms of breast tenderness	Bleeding		PMS/PMDD
Hormonal contraception	Drospirenone/ethinyl estradiol	Reduction of symptoms through mood stabilization secondary to hormonal supplementation	Chest pain, shortness of breath, leg pain, headache, eye problems, high blood pressure	Do not take if: Thromboembolic disorders, stroke, heart attack, hypertension, gallbladder disease, liver tumor, headache with focal neurologic symptoms, uncontrolled hypertension, diabetes mellitus with vascular involvement, breast- or estrogen-related cancers, pregnancy or lactating under 6 weeks postpartum, and smoking over age 35 Decreases effectiveness when taken with other liver-metabolized medications such as anticonvulsants and some antibiotics	PMS/PMDD
Selective serotonin reuptake inhibitor (SSRI)	Paroxetine	Inhibits serotonin reuptake to reduce depression or PMDD symptoms	Suicidality Depression exacerbation Abnormal bleeding	Use with caution: Alcohol use, bleeding risk, seizure history, <25, third trimester pregnancy, elderly Avoid abrupt withdrawal	PMDD or postpartum depression

PMDD, premenstrual dysphoric disorder, PMS, premenstrual syndrome.

Table 13-5

Medications to Treat Vaginal Infections That Are Not Sexually Transmitted

Class	Prototype Medication	Mechanism of Action	Major Side Effects and Adverse Effects	Critical Information	Indications
Bactericidal	Metronidazole (see Table 6-1)	Reduces metabolite formed by anaerobes Disrupts DNA	Seizures Aseptic meningitis Optic neuropathy Hypersensitivity Nausea Vomiting Epigastric discomfort Rash Headache Metallic taste	Do not use in first trimester of pregnancy Avoid alcohol use during and 14 days after Avoid disulfiram use within 14 days	Bacterial vaginosis
Antifungal	Fluconazole (see Table 6-5)	Inhibits fungal cytochrome P450 3A-dependent enzyme, decreases ergosterol synthesis, and inhibits cell membrane function	Hepatotoxicity Seizures Leukopenia Anaphylaxis Nausea Headache Rash Vomiting Taste changes		Candidiasis

Antibiotic	Mechanism of action	Side effects/adverse effects	Indication
Penicillin G (see Table 6-1)	Inhibits cell wall synthesis (bactericidal)	Anaphylaxis Superinfection *Clostridium difficile* Nausea Vomiting Diarrhea Pruritus Fever Rash	Anaphylactic reaction to beta-lactams Group B streptococcus

Table 13-6

Medication for Mastitis

Class	Prototype Medication	Mechanism of Action	Major Side Effects and Adverse Effects	Critical Information	Indications
Penicillin (see Table 6-1)	Dicloxacillin	Inhibits cell wall synthesis (bactericidal)	Anaphylaxis Hypersensitivity to drug Superinfection C. difficile Nausea Vomiting Diarrhea Pruritus Fever Rash	Anaphylactic reaction to beta-lactams Safe during lactation	Skin infections/mastitis

Table 13-7

Menopause Symptom Treatment Medications

Class	Prototype Medication	Mechanism of Action	Major Side Effects and Adverse Effects	Critical Information	Indications
Hormonal combinations Non-contraceptive	Ethinyl estradiol and nor-ethindrone	Norethindrone decreases estrogen receptors, suppresses endometrial tissue synthesis; ethinyl estradiol binds estrogen receptors	Thromboembolism Retinal thrombosis Myocardial infarction Stroke Breast cancer Ovarian cancer Endometrial cancer Endometrial hyperplasia Vaginal bleeding Spotting Breast changes Abdominal cramps Nausea/vomiting Cervical secretion changes Headache	Undiagnosed vaginal bleeding Breast cancer—past or present Estrogen or progestin-dependent CA Thromboembolism past or present Protein C or S deficiency Pregnancy	Vasomotor symptoms (hot flashes) of menopause and/or related genitourinary symptoms including atrophic vaginitis, vulvar atrophy (kraurosis vulvae) in women with an intact uterus Osteoporosis with intact uterus
Estrogens	Estradiol	Binds to estrogen receptors, developing and maintaining female sex characteristics and reproductive systems		May only be used in clients who no longer have a uterus	Vasomotor symptoms, vaginal atrophy (menopausal), osteoporosis (postmenopausal)
Vitamin	Alpha-tocopherol Vitamin E	Antioxidant	Bleeding Nausea Diarrhea Fatigue Headache Rash		Vasomotor symptoms

Table 13-8

Hormonal Contraception

Class	Prototype Medication	Mechanism of Action	Major Side and Adverse Effects	Critical information	Indications
Hormonal contraception containing estrogen and progestin	Norethindrone/ethinyl estradiol	Suppresses ovulation, thickens cervical mucus, and alters uterine lining to prevent implantation	Thrombosis Myocardial infarction Stroke Hypertension Depression Anaphylaxis Chest pain, shortness of breath, leg pain, headache, eye problems, high blood pressure	Do not take if: Thromboembolic disorders, stroke, heart attack, hypertension, gallbladder disease, liver tumor, headache with focal neurologic symptoms, uncontrolled hypertension, diabetes mellitus with vascular involvement, breast or estrogen-related cancers, pregnancy or lactating under 6 weeks postpartum, and smoking over 35 Decreases effectiveness when taken with other liver-metabolized medications such as anticonvulsants and some antibiotics All estrogen containing contraceptives must also contain a progestin to prevent endometrial hyperplasia	Contraception Irregular menses, dysmenorrhea, PCOS—anovulation, endometriosis, acne, premenstrual syndrome

		Action	Side effects	Nursing considerations	Use
Oral progestins	Norethindrone	Suppresses ovulation, thickens cervical mucus, and alters uterine lining to prevent implantation	Hypersensitivity Anaphylaxis Ectopic pregnancy Ovarian cysts Menstrual irregularities Altered menstrual flow Breakthrough bleeding Headache Breast tenderness Nausea Dizziness Acne	Do not use if: Bariatric surgery, lupus, severe cirrhosis, liver tumors, current or past breast cancer Decreases effectiveness when taken with other liver-metabolized medications such as anticonvulsants May be used without an estrogen combination	Contraception
Emergency oral contraceptive Progestin-only method	Levonorgestrel (plan B)	Alters tubal transport of ova and/or sperm Prevents fertilization from taking place Alters endometrium, preventing implantation	Severe reactions: None reported Menstrual irregularities Nausea Headache Dizziness Vomiting Diarrhea	Do not take: If pregnant or undiagnosed vaginal bleeding. May be used without an estrogen combination Repeat dose if vomiting occurs within 3 hr Best efficacy if used within 72 hr of unprotected intercourse No age restriction	Emergency contraception

(continued)

Table 13-8

Hormonal Contraception (continued)

Class	Prototype Medication	Mechanism of Action	Major Side and Adverse Effects	Critical information	Indications
Transdermal contraceptive patch	Norelgestromin (progesterone)/ethinyl estradiol	Suppresses ovulation, thickens cervical mucus, and alters uterine lining to prevent implantation	Thrombosis	Do not take: Thromboembolic disorders, stroke, heart attack, hypertension, gallbladder disease, liver tumor, headache with focal neurologic symptoms, uncontrolled hypertension, diabetes mellitus with vascular involvement, breast- or estrogen-related cancers, pregnancy or lactating under 6 weeks postpartum, and smoking over 35	Contraception
			Myocardial infarction		Irregular menses, dysmenorrhea, PCOS—anovulation, endometriosis
			Stroke		
			Hypertension		
			Depression	Decreases effectiveness when taken with other liver-metabolized medications such as anticonvulsants	
			Anaphylaxis		
			Chest pain, shortness of breath, leg pain, headache, eye problems, high blood pressure	Avoid applying to skin irritation or rashes	
			Exclude breast application	Less effective in women >198 lb (90 kg)	
			Skin reaction	All estrogen-containing contraceptives must also contain a progestin to prevent endometrial hyperplasia	
			Bleeding irregularities		
			Nausea		
			Headache		
			Weight changes		
			Libido changes		
			Acne		

			Bone density loss	Do not take if: Hypersensitivity to drug	Contraception
Injectable progestins	Medroxyprogesterone acetate	Inhibits pituitary gonadotropin release; transforms proliferative into secretory endometrium; maintains pregnancy			Endometriosis
			Osteoporosis	Pregnancy	
			Thromboembolism	Undiagnosed vaginal bleeding	
			Anaphylaxis	Breast cancer	
		Inhibits ovulation	Seizures	Thromboembolic disorders	
			Depression	Cerebrovascular disease	
			Menstrual irregularities	Hepatic tumors	
			Weight gain	May be used without an estrogen combination	
			Decreased libido		
			Acne		
			Headache		
			Amenorrhea		
			Breast tenderness		
			Depression		

(continued)

Table 13-8

Hormonal Contraception (continued)

Class	Prototype Medication	Mechanism of Action	Major Side and Adverse Effects	Critical information	Indications
Implantable progestin	Etonogestrel subdermal	Inhibits pituitary gonadotropin release; transforms proliferative into secretory endometrium; maintains pregnancy	Hypersensitivity to drug	Do not take if: Pregnant, undiagnosed vaginal bleeding, breast cancer, thromboembolic disorders, cerebrovascular disease, hepatic tumors, progestin-dependent cancers within 21 days postpartum	Contraception
			Anaphylaxis		
			Angioedema		
		Inhibits ovulation	Ectopic pregnancy	Provider training required	
			Ovarian cysts	May be used without an estrogen combination	
			Hypertension		
			Thrombosis		
			Myocardial infarction		
			Stroke		
			Depression		
			Headache		
			Vaginitis		
			Weight gain		
			Acne		
			Breast tenderness		
			Breakthrough bleeding		
			Elevated blood pressure		
			Contact lens intolerance		

			Contraception
Contraceptive vaginal ring	Etonogestrel and ethinyl estradiol	Thrombosis	Do not take if: Thromboembolic disorders, stroke, heart attack, hypertension, gallbladder disease, liver tumor, headache with focal neurologic symptoms, uncontrolled hypertension, diabetes mellitus with vascular involvement, breast- or estrogen-related cancers, pregnancy or lactating under 6 weeks postpartum, and smoking over 35
		Myocardial infarction	
		Stroke	
		Hypertension	
		Depression	Decreases effectiveness when taken with other liver-metabolized medications such as anticonvulsants and some antibiotics
		Anaphylaxis	
		Toxic shock syndrome	All estrogen-containing contraceptives must also contain a progestin to prevent endometrial hyperplasia
		Chest pain, shortness of breath, leg pain, headache, eye problems, high blood pressure	

(continued)

Table 13-8					

Hormonal Contraception *(continued)*

Class	Prototype Medication	Mechanism of Action	Major Side and Adverse Effects	Critical information	Indications
Intrauterine device (IUD)	Levonorgestrel intra-uterine device	May thicken cervical mucus preventing sperm travel, alters endometrium	Ectopic pregnancy	Do not use if: Pregnant, emergency contraception, hormone sensitive cancer, breast cancer, hepatic tumors, undiagnosed vaginal bleeding, postpartum endometritis, PID acute	Contraception
			Sepsis		.
			PID		
			Ovarian cysts	May be used without an estrogen combination	
			Myometrial embedment		
			Uterine perforation		
			Thrombosis		
			Menstrual irregularities		
			Amenorrhea		
			Vaginitis		
			Acne		
			Ovarian cysts		
			Anxiety		
			Dyspareunia		
			Back pain		
			Nausea/vomiting		
			Provider training required		

PCOS, polycystic ovarian syndrome; PID, pelvic inflammatory disease.

Table 13-9

Medications for Use During Pregnancy

Class	Prototype Medication	Mechanism of Action	Major Side Effects and Adverse Effects	Critical Information	Indications
Vitamin	Folic acid (vitamin B9)	Participates in DNA synthesis and erythropoiesis	None reported		Neural tube development
Vitamin	Calcium citrate	Essential component and participation in physiologic systems and reactions	Hypercalcemia Nephrolithiasis	Hypercalcemia	Bone and teeth formation in developing fetus
Influenza vaccine (inactivated)	Fluarix Quadrivalent	Induces antibody formulation	Anaphylaxis Guillain-Barré syndrome	Hypersensitivity to neomycin Caution if immunocompromised	Reduction of seasonal influenza
Tetanus/diphtheria/pertussis vaccine	Adacel	Induces antibody formation	Hypersensitivity Anaphylaxis Guillain-Barré syndrome Encephalopathy	Encephalopathy within 7 days after prior vaccine	Prevention of tetanus, diphtheria, and pertussis
Rho (D) immune globulin	Rho GAM	Suppresses immune response if Rh-negative clients to Rh-positive red blood cells	Anaphylaxis Viral transmission risk	Do not use in Rh-positive clients No intravenous administration Injection given with any pregnancy even if ended with miscarriage or termination. Given at 28-week prophylaxis, with chorionic villi sampling or amniocentesis. Given within 72 after birth if baby is Rh positive	Prevention of hemolytic disease of the newborn if the mother is Rh negative
Neuraminidase inhibitor	Oseltamivir	Inhibits influenza	Delirium Behavioral disturbance Anaphylaxis Nausea Vomiting Diarrhea Headache		Treatment of uncomplicated influenza A and B Prophylaxis influenza A and B May be used in pregnancy and lactation

Table 13-10

Medications Approved for Use in Various Labor and Birth Scenarios

Class	Prototype Medication	Mechanism of Action	Major Side Effects and Adverse Effects	Critical Information	Indications
Labor Induction	Oxytocin	Binds to oxytocin receptors in myo-metrium, increasing intracellular calcium and stimulating uterine contractions	Uterine hypertonicity	Use only in presence of qualified personnel	Induction of labor
			Uterine tetany	Monitor intrauterine pressure, fetal heart rate, maternal blood pressure	
			Uterine rupture		
			Abruptio placentae		
Ergot alkaloid	Methylergonovine maleate	Increases uterine contraction force and frequency	Seizures	Pregnancy	Refractory post-partum uterine bleeding
			Hypertension	Toxemia	
			Myocardial infarction	Hypertension	
			Vasospasm		
Prostaglandin E₁ analogue	Misoprostol	Produces uterine contractions	Miscarriage	Prior cesarean section	Cervical ripening
			Uterine rupture	Major uterine surgery	
			Uterine hyperstimulation		
			Anaphylaxis		
			Hypotension		
			Myocardial infarction		

Classification	Medication	Action	Contraindications/Side Effects	Nursing Considerations	Use
Tocolytic	Hydroxyprogesterone caproate	Maintains pregnancy; exact mechanism of action unknown	Current or history of thrombosis or thromboembolic disorders; Undiagnosed vaginal bleeding; Known or suspected hormone-sensitive breast cancer	Conditions aggravated by fluid retention (e.g., preeclampsia, epilepsy, migraine, asthma, cardiac, or renal dysfunction); Discontinue if depression, thromboembolic events, or allergic reactions occur	Prevention of pre-term labor
Mineral supplement	Calcium gluconate	Antidote for magnesium sulfate toxicity	Hypercalcemia; Arrhythmias; Nephrolithiasis	Hypercalcemia	Magnesium toxicity
Beta-2 agonist	Terbutaline	Tocolytic for preterm labor; stimulated beta2-adrenergic receptors to relax smooth muscle of uterus	Tachycardia, palpitations, nervousness, tremor, headache, drowsiness, nausea	Avoid excessive use; Monitor contractions; Monitor vital signs; Monitor for tremors, dizziness, headache, tachycardia, hypotension, anxiety; Do not give if client complains of chest pain	Tocolytic for pre-term labor

(continued)

Table 13-10

Medications Approved for Use in Various Labor and Birth Scenarios *(continued)*

Class	Prototype Medication	Mechanism of Action	Major Side Effects and Adverse Effects	Critical Information	Indications
Labor suppression/ tocolytic	Magnesium sulfate	Reduces muscle contractions by interfering with release of acetylcholine at myoneural junction	Stop immediately if respirations <12, loss of deep tendon reflexes, hypotension, bradycardia, altered loss of consciousness, magnesium levels above 10 mEq/L or 9 mg/dL (0.535 mmol/L) Administer calcium gluconate for signs of toxicity	Preterm labor: Monitor contractions and fetal heart rate Monitor fetal movement and fetal heart rate variability Monitor vital signs and urine output Preeclampsia: Monitor vital signs, urine output, deep tendon reflexes, and loss of consciousness Monitor magnesium levels Administer via infusion pump in diluted form Use indwelling catheter to monitor urinary elimination Contraindicated for women with myasthenia gravis	Tocolytic used for preterm labor Central nervous system depressant to prevent seizure in preeclampsia
Corticosteroid	Betamethasone sodium phosphate/ betamethasone acetate	Prevent or reduce neonatal respiratory distress syndrome in preterm infants by stimulating the production or release of lung surfactant in preterm fetus	Anaphylaxis Adrenal insufficiency Cushing syndrome Hypertension	Systemic fungal infection Thrombocytopenia purpura Assess for signs of preterm labor Monitor blood glucose levels and lung sounds	Preterm labor (24–32 weeks) Fetal lung maturation

BRIEF OVERVIEW OF MALE REPRODUCTIVE SYSTEM AND ITS DISORDERS

In the male, the organs necessary for the urinary system are connected to the reproductive system. Therefore, the male urinary system conditions can affect sexuality. Most male reproductive system disorders are treated by a urologist. The external male structures include the testes, epididymides, scrotum, and penis. The internal male genitalia include the vas deferens, ejaculatory duct, and prostatic and membranous sections of the urethra, seminal vesicles, prostate, and bulbourethral glands. Male reproductive disorders include issues with steroid production (testosterone), alterations in erectile function, abnormalities of the prostate gland, and infections. As with the female reproductive system, the nurse will be responsible for conducting a thorough history and review of systems, with the assessment being completed by the health care provider.

Testosterone Deficiency

Testosterone deficiency is a failure of the testes to produce adequate amounts of testosterone that can result in hypogonadism and delayed puberty. Male hypogonadism is usually hereditary or results from pituitary or hypothalamic failure or dysfunction of the testes. Delayed puberty is defined as failure of puberty to occur before 15 years that follows a family pattern.

Erectile Dysfunction

Erectile dysfunction (ED) is a disorder where a male has a persistent inability to achieve or maintain an erect penis for satisfactory sexual performance. ED has both psychogenic (anxiety and depression) and organic (cardiovascular diseases, diabetes, chronic kidney failure, spinal cord injury, trauma to the pelvic or genital area, alcohol, smoking, medications, and drug abuse) causes. The nurse should obtain a detailed history of the present illness, including a thorough past medical/surgical and medication history, as many medications can cause ED (e.g., beta-blockers).

Prostate Disorders

Two main types of prostate disorders are prostatitis and benign prostatic hyperplasia. Both of these conditions can affect sexual and urinary function.

- ◆ Prostatitis is an inflammation of the prostate gland that is associated with lower urinary tract symptoms and symptoms of sexual discomfort and/or dysfunction.
- ◆ Benign prostatic hyperplasia (BPH) is a nonmalignant prostate enlargement caused by overgrowth of the epithelial cells and smooth muscle cells. The overgrowth of the epithelial cells causes mechanical obstruction of the urethra, while the overgrowth of the smooth muscle cells causes dynamic obstruction of the urethra.

CLINICAL PEARLS: MALE REPRODUCTIVE DISORDERS

Testosterone Deficiency

- ◆ Assessment/Signs and Symptoms: There are many symptoms of decreased testosterone levels including but not limited to low sex drive, fatigue, decreased muscle mass and/or bone mass, and hair loss.

◆ Diagnostics: The diagnosis of testosterone deficiency is based on a thorough history and physical examination, the presence of symptoms, and a low serum testosterone level.

Erectile Dysfunction

◆ Assessment/Signs and Symptoms: Client report of inability to achieve or maintain erection.
◆ Diagnostics: If it is suggested that the ED may be caused by a medical condition, the provider may order diagnostic testing to rule out these potential causes (e.g., fasting blood glucose, hemoglobin A1c, etc.). Treatment of ED may be based solely on the client's HPI if organic causes are not suspected.

Prostate Disorders

◆ Prostatitis
  ● Assessment/Signs and Symptoms: Fever, prostate pain, urinary symptoms (dysuria, frequency, hesitancy, nocturia) are frequent clinical manifestations associated with prostatitis. The provider will perform the internal examination of the prostate gland to assess for enlargement, "bogginess," presence of nodules, or pain with palpation.
  ● Diagnostics: Urinalysis with urine culture and sensitivity.
◆ Benign prostatic hyperplasia (BPH)
  ● Assessment/Signs and Symptoms: Urinary frequency, urgency, nocturia, decreased and intermittent force of stream and sensation of incomplete bladder emptying, a decrease in the volume and force of the urinary stream, and complications of acute urinary retention and recurrent urinary tract infections (UTIs). ED often develops with BPH.
  ● Diagnostics: The provider will perform the internal examination of the prostate gland to assess for enlargement, "bogginess," presence of nodules, or pain with palpation. A prostate screening antigen (PSA) may be obtained in the evaluation of BPH to rule out prostate cancer.

MEDICATION OVERVIEW

Testosterone Deficiency

Androgen replacement therapy may be used in adult males to restore libido, increase ejaculate volume, and enhance secondary sex characteristics. Testosterone does not restore fertility. Testosterone is also used in gender reassignment or sex reassignment surgery (SRS). See Table 13-11 for an overview of treatment options for testosterone deficiency.

> **BLACK BOX WARNING:** Testosterone can increase the erythropoietic effects of the kidneys causing thrombosis development, which can lead to a stroke, myocardial infarction, and death.

Erectile Dysfunction

Treatment of this condition is directed toward improving a client's ability to achieve or maintain an erection. See Table 13-12 for an overview of treatment options for erectile dysfunction.

Table 13-11

Treatment Options for Testosterone Deficiency

Class	Prototype Medication	Mechanism of Action	Major Side Effects and Adverse Effects	Critical Information	Indications
Androgen	Testosterone	Increase secondary sex characteristics, increase muscle mass and strength in athletes	Virilization in women, girls, and boys, premature epiphyseal closure, edema, hepatotoxicity, lower high-density lipoproteins and increase low-density lipoproteins, and abuse potential	Contraindicated in pregnancy	Pubertal transformation in males, maintenance of sexual characteristics, promotion of muscle growth

BLACK BOX WARNING: Sildenafil is contraindicated for men taking organic nitrates because a life-threatening hypotension can occur.

Prostate Disorders

◆ Prostatitis treatment is based on the type of prostatitis and results of culture and sensitivity testing of the urine, summarized in Table 13-13.
◆ BPH: A pharmacologic treatment approach may be used (see Table 13-14), but surgery is another option.

BLACK BOX WARNING: Ciprofloxacin can exacerbate muscle weakness in client with myasthenia gravis (MG). Clients with MG should not be treated with ciprofloxacin.

Table 13-12

Treatment Options for Erectile Dysfunction

Class	Prototype Medication	Mechanism of Action	Major Side Effects and Adverse Effects	Critical Information	Indications
Phosphodiesterase type 4 (PDE-5) inhibitors	Sildenafil	Smooth muscle relaxant causing blood to flow into penis making the erection harder and lasting longer	Hypotension, priapism (>4 hr), headache, and diarrhea	Contraindicated with men taking nitrate medication (e.g., nitroglycerin) Caution with clients taking alpha-adrenergic antagonists and diabetic retinopathy	Erectile dysfunction

BLACK BOX WARNING: Sulfamides are contraindicated for clients with a history of severe hypersensitivity to sulfonamides and related drugs like thiazide and loop diuretics and sulfonylurea-type oral hypoglycemics (e.g., glipizide).

Table 13-13

Treatment Options for Prostatitis

Class	Prototype Medication	Mechanism of Action	Major Side Effects and Adverse Effects	Critical Information	Indications
Sulfa	Trimethoprim–sulfamethoxazole	Inhibits bacterial synthesis of folic acid, which decreases microbial activity growth	Stevens-Johnsons syndrome, hemolytic anemia, leukopenia, thrombocytopenia	Contraindicated in clients with sulfa allergies, nursing mothers, pregnant women in the first trimester and near term	Prostatitis
Fluoroquinolone	Ciprofloxacin	Inhibits DNA grown that prevents the replication of bacteria	Nausea, vomiting, diarrhea, abdominal pain, dizziness, headache, restlessness, *Candida* infections, tendon rupture, phototoxicity, *Clostridium difficile* infection	Diarrhea tested for CDI	Prostatitis

Table 13-14

Treatment Options for Benign Prostatic Hyperplasia

Class	Prototype Medication	Mechanism of Action	Major Side Effects and Adverse Effects	Critical Information	Indications
5-Alpha reductase inhibitors	Finasteride	Decreases dihydrotestosterone availability causing a decrease in mechanical obstruction; decreases size of prostate	Decreases ejaculate volume, libido, and serum levels of prostate-specific antigen Gynecomastia	Contraindicated in women who are pregnant or becoming pregnant	BPH
Alpha 1-adrenergic antagonists	Alfuzosin	Blocks alpha-1 receptors, which relaxes smooth muscle in the bladder neck, prostate capsule, and urethra decreasing dynamic obstruction of the urethra; increases urinary flow	Hypotension, fainting, dizziness, and nasal congestion	Careful with men with low blood pressure and other drugs that lower blood pressure	BPH
Phosphodiesterase type 4 (PDE-5) inhibitors	Tadalafil	Decrease in urinary frequency, urgency, and straining, assists with men with ED associated with BPH	Hypotension, priapism (>hours), headache, and diarrhea	Contraindicated with men taking nitrate medication Caution with clients taking alpha-adrenergic antagonists for BPH	ED/BPH

BPH, Benign prostatic hyperplasia; ED, erectile dysfunction.

Practice Questions and Rationales

1. A nurse is teaching the client about the treatment of trichomoniasis. Which information should the nurse include in the teaching prior to administration? Select all that apply.
    1. "You need to avoid alcohol during treatment and for 14 days after medication is stopped."
    2. "You cannot take disulfiram-containing products for 2 weeks."
    3. "Your partner(s) will not require treatment."
    4. "The medication may cause a metallic taste in your mouth."
    5. "The medication may cause nausea, vomiting, or stomach pain."

2. A nurse is caring for a client who has a uterus who would like treatment for her menopausal symptoms. Which medication will the nurse teach the client about?
    1. Estradiol
    2. Metronidazole
    3. Ethinyl estradiol and norethindrone
    4. Fluconazole

3. A nurse is caring for a 32-week pregnant client who is having contractions. The health care provider has ordered betamethasone acetate STAT. Which client finding would require the nurse to hold the medication and contact the prescriber?
    1. Uric acid level 7 mg/dL (0.416 mmol/L)
    2. Urinary protein level 25 mg/dL (1.487 mmol/L)
    3. Serum platelet count 95,000 × 10^3 μL (95,000 × 10^9/L)
    4. Serum potassium level 5.2 mEq/L (5.2 mmol/L)

4. A nurse is preparing to administer a Rho (D) immune globulin injection to the client. Which information in the client's chart would cause the nurse to question the order?
    1. A+ blood type
    2. 2+ proteinuria
    3. Blood pressure 140/90 mm Hg
    4. B− blood type

5. A nurse is counseling a 35-year-old client who smokes one pack of cigarettes per day regarding contraceptive options. She has a new partner and is concerned about an unwanted pregnancy. Which contraceptive options should the nurse discuss with the client? Select all that apply.
    1. Ethinyl estradiol
    2. Norethindrone
    3. Norelgestromin/ethinyl estradiol
    4. Condoms
    5. Etonogestrel subdermal

6. A nursing student is teaching a client about the treatment of mastitis using dicloxacillin. Which statement, if made by the nursing student, will require the nurse to intervene?
    1. "You will not need to discontinue breast-feeding while taking the medication."
    2. "You should not take the medication if you have ever had an allergic reaction to a penicillin-type drug."

3. "You should supplement with formula while using the medication and pump and discard your breast milk."

4. "This medication can be linked to superinfections such as *Clostridium difficile*."

7. A client was recently diagnosed with endometriosis and is beginning pharmacologic treatment. Which finding in the client's past medical history would require the nurse to hold the medication and notify the prescriber?

   1. Factor V Leiden
   2. Migraines without aura
   3. Diabetic ketoacidosis
   4. Breast fibroadenoma

8. The nurse is administering oxytocin to a client in labor. Which assessment finding would alert the nurse to an adverse effect of oxytocin requiring immediate intervention?

   1. Recurrent late decelerations
   2. Maternal blood pressure 162/98 mm Hg
   3. Maternal temperature of 101.4°F (38.6°C)
   4. Presence of vaginal group Beta strep bacteria

9. A nurse is counseling a client about human papillomavirus-9-valent vaccine. Which statement made by the client would indicate to the nurse that further teaching is necessary?

   1. "The vaccine is protective against the most common strains of human papillomavirus."
   2. "The vaccine can cause fainting."
   3. "The vaccine will cure any strain that I have been exposed to."
   4. "The vaccine can be administered beginning at age 9."

10. The client is receiving misoprostol for labor induction. The nurse is suddenly unable to locate the fetal heart rate. What is the **priority** nursing action at this time?

    1. Turn the client on the left side and administer oxygen.
    2. Notify the provider and locate the ultrasound machine.
    3. Administer oxygen and check the client's temperature.
    4. Administer intravenous bolus and place the client in Trendelenburg position.

11. A client is receiving intravenous magnesium sulfate. The nurse records her respiratory rate as 8 breaths per minute. Which is the **priority** nursing action based on this finding?

    1. Notify the provider.
    2. Administer intravenous calcium gluconate.
    3. Stop the infusion.
    4. Administer oxygen via nonrebreather mask.

12. A nurse is caring for a client who is postpartum that has received methylergonovine. Which client finding indicates that the medication was effective?

    1. Increase in blood pressure
    2. Report of decreased breast pain
    3. Fundus boggy to palpation
    4. Decrease in lochia

13. A client is being treated with a broad-spectrum antibiotic for an upper respiratory infection. The list of medications provided to the nurse by the client includes oral contraceptives. The nurse should include which information in the teaching plan?

    1. "You need to use a backup method of birth control while taking antibiotics."
    2. "You should avoid taking oral contraceptives and antibiotics at the same time."
    3. "It is important to have your estrogen levels monitored while taking antibiotics."
    4. "You should double your dose of oral contraceptive while taking antibiotics."

14. The student nurse is caring for a client who is 7 months postpartum. The client reports insomnia, sadness, and moodiness. The provider has prescribed paroxetine and pyridoxine. Which statement made by the student nurse would require intervention by the nurse?

    1. "If you are lactating, it is best that you wean prior to taking these medications."
    2. "Pyridoxine should be taken daily."
    3. "Do you feel any harm to yourself or your baby?"
    4. "Is there a chance you could be pregnant?"

15. A client was recently diagnosed with vulvar atrophy and dyspareunia and recently had a benign breast lump. She is currently taking ethinyl estradiol and norethindrone. She reports a red, swollen, tender area in the back of her calf. Which recommendation by the nurse is appropriate?

    1. "You must stop the medication immediately and come into the office."
    2. "You should stop the medication and see if the swelling resolves."
    3. "You can continue the medication and follow up with your provider."
    4. "You may try using an NSAID to help relieve your calf pain."

16. A postmenarchal female with visible acne is seen by the provider. She has normal menstrual cycles without dysmenorrhea and is not sexually active. Which medication does the nurse anticipate being prescribed?

    1. Norethindrone/ethinyl estradiol
    2. Medroxyprogesterone acetate
    3. Norethindrone
    4. Levonorgestrel

17. A nurse is caring for a client who is 32 weeks pregnant. She has been diagnosed with influenza A. The nurse understands that which treatments will be recommended for this client? Select all that apply.

    1. Ibuprofen
    2. Acetaminophen
    3. Oseltamivir
    4. Humidified air
    5. Guaifenesin cough syrup
    6. Increased oral fluid intake

18. The nurse is counseling a 17-year-old client with secondary amenorrhea. The client's last normal menses was 4 months ago, and she wishes to begin a contraceptive. Which recommendation by the provider does the nurse anticipate?

    1. "You should continue to wait for your period and once you get it, you may start your contraceptive."
    2. "You will need to have some laboratory testing done and then begin medroxy-progesterone to induce a withdrawal bleed."
    3. "You will need a laparoscopy to determine the cause of your amenorrhea."
    4. "You can begin the contraceptive any time."

19. The nurse is counseling a 13-year-old client regarding emergency contraception. The client took levonorgestrel last evening and vomited 2 hours later. Which information should the nurse include in client teaching?

    1. "The absorption of the drug is quick, so you should be fine."
    2. "You will need to repeat the dose."
    3. "You are too young for the medicine and should not have taken it."
    4. "You should come to the office for blood work to see if it was effective."

20. The nurse is caring for a 46-year-old client who reports continuous vaginal bleeding for the past 14 days. The client does not take any medication and has been menopausal for 2 years. Which statement made by the client would indicate that the teaching was effective?

    1. "I will call you if it happens next month."
    2. "I will schedule an appointment for an ultrasound and biopsy."
    3. "I will restart my oral contraceptive pills."
    4. "I will start my progesterone therapy."

21. A client is receiving testosterone for replacement therapy. Which statement by the client requires additional instruction?

    1. "I will make sure that I take this medication each day."
    2. "The medication does not need laboratory testing."
    3. "I will need to use protection to prevent sexually transmitted infections."
    4. "The medication will not require self-monitoring of my blood pressure."

22. A client is prescribed sildenafil. Which statement is used in the teaching of the client about the medication?

    1. "The medication lowers your blood pressure."
    2. "The medication slows your heart rate."
    3. "The medication facilitates blood flow to your penis."
    4. "The medication augments your testosterone."

23. A male client with a history of hypertension is experiencing erectile dysfunction. The client is asking about a prescription of sildenafil. Which medication in the client's history would cause the nurse concern?

    1. Nitroglycerin
    2. Lisinopril
    3. Clonidine
    4. Metoprolol

24. A nurse is reviewing the prostate-specific antigen (PSA) level of a client who has benign prostatic hyperplasia and being treated with several medications. Which statement by the nurse explains a decrease in the PSA level?

1. "Finasteride decreases the size of the prostate."
2. "Alfuzosin increases the blood pressure facilitating flow to the enlarged prostate."
3. "Tadalafil increases blood flow to the corpora cavernosum."
4. "Labetalol decreases pressure to the penis and relaxes the bladder sphincter."

25. A client presents to the primary care provider with fever and chills. The client reports having had bilateral flank pain and difficulty urinating for the past 24 hours. The nurse collects a urine specimen. Which medications does the nurse anticipate the provider to prescribe? Select all that apply.

1. Ibuprofen
2. Acetaminophen
3. Ciprofloxacin
4. Lisinopril
5. Morphine
6. Sildenafil

14

VISUAL AND AUDITORY MEDICATIONS

BRIEF PRINCIPLES OF MEDICATION ADMINISTRATION FOR VISUAL AND AUDITORY MEDICATIONS

Medications for the eyes and ears cover a large range of classes and indications. The most frequent medications used to treat eye and ear conditions are discussed separately throughout this chapter.

- ◆ The eye is responsible for providing the sense of sight. The natural defense mechanisms of the eye can present a challenge for the delivery of medications ocularly. Any medication given must be able to penetrate the layers of the eye, the sclera/cornea, the uvea, and the ciliary body. Topical administration is strongly preferred due to ease of administration, convenience, and decreased systemic absorption. Glaucoma, a progressive eye condition that results in damage to the optic nerve, can be treated with beta-blockers, prostaglandin analogs, adrenergic agonists, and carbonic anhydrase inhibitors. Antibacterials can successfully treat intraocular infections, while inflammatory conditions are best mediated by prostaglandins, mast cells, and leukocytes.
- ◆ The ear is responsible for giving the sense of hearing. It is made up of four parts: the inner (cochlea and canals), middle (tympanic membrane, malleus, incus, stapes, and eustachian tube), outer (auditory canal), and external(pinna) ear. Otitis media, an inflammation of the middle ear, is a very frequent childhood illness and can be classified as an acute, chronic, or recurrent disease. In fact, a diagnosis of acute otitis media in children results in more than 12 million antibiotic prescriptions a year in the United States alone. The focus of this section is on diseases affecting the middle and outer ear. These most commonly include bacterial and fungal infections as well as inflammatory conditions.

CLINICAL PEARLS—VISUAL AND AUDITORY MEDICATIONS

Ophthalmic Medications

- ◆ When administering eyedrops, ensure the medication is well mixed prior to administration by gently agitating the bottle before instillation. Instill the medication by placing into the space (fornix) created by gently pulling down on the lower lid of the eye.
  - Asking the client to look up during the administration of the eyedrops can help avoid the eyedrop landing on the cornea.
  - If more than one eyedrop or medication is required, separation of the drops by 5 minutes is recommended to achieve maximum benefits.

- If a client has difficulty with eyedrops, they can be administered with the client lying down with eyes closed. The drop can be administered to the closed eyelid in the nasal corner. After administration, the client should be instructed to open and close the eye slowly to let the medication absorb.
◆ When administering eye ointment, a thin ribbon of ointment should be applied to the lower fornix of the eye, while gently pulling the lower eyelid down.
  - The applicator tip should not touch the eye or eyelid, particularly with treatment of an infection, due to risk of contamination.
  - Medication may take several minutes to absorb, and client should be educated that vision may be blurry during this time.

Auditory Medications

◆ For topical otic preparations, ensure that the medication is mixed well and warmed prior to administration by rolling the bottle in the palms for a few minutes before instillation into the ear.
◆ Topical agents are recommended to treat ear conditions whenever possible. Clients with diabetes, are immunocompromised, or those who have difficulty administering topical drug should receive medication systemically instead.

Assessment/Signs and Symptoms
◆ Ophthalmic conditions
  - Assessment of the eye should include visual acuity test, pupil response, extraocular motility and alignment, intraocular pressure, external examination for any unusual eye growths or lesions, and a fundoscopic examination to assess structures including the optic nerve.
  - Glaucoma
    ▶ Common signs and symptoms include loss of peripheral vision; however, many do not notice this symptom until the disease has progressed. Other symptoms include seeing halos around lights, vision loss, redness of eye, eye pain, and narrowed vision.
  - Keratitis
    ▶ Common signs and symptoms include eye redness, eye pain, excessive discharge and/or tears from eye, blurred and/or decreased vision, difficulty opening eye related to pain, and sensitivity to light (photophobia).
  - Common signs and symptoms of other visual impairments include vision loss, elevated intraocular pressure, itching and/or burning of the eye, discharge from the eye, inflammation of the eye, and redness of the cornea or lid.
◆ Auditory conditions
  - Assessment of the ear should include a thorough past medical history and examination with a pneumatic otoscope. The lymph nodes surrounding the ears should be palpated for tenderness or enlargement as well.

- Otitis media
  - ▶ Common signs and symptoms include bulging and/or redness of the tympanic membrane, fever, pain, purulent discharge (if tympanic membrane has burst), and in younger children, pulling on the pinna of the ear.
- Otitis externa
  - ▶ Common signs and symptoms include pain at the site, ear fullness or pressure, itching, hearing loss, purulent discharge, and possible tinnitus.

> **Life Span Considerations:** The exposure to environmental risk factors may increase the risk for otitis media, particularly in children. These include exposure to secondhand smoke, day care attendance, time of year (increased prevalence in winter and early spring), and drinking while lying down (bottles and/or sippy cups).

Diagnostics

- ◆ **Ophthalmic conditions**
  - Glaucoma: A vision test, followed by pupil dilation to assess the optic nerve is done. Tonometry is done to assess intraocular pressure as will a visual field test to assess peripheral vision.
  - Keratitis: An eye exam for visual acuity should be done. A slit lamp examination may be done to assess for keratitis, and a stain may be applied to the surface of the eye to identify any surface irregularities (corneal analysis). Finally, a sample of the discharge from the eye may be collected to determine cause of keratitis.
  - For other diagnoses, depending on the signs and symptoms presented, the provider may request the following for further diagnosis:
    - ▶ Corneal imaging
    - ▶ Fluorescein imaging
    - ▶ Ocular infection diagnostics
    - ▶ Ocular pathology
    - ▶ Ocular ultrasound
- ◆ **Auditory conditions**
  - Otitis media: Otoscopy shows bulging and/or red tympanic membrane. With chronic otitis media thickening, decreased motility and some scarring of the tympanic membrane may be observed with otoscopy, while pneumotoscopy will show decreased movement of the tympanic membrane.
  - Otitis externa: Pain with palpation of the tragus or traction of the pinna is the hallmark diagnostic signs of otitis externa. On examination, erythema and edema of the auditory canal may be seen along with a purulent drainage. Hearing loss may be also present.
  - For other diagnoses, depending on the signs and symptoms presented, the provider may request the following for further diagnosis:
    - ▶ Otoscope examination
    - ▶ Hearing test
    - ▶ Tympanogram
    - ▶ Acoustic reflex testing

Pertinent Laboratory Values

- **Ophthalmic conditions:** A CBC may be ordered to rule out anemia, and antinuclear antibody (ANA) may be ordered to rule out autoimmune diseases. Tears and/or eye drainage may be cultured to determine source of an infection.
- **Auditory conditions:** If drainage from ear canal occurs, it may be cultured to determine the causative organism.

MEDICATION OVERVIEW

Ophthalmic Medications

Most medications for ophthalmic conditions are delivered intraocularly. This helps decrease systemic absorption and decrease side effects. Medications delivered intraocularly are most frequently given via drops or ointment. Drops are the simplest and most convenient to use, and measures such as waiting 5 to 10 minutes between the drops, compression of the lacrimal sac for a minute after administration, and keeping the lid closed up to 5 minutes after installation can help to increase drop absorption. Ointments will increase the contact time of ocular medications to the eye; however, it will cause vision blurring, and the medication itself must be highly lipid soluble to have full effect. Systemic medications will be used for conditions or medications that cannot be given intraocularly. See Table 14-1 for additional information.

Auditory Medications

Similarly to the ophthalmic medications, whenever possible, auditory medications are delivered directly to the site of action, the ear canal. Medications to treat otitis media are traditionally given orally if the tympanic membrane is still intact or for an otitis externa that is more extensive and involves the pinna. These oral medications, antibiotics, are covered in the chapter on Infectious Diseases. See Table 14-2 for additional information.

Table 14-1

Drugs Used in the Treatment of Ophthalmic Conditions

Class	Prototype	Mechanism of Action	Major Side and Adverse Effects	Critical Information	Indications
Beta-blockers	Timolol	Decrease the formation of aqueous humor	Local effects: eye stinging and burning, photophobia	Warn client not to touch dropper to the eye or body	Glaucoma
					Ocular hypertension
			Systemic effects: hypotension, palpitations, insomnia, headache, bronchospasm, and bradycardia	Clients should be educated to place pressure on tear ducts for 1 min after administration to limit systemic absorption	
				Client should notify provider if shortness of breath, chest pain, or irregular heart rate occurs	
				Caution should be used for clients with hypothyroidism; medication may cause thyroid storm	
Adrenergic blockers	Brimonidine	Decrease the formation of aqueous humor	Pruritus	Avoid using alcohol while taking medication	Glaucoma
			Burning and stinging of eyes		Ocular hypertension
			Photophobia	Clients must be educated not to wear contact lenses during medication administration (may be put back in after 15 min)	
			Headache		
			Dry mouth	Monitor intraocular pressure periodically (rebound elevated intraocular pressure may occur after 30 days of treatment)	
			Bradycardia		

(continued)

Table 14-1

Drugs Used in the Treatment of Ophthalmic Conditions (continued)

Class	Prototype	Mechanism of Action	Major Side and Adverse Effects	Critical Information	Indications
Carbonic anhydrase inhibitors	Dorzolamide	Prevent the action of carbonic anhydrase, thereby decreasing the production of aqueous humor	Burning or stinging in eyes	Medication given topically to eye	Glaucoma
			Blurred vision	Warn client not to touch dropper to eye or body	Ocular hypertension
			Tearing	Clients must be educated not to wear contact lenses during medication administration (may be put back in after 15 min)	
			Eye dryness		
			Photophobia	Allergic reactions (conjunctivitis and lid swelling) can occur. Medication should be discontinued in this case	
			Bitter taste in mouth		
			Aplastic anemia		
			Hypokalemia		
			Leukopenia		
Prostaglandin analogs	Latanoprost	Decrease intraocular pressure by increasing the aqueous humor outflow	Change of eye color (iris) to a brown color	Reserved for clients who do not respond to other medications that lower intraocular pressure	Glaucoma
			Visual disturbances		Ocular hypertension
			Discomfort or pain in eye	Warn client not to touch dropper to eye or body	
			Angina	Clients must be educated not to wear contact lenses during medication administration (may be put back in after 15 min)	
			Sensation of foreign body in eye		
				Clients should be educated to place pressure on tear ducts for 1 min after administration to avoid systemic absorption	

Classification	Drug	Action	Side Effects	Nursing Considerations	Uses
				Clients should be warned that iris color may become darker during treatment; eyelid and eyelash darkening may also occur Medications only good for 6 months after opening	
Antiallergic agents	Cromolyn	Decreases irritation and stabilizes mast cells	Irritation to the eye Tearing	Warn client not to touch dropper to eye or body Clients must be educated not to wear contact lenses during treatment with this medication	Allergies (symptomatic relief of itching, burning, and redness of eyes) Allergic conjunctivitis Keratitis
Antibiotics	Tobramycin	Eliminate or inhibit the growth of bacteria	Irritation to the eye Allergic reaction Secondary eye infections (with long-term use)	Warn client not to touch dropper to eye or body Clients must be educated not to wear contact lenses during treatment with this medication	Bacterial conjunctivitis Treatment of corneal ulcers
Anti-inflammatories	Dexamethasone	Diminish the infiltration of leukocytes at site of inflammation, thereby reducing edema, redness, and fluid	Irritation to the eye Corneal ulcerations Increased susceptibility to viral and fungal infections of the cornea	Warn client not to touch dropper to eye or body Clients must be educated not to wear contact lenses during treatment with this medication Clients with a systemic fungal infection should not take this medication	Inflammatory disorders of the eye

Table 14-2

Drugs Used in the Treatment of Auditory Disorders

Class	Prototype	Mechanism of Action	Major Side and Adverse Effects	Critical Information	Indications
Otic analgesics	Antipyrine/benzocaine/glycerin otic solution	Relieve pressure, reduce inflammation and congestion, decrease pain and discomfort	Allergic reaction	Given intra-aurally	Otitis media
				Medication can be warmed by hands before giving for client comfort	
				Warn client not to touch dropper to ear	
				Contraindicated if tympanic membrane is perforated	
				Recommended by American Academy of Pediatrics, however, lacks Food and Drug Administration approval	
Otic anti-inflammatory/antibiotic	Fluoroquinolone/glucocorticoid (given via ear)	Decreasing pain and swelling from inflammation	Allergic reaction	Installation of ear drops can result in dizziness; therefore, drops should be warmed in hands prior to giving	Otitis externa
			Gastrointestinal distress		
			Headache	Warn client not to touch dropper to ear	
				Risk of tendon rupture while taking fluoroquinolone is dose dependent and markedly increases with concurrent glucocorticoid use	

Practice Questions and Rationales

1. A client is prescribed a topical beta-blocker to treat glaucoma. Which statement by the client reassures the nurse that the client understands how to correctly administer the medication?
   1. "I will place pressure on the inner corner of my eye for up to 1 minute after administration of the medication to limit systemic absorption."
   2. "I will quickly rub my eyelids for up to 30 seconds after administration of the medication to ensure it is absorbed into the eye."
   3. "I will contact my provider to change the medication if I get a dry mouth or notice a decrease in urine output."
   4. "I will not drink any fluids for 30 minutes after administration of the medication to eliminate any food–drug interactions."

2. Which reported statement by the client is of greatest concern when taking a medication to treat glaucoma?
   1. "I noticed the color of my eyes is becoming a darker brown after starting the latanoprost."
   2. "I was taking dorzolamide and developed conjunctivitis."
   3. "I am experiencing sensitivity to light while taking timolol."
   4. "After starting brimonidine, I began experiencing dry mouth."

3. A nursing student is giving report on a client in the urgent care clinic being seen for allergic conjunctivitis. Which statement made about the cromolyn for allergic conjunctivitis indicates a correct understanding of the medication actions?
   1. "The benefits of the medication may take several days to develop."
   2. "The medication must be given by mouth."
   3. "Clients can continue using their contact lenses throughout treatment."
   4. "There are no known side effects to the medication."

4. The nurse is educating the client on how to administer topical eyedrops. Place the following recommended steps for administering topical eyedrops in the correct order.
   1. Avoid touching dropper tip against eye or any other part of the body.
   2. Pull down lower lid of the eye and administer one eyedrop while looking up.
   3. Tilt the head back.
   4. Keep the eye closed for up to 5 minutes and avoid blinking or squeezing eyes shut and compress the lacrimal sac for up to a minute to avoid systemic absorption.
   5. If more than one drop is prescribed, repeat the process, waiting at least 5 minutes between drops.

5. The client is prescribed dexamethasone 0.1% one drop every 8 hours to treat uveitis, an inflammatory condition of the eye. Which statement by the client would the nurse be **most** concerned about?
   1. "I was diagnosed with a systemic fungal infection last week."
   2. "Will this medication interact with the medication I take for my migraines?"
   3. "I also suffer from gout periodically. Are these two problems related?"
   4. "I am currently being treated for otitis externa as well."

6. A 4-year-old client presents with a temperature of 101.2°F (38.4°C) for the past 24 hours, right ear pain, and, on examination, middle ear inflammation and a bulging tympanic membrane in the right ear. The nurse anticipates which treatment for this client?
    1. Antibiotic therapy; amoxicillin 40 mg/kg PO twice daily for 10 days
    2. Antibiotic therapy; ceftriaxone 50 mg/kg IM for 3 days
    3. Observation and symptomatic relief; acetaminophen 10 mg/kg PO every 4 hours for 2 to 3 days as needed for right ear pain
    4. Observation with no medications for 2 to 3 days

7. An 8-year-old client with acute otitis media and a penicillin allergy is prescribed clarithromycin 7.5 mg/kg twice daily for 10 days. The client weighs 56 lb. How many milligrams of clarithromycin will the client receive with each dose? Round answer to the nearest tenth

    _____mg.

8. The client asks if there is any other option besides antibiotics to treat acute otitis media. Which is the correct response by the nurse?
    1. "Antibiotics are the only way to cure otitis media."
    2. "Pain management is also part of the treatment plan for otitis media."
    3. "Pain management is only necessary when antibiotics are prescribed."
    4. "Pain management is reserved for use when the tympanic membrane is burst."

9. A client diagnosed with otitis externa and taking a fluoroquinolone/glucocorticoid combination medication asks the nurse what the benefit is to taking the medications together. Which information should the nurse provide the client?
    1. "The glucocorticoid decreases the adverse effects of the fluoroquinolone."
    2. "The two medications are contraindicated for use together."
    3. "The glucocorticoid reduces the swelling caused by the inflammation and decreases pain, while the fluoroquinolone treats the infection."
    4. "The glucocorticoid decreases the likelihood of antibiotic resistance developing to the fluoroquinolone."

10. A client is diagnosed with otitis externa. Comorbidities include diabetes mellitus, hypertension, and advanced multiple sclerosis. Which type of education regarding medication administration would the nurse provide?
    1. the administration of topical medications for a prescription of alcohol plus acetic acid solution
    2. the administration of topical combination medications for a prescription of fluoroquinolone/glucocorticoid combination solution
    3. the oral administration of a prescription for hydrocortisone/neomycin/polymyxin B combination solution
    4. the oral administration of a prescription for fluoroquinolone

15

MUSCULOSKELETAL MEDICATIONS

BRIEF OVERVIEW OF MUSCULOSKELETAL DISORDERS

There are a variety of musculoskeletal disorders ranging from inflammatory conditions, such as rheumatoid arthritis, to bone loss in osteoporosis. Most disorders of the musculoskeletal system do not have a cure, and treatment is targeted at reducing pain and inflammation or slowing bone loss. The nurse's role beyond medication administration is providing client comfort and helping clients maintain their ability to perform activities of daily living.

◆ **Rheumatoid arthritis:** An autoimmune disorder with an inflammatory component. This disorder usually presents around age 40, more commonly in women. Symptoms include swelling and pain of joints bilaterally. As the disease progresses, more systemic symptoms may occur, including fever, inflamed sclera, and weakness. Treatment is aimed at reducing inflammation and pain, maintaining joint function, and reducing the speed of disease progression.

◆ **Osteoporosis:** A disorder characterized by a decrease in bone mass and increased risk of fracture. Bone resorption is the breakdown of bone by osteoclasts, which increases in the setting of osteoporosis. The bones become so frail that simple actions (coughing) can lead to a bone fracture. Osteoporosis occurs most commonly in women. Risk factors include smoking, increased age (>65 years), small body frame, and family history. Secondary osteoporosis is bone loss caused by another factor. These factors include chronic use of oral glucocorticoids, malnutrition, and long-term use of proton pump inhibitors (i.e., omeprazole). The goal of pharmacologic treatment is to increase bone strength. Medications approved for treatment either increase the formation of bone or decrease resorption of bone. A goal is to reduce the risk of developing osteoporosis, which includes intake of sufficient amounts of calcium and vitamin D. In addition, clients should be encouraged to participate in weight-bearing exercise most days of the week and stop smoking, if applicable.

◆ **Gout:** An anti-inflammatory condition caused by elevated blood levels of uric acid >6 mg/dL (356.91 µmol/L). The high uric acid levels lead to accumulation in joint spaces, most commonly in the hands and feet, which presents as redness, swelling, and extreme tenderness to palpation. Chronic gout can lead to the formation of tophi, which are hard deposits of uric acid under the skin that can impact joint mobility. Pharmacologic treatment can be used during acute episodes and/or for prophylactic therapy if symptoms occur more than three times per year. Medications used to treat gout are aimed at decreasing inflammation during acute attacks and decreasing uric acid levels for long-term prevention of flares.

CLINICAL PEARLS: MUSCULOSKELETAL DISORDERS

Rheumatoid Arthritis

Assessment/Signs and Symptoms

◆ Signs and symptoms include pain, swelling, and limited range of motion of joints (usually small joints of fingers and hands) that occurs symmetrically. Pain is worse after long periods of rest, such as on waking in the morning, and generally becomes less intense throughout the course of the day. There is a characteristic change in the joint appearance, known as swan neck deformity (Fig. 15-1).

Nonpharmacologic therapy is provided to improve joint function and may include physical therapy, application of heat to affected joints, and exercise. There must be a balance between exercise and rest. Vigorous activity may increase swelling and pain, whereas too little activity will lead to more joint stiffness.

Diagnostics

◆ Diagnosis is by history and physical examination as well as laboratory results, including elevation of studies specific to inflammation: antinuclear antibody (ANA), erythrocyte sedimentation rate (ESR), and C-reactive protein (CRP), as well as rheumatoid factor (RF).

Pertinent Laboratory Values

◆ Elevation in laboratory values may represent increase in inflammation.
◆ For clients started on disease-modifying antirheumatic drugs (DMARDs; a class of medication), renal and liver function as well as complete blood counts should be assessed at baseline and periodically during treatment.

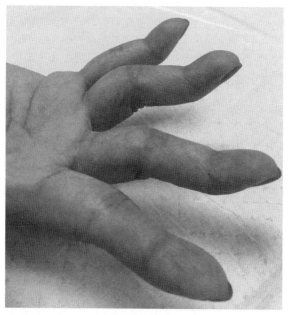

■ **Figure 15-1** Clinical presentation of rheumatic hand with prominent swan neck deformities. (Reprinted with permission from Egol K. *The Orthopaedic Manual: From the Office to the OR*, first edition. Philadelphia: Wolters Kluwer Health, 2017.)

Osteoporosis

Assessment/Signs and Symptoms
◆ Physical examination findings include loss of height and bone fractures, most commonly of the spine.

Diagnostics
◆ Osteoporosis frequently goes undiagnosed until fracture occurs.
◆ Screening may occur for individuals with known risk factors for development of osteoporosis. Bone loss is not seen on routine x-rays.
◆ The gold standard to diagnose is a bone mineral density (BMD) test. Management includes safety precautions to prevent injury and fracture, along with pharmacology therapy. Treatment begins when osteoporosis is diagnosed.

Pertinent Laboratory Values
◆ There are no lab values that indicate osteoporosis. Calcium and vitamin D levels may be low.
◆ Normal calcium level is 8.6 to 10.2 mg/dL (2.15 to 2.55 mmol/L).
◆ Normal vitamin D level is 20 to 50 pg/mL (52 to 130 pmol/L).

Gout

Assessment/Signs and Symptoms
◆ Symptoms occur acutely and include pain, swelling, redness, and limited range of motion of the joints affected. A low-grade fever may also be present.
◆ For clients diagnosed with gout, nursing management should focus on education about ways to reduce uric acid levels, which includes reduction of purine intake.
  ● Foods high in purine include red meats, organ meats, shellfish, and beverages containing fructose (i.e., soda).
  ● Factors that lead to elevated uric acid beyond purine intake include alcohol intake, hypertension, hyperlipidemia, obesity, and use of some commonly prescribed medications. Aspirin and diuretics (loop [i.e., furosemide] and thiazide [i.e., hydrochlorothiazide]) have been implicated in causing hyperuricemia.

Diagnostics
◆ The development of gout is caused by elevated serum uric acid levels. Uric acid is a byproduct of purine. Usually less than four joints are involved in a flare of the disease.
◆ The gold standard for diagnosis of gout is a fluid aspiration of the joint space. However, the condition is most commonly diagnosed by history and physical examination.

Pertinent Laboratory Values
◆ A uric acid level >6 mg/dL (356.91 µmol/L) is diagnostic of gout.

MEDICATION OVERVIEW

Rheumatoid Arthritis (Table 15-1)

Medications are used to decrease inflammation (nonsteroidal anti-inflammatory drugs [NSAIDs] and glucocorticoids) and slow the progression of the disease (DMARDs). The DMARDs are classified

Table 15-1

Drugs Used to Treat Rheumatoid Arthritis

Class	Prototype	Mechanism of Action	Major Side and Adverse Effects	Critical Information	Indications
Nonsteroidal anti-inflammatory drugs (NSAIDs) (oral agents)	Aspirin: first-generation NSAID Celecoxib: second-generation NSAID	Decrease inflammation via inhibition of cyclooxygenase	First generation: risk of clot formation (except with aspirin), risk of bleeding (aspirin), gastric irritation that may progress to ulceration Second generation: risk of clot formation, heightened risk of stroke and myocardial infarction, less risk of gastric irritation	NSAIDs will not alter disease progression Risk vs. benefit due to complications such as bleeding and gastrointestinal ulceration	Inflammation and pain
Glucocorticoids (oral or injectable agents)	Prednisone	Decrease inflammation	Short term (oral): weight gain, fluid retention, insomnia, hyperglycemia Long term (oral): bone loss leading to osteoporosis, adrenal suppression, gastric ulceration, exogenous glucocorticoid—excess leading to Cushing syndrome	Use oral form for shortest possible duration, as long-term side and adverse effects are numerous and many are severe Injectable agents are injected into the joint space: used if fewer joints are affected Monitor blood sugar in clients with diabetes mellitus; hypoglycemic medication doses may need to be increased while taking glucocorticoids If taken long term, during episodes of illness, dosage may be increased to compensate for adrenal suppression	Inflammation, slowing of disease progression

Nonbiologic disease-modifying antirheumatic drugs (DMARDs)	Methotrexate	Slow disease progression via decreasing joint destruction through decreased activity of B and T lymphocytes, which results in immune suppression	Common side effects include nausea, diarrhea, fatigue, and photosensitivity Severe adverse reactions include hepatic and pulmonary fibrosis, hepatotoxicity, nephrotoxicity, leukopenia, and thrombocytopenia	Administered orally or by injection Pregnancy category X Liver and renal function monitoring is required Complete blood count monitoring and assessing for signs of infection secondary to leukopenia or bleeding secondary to thrombocytopenia Clients on immunosuppressants should receive annual influenza vaccinations, avoid sick contacts, and engage in frequent handwashing	Immune suppression to slow disease progression
Biologic DMARDs	Etanercept	Blocks (antagonist) to tumor necrosis factor (TNF); TNF leads to joint destruction	Common side effects: injection site reactions such as redness and pain Severe adverse reactions: increased risk of serious infection due to immune suppression, thrombocytopenia, and leukopenia Less risk of liver injury when compared with nonbiologic DMARDs By blocking tumor necrosis factor, risk of cancer increases	More expensive than nonbiologic DMARDs Administered by subcutaneous injection once weekly Immune suppression increases risk of infection Clients must be screened for tuberculosis prior to start a treatment May worsen heart failure; monitor for signs and symptoms (dyspnea, edema, crackles in the lungs)	Immune suppression to slow disease progression

as Nonbiologic or biologic based on how they are manufactured. Nonbiologic are synthetically created medications; biologic are created using DNA. DMARDs have a delayed onset of action when compared to NSAIDs and have more serious side and adverse effects. Rheumatoid arthritis typically goes through remissions and flares; treatment is frequently long term.

> **BLACK BOX WARNING:** Etanercept has black box warnings to consider risk versus benefit of use due to potential for the development of serious infections such as tuberculosis, systemic fungal and opportunistic infections, and malignancies.

> **BLACK BOX WARNING:** Methotrexate has several black box warnings related to organ-specific toxicities of the liver, lungs, and gastrointestinal system. Potentially fatal skin reactions can also occur.

Osteoporosis

Medications are used to increase bone formation and slow bone resorption (Table 15-2). See Table 15-3 for information regarding drugs used to treat osteoporosis.

> **BLACK BOX WARNING:** Raloxifene has a black box warning for the potential development of venous thrombosis and an increased risk of death caused by stroke.

Table 15-2

Drugs Used to Prevent Osteoporosis

Class	Prototype	Mechanism of Action	Major Side and Adverse Effects	Critical Information	Indications
Calcium salts	Calcium citrate	Absorbed in the small intestine, deposited in bone	If taken in excessive doses, there is a risk of hypercalcemia	Absorbed best in the presence of sufficient vitamin D and parathyroid hormone Signs of toxicity include nausea, vomiting, constipation, and cardiac dysrhythmias	Prevention of osteoporosis
Vitamin D	Ergocalciferol	Increases bone absorption of calcium	Fat-soluble vitamin that can accumulate to toxic levels, usually occurs in conjunction with hypercalcemia	Signs of toxicity include nausea, vomiting, and weakness	Supplementation for increased absorption of calcium to prevent osteoporosis

Table 15-3

Drugs Used to Treat Osteoporosis

Class	Prototype	Mechanism of Action	Major Side and Adverse Effects	Critical Information	Indications
Bisphosphonates	Alendronate	Decrease osteoclast activity, which decreases bone resorption	Well tolerated Serious adverse effect is inflammation of esophageal tissue that can lead to ulceration	Must be taken with a full glass of water, and the client must remain in the upright position for at least 30 minutes to reduce esophageal contact and potential irritation Must be taken on an empty stomach	Osteoporosis, including bone loss caused by glucocorticoids
Selective estrogen receptor modulators	Raloxifene	Acts like estrogen, decreases number of osteoclasts to decrease bone resorption	Severe adverse effects due to excessive clotting. The risk of deep vein thrombosis, pulmonary embolism, and stroke	Pregnancy category X Clients should stop taking this medication if they are immobile or plan to be immobile (travel, surgery) to reduce risk of clot formation	Prevention and treatment of osteoporosis that occurs after menopause when estrogen levels decline

Gout

Medications are used to relieve pain and inflammation in an acute flare and to reduce the number of flares for clients who experience more than three acute gout episodes in 1 year (Table 15-4).

BLACK BOX WARNING: First- and second-generation NSAIDs (indomethacin, aspirin, and celecoxib) black box warnings represent the potential for an increased risk for heart attack, stroke, and potentially fatal bleeding within the gastrointestinal system.

Table 15-4

Drugs Used to Treat Gout

Class	Prototype	Mechanism of Action	Major Side and Adverse Effects	Critical Information	Indications
Nonsteroidal anti-inflammatory drugs (NSAIDs)	Indomethacin	Decrease inflammation via inhibition of cyclooxygenase	Gastric irritation and ulceration, renal impairment	First choice for gout flare, used short term only	Acute gout
Glucocorticoids	Prednisone	Decrease inflammation	Short term (oral): weight gain, fluid retention, insomnia, hyperglycemia	Second choice for gout flare for clients who cannot take NSAIDs, used short term only	Acute gout
Anti-inflammatory	Colchicine	Exact mechanism of action unknown. Approved only for the treatment of acute gout	Common side effects: nausea, vomiting, diarrhea, fatigue Serious adverse effects: pancytopenia, severe diarrhea, rhabdomyolysis (when used long term)	Can be used short term for acute gout or long term for prophylaxis Long term use is not recommended based on adverse effects Monitor for muscle pain or injury. The risk is increased if client is also taking a statin If gastrointestinal symptoms occur, the medication must be stopped immediately	Acute gout or prophylaxis
Xanthine oxidase inhibitors	Allopurinol	Prevent the formation of uric acid by inhibiting xanthine oxidase, which is the enzyme that produces uric acid	Common side effects: nausea, vomiting, fatigue Severe adverse effects: hypersensitivity reaction resulting in rash, fever, hepatotoxicity, and nephrotoxicity	If rash or fever develop, allopurinol must be stopped immediately Allopurinol increases the effects of warfarin, which promotes bleeding; warfarin dosage should be decreased	Prophylaxis
Uricosuric agents	Probenecid	Increases excretion of uric acid via kidneys through urine by preventing uric acid absorption in the nephron	Common side effects: nausea, vomiting Kidney injury can occur from excess uric acid in the nephrons	Probenecid can be taken with food to decrease nausea Increase fluid intake to keep uric acid flushed out of kidneys	Prophylaxis

Practice Questions and Rationales

1. A client is admitted to the medical unit and is prescribed allopurinol and ciprofloxacin. Following administration of the medications, the client's temperature is 101.2°F (38.4°C). What is the **priority** nursing action?
   1. Request an order for a complete blood count (CBC).
   2. Hold the allopurinol and notify the provider.
   3. Administer a dose of acetaminophen as ordered.
   4. Document the findings and reassess the client in 30 minutes.

2. The nurse is caring for a client who is experiencing increasingly worse indigestion. Which medication prescribed to the client would be of **greatest** concern to the nurse?
   1. Aspirin
   2. Prednisone
   3. Allopurinol
   4. Alendronate

3. The nurse is preparing to administer etanercept to a client with rheumatoid arthritis. Which assessment finding(s) would alert the nurse to potential contraindications to this medication? Select all that apply.
   1. Bilateral crackles in the lung bases
   2. 2+ pitting edema of the right lower extremity
   3. A tuberculin skin test with induration measuring 10 mm
   4. Hyperactive bowel sounds in all four abdominal quadrants
   5. Platelet count of 135,000 × 10³/μL (135 × 10⁹/L)

4. A client with rheumatoid arthritis who has been taking prednisone for the past 6 months develops influenza. Which statement made by the client indicates proper understanding of the dosage requirements of prednisone during an acute illness?
   1. "I will stop taking my prednisone until my fever is gone."
   2. "I need to slowly taper off of my prednisone to reduce the severity of my flu symptoms."
   3. "I should increase my prednisone dose until my flu symptoms resolve."
   4. "I should continue taking my prednisone as prescribed, even while sick."

5. A 30-year-old woman has been diagnosed with rheumatoid arthritis and prescribed methotrexate. Which diagnostic studies does the nurse anticipate obtaining prior to starting the medication? Select all that apply.
   1. Creatinine
   2. Serum uric acid
   3. Urine pregnancy test
   4. Serum electrolyte levels
   5. Aspartate aminotransferase

6. A client with osteoporosis has been prescribed raloxifene. Which statement made by the client requires **immediate** intervention by the nurse?
   1. "I have been bruising much more easily over the past several months."
   2. "My breast cancer has been in remission for several years now."

3. "I have developed a cough that seems to have some blood in it."

4. "When I sit for prolonged periods of time, my feet begin to tingle and hurt."

7. A client with an acute gout flare reports severe nausea when taking colchicine. Which medications would be an acceptable alternative for the client's treatment? Select all that apply.

1. Allopurinol

2. Acetaminophen

3. Prednisone

4. Naproxen

5. Indomethacin

8. A client has been prescribed methotrexate 30 mg intramuscularly once weekly. The medication is supplied as 200 mg/8 mL. How many milliliters should the nurse administer? Round the answer to the nearest tenth.

_____ mL

9. A client has been taking calcium citrate with vitamin D for the prevention of osteoporosis. What signs or symptoms assessed by the nurse may indicate toxicity of these medications? Select all that apply.

1. Diarrhea

2. Flank pain

3. Hypotension

4. Anxiety

5. Leg pain

10. A client taking aspirin for rheumatoid arthritis has recently been prescribed misoprostol. The client asks why they are now taking a second medication. What is the correct response by the nurse?

1. "Misoprostol will increase the effectiveness of the aspirin."

2. "This seems to be an error, let me check with your prescriber."

3. "The misoprostol will help protect your stomach from ulceration."

4. "The combination of these two medications decreases joint stiffness."

16

PALLIATIVE CARE MEDICATIONS

BRIEF OVERVIEW OF PALLIATIVE CARE

Palliative care is holistic care that focuses on relieving distressing symptoms of disease processes and treatments. In providing palliative care, a thorough assessment needs to be completed. Then, symptoms are addressed and treated. Lab work and diagnostic tests are not typically ordered prior to treating symptoms. Palliative care can be used concurrently with curative treatments for chronic disease, or as the primary treatment for clients with end-stage disease. Hospice is under the umbrella of palliative care, but the care is specific to clients with end-stage/terminal disease, who have 6 months or less to live. Drugs that help alleviate symptoms are used in the palliative care setting.

- ◆ **Pain:** Most clients with severe disease experience pain. Pain has adverse consequences and should be treated adequately, as unrelieved pain can cause disruptive physiologic changes.
- ◆ **Respiratory symptoms:** Dyspnea is an anxiety-producing symptom of many different disease processes, such as lung disease, heart failure, renal failure, and many types of cancers. Dyspnea and upper airway congestion are common in end-stage disease.
- ◆ **Neurologic symptoms:** Disease processes that affect the central nervous system (CNS) can cause delirium. At end of life, clients can experience terminal agitation. Prescribed medications and client discomfort can also cause these symptoms. To treat these neurologic issues, neuroleptics and benzodiazepines are used.
- ◆ **Gastrointestinal symptoms:** Gastrointestinal issues often accompany chronic and end-stage diseases and treatments. Nausea, anorexia/cachexia, constipation, and diarrhea are common gastrointestinal symptoms treated in palliative care.
- ◆ **Anxiety:** With chronic and end-stage disease, psychological and emotional distress are occur frequently and can exacerbate symptoms, such as dyspnea, pain, and nausea. Benzodiazepines are standard treatments for anxiety.

CLINICAL PEARLS: PALLIATIVE CARE SYMPTOM MANAGEMENT

Pain

Many chronic and end-stage disease processes and treatments may result in some degree of pain.

Types of Pain
- ◆ Acute
- ◆ Chronic
- ◆ Acute-on-chronic

- Nociceptive
- Somatic
- Visceral
- Neuropathic
- Referred
- Breakthrough

Assessment/Signs and Symptoms

- Assess vital signs: Heart rate, respiratory rate, and blood pressure are often elevated with pain.
- Assess for pain frequently and encourage clients to report pain. Pain is subjective, and self-report of pain is the best indicator.
  - In a pain assessment, include onset, location, duration, pain characteristics, intensity, and aggravating/relieving factors.
  - In addition, use visual and behavioral assessments. If a client is nonverbal, visual assessment is key, along with observational pain scales.
- When assessing both verbal and nonverbal clients, note guarding, frowning, agitation, moaning, and furrowing of the brow, as they can all be signs of pain.
- Examine the client's pain regimen and find out what has been taken and what has worked before.
- Address psychological, spiritual, and cultural aspects of pain.

Pharmacologic Interventions

- Nonsteroidal anti-inflammatory drugs (NSAIDs) and acetaminophen can be used for mild pain or as adjuvants.
- Opioids are commonly used to treat moderate to severe pain.
- Tricyclic antidepressants and anticonvulsants are used as adjuvants for neuropathic pain.
- Corticosteroids are used as adjuvants to decrease bone pain and inflammation.

Nursing Considerations

- Administer medications in a timely manner in order to stay ahead of the pain.
  - Deliver pain medication as noninvasively as possible. The oral route is preferred.
- Continue pain regimens when a client is no longer conscious. Unconscious clients can still feel pain.
- Recognize that pain tolerance levels are different for each person.
- Do not withhold pain medications from clients with a history of drug or alcohol use. These clients may have higher tolerances for pain medications and may need higher dosing for relief.
- Monitor for side/adverse effects.
- Reassess pain after medication administration to ensure effectiveness of dosing.
  - Reassessment after 30 minutes with intravenous medication administration and after 1 hour for oral administration of medications

Safety Concerns

- There is no ceiling for opioid medications, but they need to be titrated slowly. "Start low, go slow."
- Opioids can cause respiratory depression.

- ◆ The reversal agent for opioid overdose is naloxone.
  - ● Naloxone should only be given in cases of severe respiratory depression (respiratory rate < 8 breaths per minute) due to opioid overdose.
  - ● The goal should be to give enough of a dose to reverse adverse symptoms, but not completely reverse the effects of the medication, as this would cause client discomfort and distress.
  - ● Abrupt cessation of the opioid effect may cause severe withdrawal symptoms.
  - ● Clients need to be monitored for the recurrence of respiratory depression for at least 2 hours after naloxone administration.
  - ● Retreatment with naloxone may be necessary with return of respiratory depression.
- ◆ Clients who are taking opioid medications are at high risk for confusion, sedation, and falls.
- ◆ Corticosteroids must be tapered to avoid adrenal insufficiency.
- ◆ If taking tricyclic antidepressants as an adjuvant, watch for serotonin syndrome, neuroleptic malignant syndrome, and extrapyramidal symptoms.

Respiratory Symptoms

Causes of respiratory symptoms include cancer, lung disease or injury, heart failure, renal failure, neurologic disorders (amyotrophic lateral sclerosis), and anemia

Assessment/Signs and Symptoms

- ◆ Assess client history.
- ◆ Take vital signs: heart rate, respiratory rate and blood pressure may be elevated with dyspnea. Oxygen saturation may be low.
- ◆ Assess dyspnea on a dyspnea scale.
- ◆ Auscultate lung sounds (stridor, wheezing, crackles, and rhonchi).
- ◆ Evaluate accessory muscle use, cough, phlegm, and congestion.
- ◆ Assess for:
  - ● Pallor, cyanosis, edema, pain
  - ● Anxiety, which may worsen dyspnea
  - ● Aggrevating and alleviating factors
  - ● Medications and/or treatments that have been used to treat dyspnea
- ◆ Find out which medications/treatments have been taken to treat the dyspnea, as well as which medications/treatments have worked previously.
- ◆ Thorough assessment may lead to the specific cause of dyspnea and, therefore, more effective treatment.

Pharmacologic Interventions

- ◆ Anxiolytics (lorazepam) can be used to treat anxiety.
- ◆ Oxygen should be used as ordered.
  - ● With chronic obstructive pulmonary disease (COPD), clients may be carbon dioxide retainers, so caution must be taken with oxygen delivery rates.
  - ● Encourage pursed lip breathing for clients with COPD.

- Low-dose opioids can help decrease the sensation of dyspnea.
- Diuretics (furosemide) can decrease fluid retention, easing breathing.
- Bronchodilators (albuterol), steroids (prednisone), and antibiotics may help to relieve dyspnea for COPD clients.

Nursing Considerations

- Reassess effectiveness of medications/treatments in a timely manner.
- Reassess efficacy of dyspnea treatment plan.
- Monitor for side effects caused by medications.
- Understand that at end of life, clients may lose respiratory muscle tone, and upper airway congestion may be seen.
  - Secretions may collect in the back of the throat and upper airways, causing a "rattling" sound (death rattle). This can be treated with anticholinergics to help dry up secretions.
- If both anxiolytics and opioids are ordered for dyspnea, care must be taken to give one medication first and assess for effect. If there is no effect, give the second medication and reassess.
- Clients on opioid pain medications and/or benzodiazepines are at high risk for confusion, sedation, and falls.
- Taper corticosteroids to avoid adrenal insufficiency.

Neurologic Disorders

Causes of neurologic disorders include hypoxia, medications, pain, constipation, urinary retention/need to urinate, constipation/need to defecate, fever, insomnia, CNS disorders/malignancies, fear/anxiety, spiritual unrest, and terminal agitation.

Types of Disorders

- Delirium
  - Delirium can manifest as cognitive changes, hallucinations, agitation, incoherence, delusions, paranoia, decreased or increased psychomotor activity, and sleep disturbances.
  - Changes that occur with delirium take place over a short period of time, and can be reversible, unlike dementia, which is progressive.
- Terminal agitation/terminal restlessness
  - Terminal agitation occurs at the end of life as part of the dying process and manifests as emotional and physical restlessness and delirium.
  - It is not reversible, though it can wax and wane.
  - A thorough assessment must be done in order to differentiate between reversible causes of delirium and terminal agitation.

Assessment/Signs and Symptoms

- Assess for:
  - Case of delirium or terminal agitation
  - Dyspnea
  - Vital signs, lung sounds and breathing effort
  - Pain

- Medications that may be altering mental status
- Psychosocial and spiritual unrest
◆ Assess abdomen for bladder distension or constipation.
  - Catheterize if there is urinary retention.
  - Establish a bowel regimen and disimpact if necessary.
◆ Treat fever as indicated.

Pharmacologic Interventions
◆ Neuroleptics and anxiolytics are used to treat terminal agitation.

Nursing Considerations
◆ Before treating terminal agitation, rule out reversible causes of delirium.
◆ Know that benzodiazepines can address agitation but can also cause a paradoxical effect.
◆ Understand that medications used to treat terminal agitation and delirium may cause sedation and worsen delirium.
◆ Reassess medication for effectiveness and for adverse/side effects.
◆ Clients taking benzodiazepines and/or neuroleptics are at high risk for confusion, sedation, and falls.
◆ Watch for serotonin syndrome, a medical emergency causing high body temperature, agitation, tremors, hyperreflexia, and tachycardia.
  - Serotonin syndrome can be treated with benzodiazepines and cyproheptadine (blocks serotonin production).
◆ Watch for extrapyramidal symptoms: dystonia, akathisia, parkinsonism, tardive dyskinesia, and bradykinesia.
  - Tardive dyskinesia includes jerking movements of face, neck, and tongue (lip smacking, sticking out the tongue, and facial grimacing and may be irreversible.
  - Treated with benzodiazepines or anticholinergics.
◆ Watch for neuroleptic malignant syndrome, a medical emergency causing dangerously high fever and rigidity.
  - Treated with dantrolene sodium.
◆ Watch for anticholinergic effects: dry mouth, dry eyes, blurry vision, sedation, constipation, urinary retention, tachycardia, and increased body temperature.
◆ Watch for Stevens-Johnson syndrome: a side effect of quetiapine that is a medical emergency.
  - A severe red or purple skin rash develops on the face and chest, then spreads, blisters, and peels.
  - Treatment is supportive care and discontinuation of the offending agent.

Gastrointestinal Disorders

Nausea and Vomiting
Many different disease processes can cause nausea and vomiting. Nausea and vomiting can also result from pain, constipation, anxiety, medications, and chemotherapy. Treatments for nausea and vomiting can differ based on cause.

Assessment/Signs and Symptoms

- ◆ Assess client history of nausea and vomiting.
  - • Considerations include onset, pattern, factors that alleviate/exacerbate, and treatments
- ◆ Assess vital signs and hydration status.
  - • Signs of dehydration may include weight loss, fever, tachycardia, tachypnea, hypotension, delayed capillary refill, and skin tenting.
- ◆ Assess the abdomen for pain, distension, and bowel sounds.
- ◆ Examine vomitus for blood, color, content, and amount.
- ◆ Assess for possible constipation or obstruction as causes.
- ◆ Look at other factors such as pain, medications, and fear/anxiety.
- ◆ Assess diet and fluid intake.

Pharmacologic Interventions

- ◆ Antiemetics (ondansetron) are used to treat nausea and vomiting.
- ◆ Prokinetic agents (metoclopramide) can be used to treat nausea and vomiting due to decreased gastrointestinal motility.
- ◆ Benzodiazepines (lorazepam) may be used to treat nausea and vomiting related to anxiety.

Nursing Considerations

- ◆ Reassess efficacy of medication regimen in controlling nausea and vomiting.
- ◆ Monitor for side and adverse effects of medication.
- ◆ Understand that treatments for nausea and vomiting may differ based on etiology.
- ◆ Assess for bowel obstruction prior to giving prokinetic agents. Failure to do so may result in a perforated or ruptured bowel.
- ◆ Use of benzodiazepines may result in higher risk for confusion and falls.

Anorexia/Cachexia

Causes of anorexia/cachexia include complications of disease, medications, chemotherapy, radiation, and/or the dying process.

Assessment/Signs and Symptoms

- ◆ Assess for:
  - • Onset and cause of loss of appetite
  - • Mucositis or poor dentition
  - • Altered taste sensation
  - • Nausea and vomiting
  - • Pain
  - • Fatigue and lethargy
  - • Medications that may cause nausea or loss of appetite
  - • Vital signs and hydration status
  - • Abdominal pain, distension, and the presence of bowel sounds
- ◆ Determine client food preferences.
  - • Encourage smaller, more frequent meals.
  - • Consider nutritional supplements.
  - • Encourage oral hygiene.
  - • Add fiber intake, if tolerated.

Pharmacologic Interventions

- ◆ Appetite stimulants can be used short-term.
- ◆ Short-term parenteral or enteral feeding is possible depending on the etiology and progression of disease.

Nursing Considerations

- ◆ Understand that prior to treating with appetite stimulants, prokinetic agents should be considered to address possible delayed gastric emptying.
- ◆ Note that when appetite stimulants are used, effects are variable and time-limited.
- ◆ Monitor medication effectiveness and taper or stop medications if there is no effect within 4 to 6 weeks.
- ◆ Taper cannabinoids to avoid withdrawal syndrome.

Constipation

Causes of constipation include medications, pain, diet, immobility, tumors, ascites, fluid and electrolyte imbalances, intestinal obstructions, surgical procedures, and psychosocial issues. Unmanaged constipation can lead to obstipation and obstruction.

Assessment/Signs and Symptoms

- ◆ Determine history, onset, and cause of constipation.
- ◆ Assess vital signs, pain, nausea/vomiting, abdominal distension, and bowel sounds.
  - • Bowel sounds may be hypoactive or absent; if there is a mechanical obstruction, bowel sounds may be hyperactive above the obstruction and hypoactive below.
- ◆ Assess bowel movements for frequency, amount, color, consistency, and presence of blood.
- ◆ Examine rectal area for impaction, hemorrhoids, anal fissures, and injury.
- ◆ Examine diet and fluid intake. Assess for possible dehydration.
- ◆ Assess mobility.
- ◆ Review medication list to see if there are any medications taken that cause constipation (opioids).
- ◆ Determine if the client has a bowel regimen.

Pharmacologic Interventions

- ◆ Medications that increase the amount of fluid absorbed by feces, increase gastric motility and peristalsis can be used to treat constipation.

Nursing Considerations

- ◆ Have a bowel regimen in place if the client is taking opioids.
- ◆ Prophylactic treatment with start of medications with the side effect of constipation is recommended.
- ◆ Bulk-forming agents are not typically used for constipation in palliative care, as they can exacerbate constipation and cause dehydration.
- ◆ If there has been no bowel movement for 5 days or more, assess for impaction with a digital rectal exam.
- ◆ Know that diarrhea may result from the use of bowel medications.
- ◆ Understand that frequent use of suppositories and enemas may cause dependence.

Diarrhea

Causes of diarrhea include cancer, infection, inflammatory bowel disease, laxative use, medications and treatments (chemotherapy), diet, tube feedings, metabolic disease, and gastrointestinal surgery.

Assessment/Signs and Symptoms

◆ Determine the client's medical history.
◆ Assess:
  ● Vital signs and hydration status
  ● Diet and fluid intake
  ● Skin for any breakdown
  ● Bowel movements for frequency, color, consistency, and presence of blood
  ● Abdomen for tenderness, distension, and bowel sounds
  ● Bowel sounds may be hyperactive during episodes of diarrhea

Pharmacologic Interventions

◆ Diarrhea may not be treated initially in order to allow toxins to be excreted. However, if diarrhea persists, it may be treated with opioids and bulk-forming agents.
◆ If the diarrhea is due to an infectious process, it is treated with antibiotics.
◆ If the cause of diarrhea is an inflammatory bowel disease, it is treated with steroids.

Nursing Considerations

◆ Reassess medication effectiveness and evaluate for improvement.
  ● Monitor for medication adverse and side effects.
  ● Taking opioids for diarrhea may result in constipation.

Anxiety

Causes of anxiety include chronic or terminal disease diagnoses, major procedures and treatments, pain, dyspnea, uncontrolled nausea and vomiting, change in mental status, fear of death, psychosocial and/or spiritual distress, and medications.

Assessment/Signs and Symptoms

◆ Assess client and family comprehension of diagnosis and prognosis, client and family roles, functions, and needs.
  ● Client and family coping strategies
  ● Risk factors for client and family (mental illness, substance use, and history of suicidal ideation)
◆ Identify values, hopes, fears, goals, and quality of life desired.

Pharmacologic Intervention

◆ Benzodiazepines (lorazepam) are typically used to reduce anxiety.

Nursing Considerations

◆ Assess medication effectiveness.
◆ Monitor medication for side effects, such as sedation and confusion.
  ● Use of benzodiazepines may have a paradoxical effect.

SAFETY ALERT! Clients taking benzodiazepines are at higher risk for confusion, sedation, and falls.

PALLIATIVE CARE MEDICATION OVERVIEW

Palliative Care Medications for Pain

A wide variety of medications are available for pain management in palliative care (see Table 16-1).

Palliative Care Medications for Respiratory Symptoms

Several medications are approved for the treatment of respiratory concerns in palliative care (see Table 16-2).

Palliative Care Medications for Neurologic Symptoms

Delirium, agitation, and psychosis are treated with a variety of medications (see Table 16-3).

Palliative Care Medications for Gastrointestinal Symptoms

Antiemetics
A common concern in palliative care is relief of nausea and vomiting (see Table 16-4).

Appetite Stimulants
Various classes of medications can be used to increase appetite (see Table 16-5).

Constipation Medications and Antidiarrheals
Many disorders can cause diarrhea and/or constipation in palliative care, requiring treatment (see Table 16-6).

Palliative Care Medications for Anxiety

Benzodiazepines are the mainstay of anxiety treatment in palliative care (see Table 16-7).

Table 16-1

Types of Pain Medications Used in Palliative Care

Class	Prototype Medication	Mechanism of Action	Major Side and Adverse Effects	Critical Information	Indications
Opioids	Morphine Hydrocodone	Exact mechanism is unknown. Is thought to activate the mu and kappa receptors in the central nervous system, resulting in pain relief	Constipation, urinary retention Nausea and vomiting Sedation, respiratory depression Dizziness, hypotension Rash Myoclonus	Monitor vital signs for respiratory rate and blood pressure Monitor urine output Establish a bowel regimen If myoclonus is observed, decreasing or switching pain medications may be helpful Watch for allergic reactions Use with caution with clients in renal failure and in clients taking benzodiazepines Be aware of potential for addiction, tolerance, physical dependence, and pseudo addiction	Moderate to severe somatic and visceral pain
Nonsteroidal anti-inflammatory drugs (NSAIDs)	Ibuprofen	Inhibits synthesis of prostaglandins, which mediate pain, fever, and inflammation	Gastrointestinal discomfort and bleeding Renal insufficiency, Dizziness Tinnitus Headache	Advise clients to eat with NSAID medication, as it can cause gastrointestinal discomfort Taking steroids concurrently increases risk of gastrointestinal bleeding Clients with history of gastrointestinal bleeding, or coagulopathies, should not take NSAIDs	Mild to moderate pain, can be used as an adjuvant with severe pain Fever

Class	Medication	Action	Side Effects	Nursing Considerations	Use
Analgesic and antipyretic	Acetaminophen	Indirectly blocks prostaglandin synthesis in central nervous system. Has analgesic and antipyretic effects	Hepatotoxicity in large doses	The maximum dose is 4 g/day. Acetaminophen may already be included in other pain medication and must be included in dosing totals. Medication must be used with caution with clients who are older adults or have liver disease	Mild to moderate pain, can be used as adjuvant in severe pain. Fever
Anticonvulsants	Gabapentin	Act on nervous system by inhibiting neurons from firing	Dizziness. Somnolence. Visual changes. Fatigue. Bone marrow suppression	Monitor labs for toxicity	Neuropathic pain adjuvant
Tricyclic antidepressants	Nortriptyline	Prevent reuptake of serotonin and norepinephrine	Anticholinergic effects. Drowsiness. Fatigue and lethargy. Extrapyramidal symptoms. Neuroleptic malignant syndrome	Monitor for serotonin syndrome, as it can be life threatening. Monitor for neuroleptic malignant syndrome medical emergency. Monitor for extrapyramidal symptoms. Tardive dyskinesia may be irreversible	Neuropathic pain adjuvant

(continued)

Table 16-1

Types of Pain Medications Used in Palliative Care *(continued)*

Class	Prototype Medication	Mechanism of Action	Major Side and Adverse Effects	Critical Information	Indications
Corticosteroids	Dexamethasone	Suppresses inflammation and immune response, block nociceptive stimuli	Hyperglycemia	Steroids should be given in the morning, or in split doses in morning and afternoon, as they cause insomnia	Somatic pain adjuvant
			Hypertension		
			Increased appetite	Taking NSAIDs concurrently increases risk of gastrointestinal bleeding	
			Weight gain		
			Mood changes	Monitor for fever and infection, as steroids cause immunosuppression	
			Peptic ulcers		
			Immunosuppression	Medication must be tapered when discontinuing, otherwise there is a risk for adrenal insufficiency	
			Cushing syndrome		
Opioid antagonist	Naloxone	Acts as a competitive inhibitor. Blocks opiates from binding to opiate receptors	Nausea, vomiting, diaphoresis	Abrupt reversal of opioids by naloxone can lead to narcotic withdrawal	Severe respiratory depression due to opioid overdose
			Hypertension, tremors, pulmonary edema	The duration of action of naloxone is shorter than that of opioids	
			Seizures, ventricular arrhythmias, cardiac arrest	Monitor for 2 hours after administration	
				Retreatment may be necessary if symptoms return	

Table 16-2

Palliative Care Medications for Respiratory Symptoms

Class	Prototype Medication	Mechanism of Action	Major Side and Adverse Effects	Critical Information	Indications
Opioids	Morphine	Exact mechanism is unknown. Is thought to activate the mu and kappa receptors in the central nervous system. Depresses respiration and cough reflex	Constipation	Monitor respiratory rate and blood pressure	Dyspnea
			Nausea	Monitor urine output	Increased work of breathing
			Vomiting	Establish a bowel regimen	
			Urinary retention	If myoclonus is observed, decreasing or switching pain medications may be helpful	
			Sedation, respiratory depression Dizziness	Use with caution with clients in renal failure and clients taking benzodiazepines	
			Hypotension		
			Myoclonus	Potential for addiction, tolerance, physical dependence, and pseudo addiction	
Bronchodilators	Albuterol sulfate	Causes smooth muscle in airways to relax and dilate.	Tachycardia	Bronchodilators should be used with caution in clients with cardiac issues	Chronic obstructive pulmonary disease
	Ipratropium bromide		Anxiety		Asthma
			Tremors		
			Hypertension		

(continued)

Table 16-2

Palliative Care Medications for Respiratory Symptoms (continued)

Class	Prototype Medication	Mechanism of Action	Major Side and Adverse Effects	Critical Information	Indications
Corticosteroids	Prednisone	Suppresses inflammation and immune responses, decreases inflammation and opens airways	Hyperglycemia	Steroids should be given in the morning, or in split doses in morning and afternoon, as they cause insomnia	Chronic obstructive pulmonary disease
			Hypertension		Asthma
			Mood changes	Taking NSAIDs concurrently increases risk of gastrointestinal bleeding	Inflammatory lung disease
			Increased appetite	Monitor for fever and infection, as steroids cause immunosuppression	
			Weight gain		
			Peptic ulcers	Steroids must be tapered when discontinuing, otherwise there is a risk for adrenal insufficiency	
			Immunosuppression		
			Cushing syndrome		
Antibiotics	Ceftriaxone	Dependent on medication used	Adverse/side effects dependent on antibiotic used	Monitor for hypersensitivity and allergic reaction	Lung infection
					Pneumonia
Diuretics	Furosemide	Inhibits water and electrolyte reabsorption in the ascending limb of the loop of Henle	Dehydration	Monitor for dehydration and hypokalemia	Edema
			Hypokalemia		Ascites
			Tinnitus		Heart failure Fluid overload
			Hearing loss		
			Increased urination		
			Thirst		

Anticholinergics	Scopolamine	Interferes with nerve transmission by blocking acetylcholine receptors	Anticholinergic effects: Dry mouth Dry eyes, blurred vision Sedation Constipation Urinary retention Tachycardia Increased body temperature	Scopolamine also treats nausea and vomiting	Upper airway secretions

NSAID, nonsteroidal anti-inflammatory drug.

Table 16-3

Palliative Care Medications for Neurologic Symptoms

Class	Prototype Medication	Mechanism of Action	Major Side and Adverse Effects	Critical Information	Indications
Butyrophenones	Haloperidol	Blocks dopamine receptors	Extrapyramidal symptoms	Monitor for extrapyramidal symptoms and neuroleptic malignant syndrome	Delirium
			Neuroleptic malignant syndrome	Tardive dyskinesia may be irreversible	Terminal agitation
			Sedation	Monitor for neuroleptic malignant syndrome, as it is a medical emergency	Psychosis
			Seizures	Haloperidol lowers seizure threshold in Parkinson's clients and should not be used	
Phenothiazines	Chlorpromazine	Blocks the actions of dopamine	Extrapyramidal symptoms	Monitor for extrapyramidal symptoms and neuroleptic malignant syndrome	Delirium
			Urinary retention	Neuroleptic syndrome is a medical emergency	Terminal agitation
			Constipation	Tardive dyskinesia may be irreversible	
			Dizziness	Monitor for neuroleptic malignant syndrome, a medical emergency	
			Drowsiness		
			Neuroleptic malignant syndrome		
			Anticholinergic effects		

Classification	Medication	Action	Side Effects	Nursing Considerations	Uses
Selective serotonin reuptake inhibitor	Olanzapine	Blocks serotonin and dopamine receptors	Weight gain Constipation Sedation Drowsiness Dizziness Suicidal ideation Extrapyramidal symptoms Neuroleptic malignant syndrome	Monitor for suicidal ideation Monitor for neuroleptic malignant syndrome and extrapyramidal symptoms If tardive dyskinesia develops, it may be irreversible	Delirium and terminal agitation in older adult clients Depression Psychosis
Antipsychotic	Quetiapine	Blocks serotonin and dopamine receptors	Drowsiness Dizziness Constipation Extrapyramidal symptoms Neuroleptic malignant syndrome	Quetiapine may cause Stevens-Johnson syndrome, which is a medical emergency Monitor for suicidal ideation If tardive dyskinesia develops, it may be irreversible Monitor for neuroleptic malignant syndrome and extrapyramidal symptoms Neuroleptic malignant syndrome is a medical emergency	Delirium and terminal agitation Sedation Insomnia
Benzodiazepine	Lorazepam	Binds with GABA receptors in central nervous system, which decrease brain stimulation	Drowsiness Dizziness Weakness Hypotension Respiratory depression Paradoxical reaction—restlessness and agitation	Benzodiazepines can cause a paradoxical reaction Be aware of tolerance, physical, and psychological dependence	Delirium Terminal agitation Anxiety

GABA, gamma aminobutyric acid.

Table 16-4

Treatment of Nausea and Vomiting

Class	Prototype Medication	Mechanism of Action	Major Side and Adverse Effects	Critical Information	Indications
Prokinetic agent	Metoclopramide	Inhibits smooth GI muscle relaxation produced by dopamine and decreases gastric emptying time	Drowsiness Dizziness Diarrhea	Do not use in case of complete bowel obstruction, as it may cause perforation or rupture	Nausea and vomiting due to decreased gastrointestinal motility, partial bowel obstruction
Serotonin 5HT$_3$ antagonist	Ondansetron	Blocks the action of serotonin, which may cause nausea and vomiting	Constipation	Ondansetron is especially effective with chemotherapy-induced nausea	Nausea and vomiting
Butyrophenone	Haloperidol	Blocks dopamine receptors	Sedation Drowsiness Extrapyramidal symptoms Neuroleptic malignant syndrome Seizures	Haloperidol is helpful with opioid-induced nausea and vomiting Haloperidol lowers seizure threshold Should not be used in clients with Parkinson disease Monitor for extrapyramidal symptoms and neuroleptic malignant syndrome If tardive dyskinesia develops, it may be irreversible Neuroleptic malignant syndrome is a medical emergency	Nausea and vomiting

Classification	Medication	Action	Side Effects	Nursing Considerations	Use
Phenothiazine	Promethazine	Inhibits histamine, dopamine, and acetylcholine effects, which cause nausea	Extrapyramidal symptoms Urinary retention Constipation Dizziness Drowsiness Neuroleptic malignant syndrome Anticholinergic effects	Promethazine is helpful with nausea and vomiting due to motion sickness and allergic response Monitor for extrapyramidal symptoms and neuroleptic malignant syndrome If tardive dyskinesia develops, it may be irreversible Neuroleptic malignant syndrome is a medical emergency	Nausea and vomiting
Benzodiazepine	Lorazepam	Binds with GABA receptors in central nervous system, which decrease brain stimulation	Drowsiness Dizziness Lethargy Respiratory depression Hypotension Paradoxical reaction—hallucinations Restlessness	Benzodiazepines can cause a paradoxical reaction Use can result in addiction, tolerance, and physical dependence	Nausea and vomiting caused by fear/anxiety

GABA, gamma aminobutyric acid; GI, gastrointestinal.

Table 16-5

Appetite Stimulants

Class	Prototype Medication	Mechanism of Action	Major Side and Adverse Effects	Critical Information	Indications
Tricyclic antidepressant	Mirtazapine	Prevents reuptake of serotonin and dopamine	Anticholinergic effects	Monitor mental status	Anorexia
			Suicidal ideation	Monitor for serotonin syndrome, as it can be life threatening	
			Neuroleptic malignant syndrome	Monitor for extrapyramidal symptoms and neuroleptic malignant syndrome	
			Extrapyramidal symptoms		
			Lethargy	If tardive dyskinesia develops, it may be irreversible	
			Weight gain	Neuroleptic malignant syndrome is a medical emergency	
				Mirtazapine should be discontinued if there is no effect within 4–6 weeks	
				Mirtazapine may cause serotonin syndrome, which is life threatening	
Progesterone	Megestrol	Exact mechanism for appetite stimulation is unknown	Hyperglycemia	Megestrol should be discontinued if there is no effect within 4–6 weeks	Anorexia
			Hypertension		
			Weakness		
			Dizziness		
			Vaginal bleeding		

| Corticosteroids | Dexamethasone | Primarily suppresses inflammation and immune responses; also blocks nociceptive stimuli, and has the effect of increasing appetite | Hyperglycemia

Hypertension

Mood changes

Weight gain

Peptic ulcers

Immunosuppression

Cushing syndrome | Steroids should be given in the morning, or in split doses in morning and afternoon, as they cause insomnia

Taking NSAIDs concurrently increases risk of gastrointestinal bleeding

Monitor for fever and infection, as steroids cause immunosuppression

Discontinue the steroids if there is no effect within 4–6 weeks

Steroids must be tapered when discontinuing, otherwise there is a risk for adrenal insufficiency | Anorexia

Nausea and vomiting |
| Cannabinoids | Dronabinol | Not completely understood. Possibly mediated by cannabinoid receptors in central nervous system | Sedation

Cognitive changes

Anxiety

Delusions

Paranoia | Cannabinoids have low toxicity; there is no lethal dose

Can cause tolerance and physical dependence

Stopping the medication suddenly may cause agitation, anxiety, insomnia, and tremors.

Cannabinoids should be discontinued if there is no effect on appetite | Anorexia

Nausea and vomiting |

NSAID, nonsteroidal anti-inflammatory drug.

Table 16-6

Medications for Constipation and Diarrhea

Class	Prototype Medication	Mechanism of Action	Major Side and Adverse Effects	Critical Information	Indications
Bulk-forming agents	Psyllium	Helps intestinal content absorb water, promotes peristalsis and expulsion of feces	Constipation Dehydration	Psyllium is also used for constipation but may exacerbate constipation Take with a full glass of water	Diarrhea
Laxatives	Sennosides	Causes the large intestine to absorb more water and increases peristalsis	Cramping Diarrhea Nausea	Overuse can result in laxative dependence	Constipation
Suppositories	Bisacodyl	Stimulates peristalsis and water reabsorption in large intestine	Cramping Diarrhea	Overuse can result in dependence	Constipation
Stool softeners	Docusate sodium	Causes feces to absorb water for easier and faster transit	Cramping Diarrhea Nausea	Overuse can cause dependence	Constipation
Enemas	Sodium phosphate enema	Stimulates bowel movement by intestinal water retention and increased peristalsis	Cramping Bloating Nausea Vomiting Electrolyte imbalance	Excessive use can cause dependence and severe electrolyte imbalance	Constipation
Opioids	Loperamide	Inhibits peristalsis and prolongs intestinal transit time	Constipation Drowsiness Nausea Vomiting	Use loperamide cautiously as use may cause retention of infectious organisms/toxins May cause constipation	Diarrhea

		Mechanism of action depends on antibiotic used	Hypersensitivity and allergic reaction	Effects depend on antibiotic used	Infectious diarrhea
Antibiotics	Metronidazole Vancomycin				
Corticosteroids	Dexamethasone	Suppresses inflammation and immune response	Hyperglycemia, Hypertension Mood changes Increased appetite Weight gain Peptic ulcers Immunosuppression, Cushing syndrome	Steroids should be given in the morning, or in split doses in morning and afternoon, as they cause insomnia Taking NSAIDs concurrently increases risk of gastrointestinal bleeding Monitor for fever and infection, as steroids cause immunosuppression Steroids must be tapered when discontinuing, otherwise there is a risk for adrenal insufficiency	Inflammatory bowel disease

NSAID, nonsteroidal anti-inflammatory drug.

Table 16-7

Treatment of Anxiety

Class	Prototype Medication	Mechanism of Action	Major Side and Adverse Effects	Critical Information	Indications
Benzodiazepine	Lorazepam	Binds with GABA receptors in central nervous system, which decrease brain stimulation	Drowsiness	Benzodiazepines can cause paradoxical reaction	Anxiety
			Dizziness		Dyspnea
			Lethargy	Benzodiazepines can result in addiction, tolerance, and physical dependence	
			Respiratory depression		
			Hypotension		
			Paradoxical effect—restlessness and agitation		

GABA, gamma aminobutyric acid.

Practice Questions and Rationales

1. A nurse is teaching a nursing student about a palliative care client's opioid medication. Which statement by the nursing student indicates a need for additional teaching?
    1. "I will need to make sure to stay ahead of the pain."
    2. "I will request a bowel regimen when my client becomes constipated."
    3. "My client has a history of drug and alcohol use, but this does not mean that we withhold pain medications."
    4. "There is no ceiling for opioid medications, but they must be titrated."

2. The nurse is assessing a client, who has lung cancer with spinal metastasis, for pain. The client tells the nurse that the ordered opioid medication helps, but there is still a shooting pain down the client's left leg. Identify the **best** pharmacologic measure to address this pain.
    1. A higher dose of the opioid
    2. An adjuvant, such as ibuprofen
    3. An adjuvant, such as gabapentin
    4. A different opioid medication

3. The nurse is assessing a client who takes nonsteroidal anti-inflammatory drugs (NSAIDs) for joint pain. Which statement by the client would be a **priority** concern for the nurse?
    1. "I have been eating more than usual."
    2. "I notice that I get a headache after I take the medication."
    3. "The medication helps, but I can still feel some pain."
    4. "I've been having severe stomach cramps and my stools are darker than usual."

4. A nurse assesses a client with end-stage chronic obstructive pulmonary disease (COPD) who is having severe dyspnea. Which action(s) should the nurse take? Select all that apply.
    1. Place the client in high Fowler position.
    2. Administer ordered anxiolytics.
    3. Administer high flow oxygen.
    4. Administer ordered opioids.
    5. Place the client in reverse Trendelenburg position.

5. The nurse is making medication rounds. Which client should the nurse **prioritize**?
    1. A client with diffuse inspiratory and expiratory wheezing, accessory muscle use, and a respiratory rate of 28.
    2. A client with bilateral crackles in the lung bases, lower extremity edema, and a respiratory rate of 22.
    3. A client who is anxious about a new terminal diagnosis with a respiratory rate of 28.
    4. A client with a history of emphysema and a respiratory rate of 24.

6. The nurse assesses a hospice client and finds that the client is breathing rapidly with accessory muscle use, has diffuse crackles and rhonchi, is sitting upright, and is diaphoretic. Which medication(s) will the nurse prepare to administer to relieve the client's symptoms? Select all that apply.

    1. Bronchodilators
    2. Morphine
    3. Prednisone
    4. Furosemide
    5. Scopolamine

7. The nurse notices that an actively dying client is suddenly agitated, restless, and hallucinating. What is the nurse's **priority** in this situation?

    1. Administer ordered neuroleptics immediately to treat delirium.
    2. Assess for dementia and possible causes.
    3. Assess for reversible causes of delirium.
    4. Administer pain medications, as pain often causes delirium.

8. The nurse sees that a hospice client, who is taking haloperidol, is grimacing and lip smacking. The client's family asks the nurse why this is happening. What is the correct response by the nurse?

    1. "This is called tardive dyskinesia. It is a side effect of haloperidol."
    2. "The dose of haloperidol needs to be increased to treat this."
    3. "I will contact the health care provider to discuss this finding with you."
    4. "This is a sign of worsening pain, I will request additional pain medications."

9. A client is taking quetiapine for sleep and for agitation. Which assessment finding would require **immediate** intervention by the nurse?

    1. A red, blistering rash
    2. Systolic blood pressure 98 mm Hg
    3. Heart rate 115 beats per minute
    4. Urinary output 30 mL over the past 2 hours

10. The nurse is assessing a palliative care client who has nausea and vomiting. The nurse finds that the client has hypoactive bowel sounds in all four quadrants. Which antiemetic would be the **best** choice for the nurse to administer?

    1. Ondansetron
    2. Metoclopramide
    3. Haloperidol
    4. Promethazine

11. The nurse educates a palliative care client about starting an appetite stimulant. Which statement indicates that the client has correctly understood the education?

    1. "The medication will help me gain all of the weight back that I lost."
    2. "The medication is a short-term measure to help me increase my appetite."
    3. "Appetite stimulants should be avoided, as they can be addicting."
    4. "If the medication does not work in a few weeks, I should keep taking it."

12. A hospice client has not had a normal bowel movement for the last 4 days, beyond a small amount of liquid stool. The nurse assesses the client's abdomen and finds bowel sounds present in all four quadrants, slight distension, and no pain. What is the nurse's **priority** action?

    1. Encourage the client to increase fiber and fluid intake.
    2. Administer ordered sennosides and docusate sodium.
    3. Check for impaction with a digital rectal exam.
    4. Administer an enema.

13. The nurse is teaching a palliative care client taking opioids about preventing constipation. Which statement(s) by the client indicates that the education has been successful? Select all that apply.

    1. "I should take suppositories daily to prevent constipation."
    2. "I should start a bowel regimen right away, as opioids cause constipation."
    3. "I should increase my fluid intake."
    4. "Immobility can worsen constipation."
    5. "I should use bulk-forming agents to help relieve my constipation."

14. The nurse is talking with the client about a recent terminal diagnosis. During the conversation, the nurse notices that the client is not paying attention, is pacing, and is breathing more rapidly. What do the client's actions indicate to the nurse?

    1. Anxiety.
    2. Terminal agitation.
    3. Psychosis.
    4. Nausea.

15. A palliative care client comes to the emergency department with nausea and vomiting on New Year's Eve. During the assessment, the nurse learns that the client lives alone and frequently comes to the emergency department on holidays with episodes of nausea and vomiting. Which medication does the nurse anticipate administering?

    1. Metoclopramide
    2. Benzodiazepines
    3. Ondansetron
    4. Haloperidol

17 HERBAL REMEDIES

BRIEF PRINCIPLES OF USE OF HERBAL REMEDIES

Herbal remedies have been used for thousands of years to treat ailments and diseases. Today their focus is more on overall well-being and health promotion rather than the treatment of a particular disease. Herbal remedies are becoming more common and frequently used among clients. The part they now play within the health care field cannot be ignored. The term "herbal remedies" refer to medications that are exclusively prepared using plants and sold over the counter as "supplements."

It is important to recognize that herbal remedies are not regulated for quality or potency as traditional medications are. In addition, these remedies are not subjected to the same rigorous studies to determine their efficacy and side effects. However, this is not to say these products are not beneficial for a client, and in fact, many clients take them and will attest to their benefits. Research is slow to come, but in some cases, evidence does exist to support the beneficial claims.

CLINICAL PEARLS: HERBAL REMEDIES

◆ Companies that produce herbal remedies can state the herbal remedy has any health benefit they choose; however, they can NOT claim that it treats any disease. For example, companies can state that raw garlic can help fight inflammation; however, they cannot state that raw garlic can be used to treat diabetes or lower cholesterol levels.

◆ As herbal remedies are not regulated in the same way other medications are, pregnant clients are not recommended to use them due to the unknown risk to themselves and the fetus.

◆ "Natural" is not synonymous with "safe." Herbal remedies can have dangerous side effects just as other medications can. Communication with the client's provider is essential for ensuring herbal-to-drug interactions do not occur and monitoring for potential side effects.

Assessment/Signs and Symptoms

◆ Client's past medical history as well as their current symptoms should be assessed.
◆ Signs and symptoms will vary depending on the condition the client is using the herbal remedy to treat.

Diagnostics

- ◆ Blood tests and/or cultures may be indicated for certain conditions or to determine the client's health status.

MEDICATION OVERVIEW: SPECIFIC HERBAL REMEDIES

There are many herbal remedies that clients may use. The most common ones are discussed here, with a focus on potential indications for use and critical information to know about the herbal remedy (see Table 17-1). In 1994, the Dietary Supplement Health and Education Act (DSHEA) was created and defined herbal remedies as dietary supplements. This means they are not treated in the same way as other medications and are not subjected to the same rigorous testing for safety and efficacy. In addition, the DSHEA gave the Food and Drug Administration (FDA) the authority to take any product that poses a significant risk to the public off the market, helping in some part to ensure client safety. Since that time, two other major rulings have been made pertaining to herbal remedies; in 2006, the Dietary Supplement and Nonprescription Drug Consumer Protection Act was passed mandating the reporting of serious adverse reactions for dietary supplements and nonprescription drugs, and in 2007, the FDA ruled that standardized manufacturing and labeling of dietary supplements must occur, along with quality control procedures clearly outlined.

SAFETY ALERT! Ginseng, St. John's wort, and several other herbal remedies affect the cytochrome P-450 drug metabolizing enzymes. Caution should be taken, and clients should be closely monitored when concurrently taking any other medication that also affects the cytochrome P-450 system.

Table 17-1

Herbal Remedies and Their Uses

Class	Properties of the Plant	Major Side and Adverse Effects	Critical Information	Potential Indications
Aloe vera	Two substances, the clear gel (topical or oral) and yellow latex (oral), are both used More than 75 biologically active compounds have been identified	Abdominal cramping and diarrhea (oral dose)	Aloe yellow latex contains potent laxative properties. Removed from over the counter in 2002 by the FDA due to safety concerns Use of topical aloe appears to be safe Caution used for clients with diabetes as aloe may decrease blood glucose levels	Yellow latex: constipation Clear gel: sunburns and other skin irritations, skin moisturizer, and reduction of inflammation
Black cohosh	Root or underground stem is active part of plant	Headache GI distress Weight gain Skin rashes Hepatotoxicity (rare)	Although research is inconclusive, some evidence suggests a safety risk for those with breast cancer taking this herbal remedy Isolated incidences of liver damage have been reported—clients with a history of liver disease should not use black cohosh Can be used in dried format, tablets, capsules, or as an extract No not confuse with blue cohosh, which has very different indications and may not be as safe to use	Rheumatoid arthritis Menopause symptoms Menstrual cycle irregularities Induction of labor
Echinacea	The entire plant, including root is used fresh or dried to produce effects	Allergic reactions (increased risk for those with other plant allergies) GI effects (nausea and stomach pain)	Can be used in extracts, capsules, tablets, and teas. Topical preparations also available Individuals with autoimmune disorders, tuberculosis and young children should avoid this herbal remedy Side effect severity and frequency increases when herbal remedy is used for >8 weeks	Viruses such as the common cold and influenza Improving the immune system May help treat infections including wounds and skin conditions (acne or boils)

Feverfew	Dried leaves, including flowers and stems are active parts of plant Pain relief properties come from parthenolides	Nausea Bloating When discontinued after long-term use, client may experience insomnia, headaches, and anxiety	Available in capsule form, as tablets, or liquid extract If fresh leaves are chewed, may cause sores and irritation in the mouth. Likewise, handling the plant may cause skin irritation—clients should wear gloves if handling fresh plant May affect uterine contraction in pregnant clients	To treat fevers Migraine headaches Menstrual irregularities Pain related to arthritis Anticoagulant Relief from seasonal allergies
Garlic	Garlic cloves are active parts of plant Can block lipid synthesis enzymes, decrease platelet aggregation, decrease LDL cholesterol, and inhibit angiotensin-converting enzyme Can also increase antioxidant status	Body odor Halitosis GI upset Increased risk of bleeding Allergic reactions are possible	Must be taken in raw form, cooking significantly weakens effects Supplements sold in tablet or capsule form Caution should be used for clients taking anticoagulants as garlic may increase risk of bleeding May interfere with medications used to treat HIV, clients should discuss use with provider	Increases client's antioxidant status Decreased platelet aggregation May have small effects on decreasing blood pressure Reduction in LDL cholesterol (Rahman & Lowe, 2006)
Ginger	Root of ginger plant is used for medicinal purposes Gingerol (oily resin in the root of the plant) has antioxidant and anti-inflammatory properties	GI distress including abdominal discomfort, heartburn, diarrhea, and flatulence	Can be eaten raw, used in powder or supplement, used as a liquid or oil Some evidence indicates that ginger may be helpful for nausea and vomiting related to pregnancy and cancer chemotherapy Researchers have not found harm in taking ginger while pregnant, however, clients should discuss with their provider	GI upset including indigestion and nausea Bacterial and fungal infections Support immune system Inhibit growth of certain cancer cells (Mashhadi et al., 2013)

(continued)

Table 17-1

Herbal Remedies and Their Uses (continued)

Class	Properties of the Plant	Major Side and Adverse Effects	Critical Information	Potential Indications
Ginkgo biloba	Flavonoids and terpenoids are active substances in the plant's leaves	Headache	Clients who are taking anticoagulants or are diagnosed with a bleeding disorder should not be using	Asthma
		Nausea		Bronchitis
		Diarrhea	Clients should discontinue use prior to surgery	Tinnitus
		Dizziness		Memory improvement
		Increase bleeding risk	May be taken in capsule, liquid extract, tablet, or capsule form	Intermittent claudication
		Seizures	Eating raw ginkgo seeds may be poisonous	
		Allergic reaction		
		Increased risk of bleeding		
Ginseng	The root of the plant is used for medicinal purposes	Headaches	May be taken in powdered format, tea, capsule, or tablet	May help to increase immune system, increase energy and stamina
		Nausea, vomiting, and diarrhea	Clients with diabetes already taking medications to lower their blood sugar should use with caution	Headaches
		Breast tenderness and menstrual irregularities		Erectile dysfunction
		Elevated blood pressure		Menopausal symptoms
		Decreased blood sugar		May help decrease blood sugar and lower blood pressure
				Dyspepsia
Milk thistle	Seeds from the plant contain the lipophilic extracts, known as silymarin	GI upset	Most commonly found in capsules	Liver disease such as hepatitis and cirrhosis
	Helps prevent liver from damage due to high lipophilic extract levels. These extracts help to increase immunity and decrease oxidative stress	Allergic reactions (more common in clients who have other plant allergies)	Clients with diabetes already taking medications to lower their blood sugar should use with caution	Lower cholesterol levels
		Decreased blood sugar		Anti-inflammatory

	Description	Side effects	Nursing considerations	Uses
Saw palmetto	Extracts of the saw palmetto fruit are used	GI distress Headache	Used in tablet or capsule form. May also be dried, made into a tea or taken raw as a whole berries Male clients have reported tender breasts and decreased sexual drive while taking saw palmetto	Urinary symptoms associated with benign prostatic syndrome Bladder and urinary disorders Hormone imbalances Migraine headaches
Soy	Soy bean used as a whole or isoflavones extracted to be used as a supplement Soy protein and isoflavones produce effects	GI upset, including diarrhea	Can be used in its' traditional use, as a food Also available as a dietary supplement, tablet, capsule, or powder Caution should be used giving isoflavones to clients with history of breast cancer	Menopausal symptoms (hot flashes) Treat high blood pressure and elevated LDL cholesterol levels Memory improvement
St. John's wort	The yellow flowers of the plant is used for medicinal purposes Produces hypericin and hyperforin, biologically active products	Anxiety Dry mouth Dizziness GI distress including nausea, vomiting diarrhea Fatigue Headache Photosensitivity	May be taken as tablet, capsule, liquid extract, or tea May decrease the effectiveness of many medications—use with caution and ensure the client's provider is aware of use Clients already taking antidepressants, oral contraceptives, digoxin, warfarin, or antiepileptics should not be taking due to risk of herbal–drug interactions Clients who are immunocompromised (e.g., individuals with HIV or recipients of a transplant) should not take this herbal remedy Interferes with the absorption of iron—should be taken separately from iron products	Depression Anxiety Premenstrual symptoms (Canning et al., 2010) Sleep disorders Nerve pain Anti-inflammatory processes including wound healing (topically)
Turmeric	Curcuminoids are the primary active ingredient and are found primarily in the plant's underground stems, or rhizomes Has antioxidant and antiinflammatory as well as antimicrobial properties	GI distress	Can be taken as a supplement (tablets or capsules), teas, or extracts Not to be confused with Japanese turmeric, an entirely different plant. This is a very common spice and a main ingredient of curry powder	Slow blood clotting Depression Reduce inflammation (cardiac and skin) Relieve pain associated with arthritis Help lower cholesterol Lower blood sugar

(continued)

Table 17-1

Herbal Remedies and Their Uses *(continued)*

Class	Properties of the Plant	Major Side and Adverse Effects	Critical Information	Potential Indications
Kava	Root and underground stem are used for medicinal purposes	Hepatotoxic	May be taken as extracts, tablets, capsules, or prepared into a liquid	Anxiety
		Dystonia		Insomnia
		Hypertension	Individuals with any history of liver disease or hypertension should avoid taking this herbal remedy	Menopause symptoms
		Skin problems (yellowed, scaly skin with long-term use)	The FDA has issued a warning in 2002 that using kava supplements may result in liver damage; all further government-funded studies were discontinued after this	Asthma
				Urinary tract infections
			Combination with alcohol may increase risk for liver damage	
Ma huang (ephedra) ****BANNED****	Dried stems and leaves of plants are used for medicinal purposes	Anxiety	Can be used in capsules, tablets, and extracts	Promote weight loss
		Dizziness		Increase energy levels
	The active ingredient, ephedrine, acts like an amphetamine with the ability to stimulate the nervous system and heart	Decreased urination	Banned by FDA in 2004 due to elevated risk for cardiovascular complications and stroke; risks outweighed any potential weight loss benefit	
		Nausea		
		Restlessness	Clients with history of seizure disorder have increased risk of worsening seizures if taking ephedra	
		Tremors		
		Psychosis	Clients should avoid using with caffeine	
			Clients with diabetes must avoid due to potential increase in blood sugar	

FDA, Food and Drug Administration; GI, gastrointestinal; LDL, low-density lipoprotein.

Practice Questions and Rationales

1. A male client reports using saw palmetto for an increased frequency of urination and asks the nurse about its use. What is the correct response by the nurse?

    1. "Saw palmetto has been banned for use by the FDA due to an increased risk of benign prostatic hyperplasia."
    2. "An increased frequency of urination can be caused by a number of factors. It is important to be assessed by your provider before starting the use of any herbal remedy."
    3. "It is important to ensure you have your prostate-specific antigen (PSA) levels drawn periodically while using saw palmetto."
    4. "Saw palmetto may cause a decreased sexual drive in male clients."

2. The nurse asks a nursing student about the risks associated with St. John's wort. Which statement by the student is correct?

    1. "St. John's wort cannot be taken with methylphenidate due to serious drug–drug interactions."
    2. "The use of St. John's wort is contraindicated for use by any female client of childbearing age."
    3. "The use of serotonin-specific reuptake inhibitors (SSRIs) and St. John's wort is contraindicated due to the risk of serotonin-related side effects."
    4. "St. John's wort is contraindicated for use in all elderly patients due to confusion and postural hypotension."

3. Which symptom would the nurse be **most** concerned with for a client taking kava supplements?

    1. Headache
    2. Skin rash
    3. Loss of peripheral vision
    4. A yellowing of skin

4. A client reports taking milk thistle as part of a treatment regimen for hepatitis C. The nurse is reviewing the client's medical history. Which condition in the client's history would concern the nurse?

    1. Gout
    2. Ragweed allergy
    3. Cooley's anemia
    4. Gallstones

5. A client reports taking echinacea to help stimulate her immune system and reduce the chance of catching a cold. The client reports taking a 300-mg capsule three times a day. If the client can purchase the herbal remedy only in 100-mg capsules, how many capsules does the client need to take with each dose?

    _____ capsules

6. A client with migraine headaches is taking feverfew to help with symptoms. The client reports recently starting a garden and plans to use the raw leaves in a salad daily. Which response by the nurse is appropriate?

    1. "Some people experience mouth ulcers and skin irritation when handling and ingesting raw leaves. Caution should be made when handling or eating raw leaves."
    2. "Raw leaves are contraindicated for use. You must boil the leaves before they are ingested."
    3. "The leaves are not the active part of the feverfew plant. You must use the root of the plant to achieve desired effects."
    4. "Feverfew must be grown in a lab environment to ensure its safety for use."

7. A client asks how herbal remedies are currently regulated to help ensure their quality and safety. Which is the **best** response by the nurse?

    1. "The measures of safety or quality put in place for herbal remedies in the United States are not subject to the same standards as conventional medications are. Use the products at your own risk."
    2. "The US Food and Drug Administration (FDA) has put several measures in place to help improve the quality and safety of herbal remedies, including manufacturing and labeling standards."
    3. "Herbal remedies are placed under the same rigorous standards for quality and safety as conventional medications are."
    4. "Manufacturers do not have to seek FDA approval before selling dietary supplements, and there is no guarantee herbal remedies are safe to use."

8. The client asks the nurse why it is important to keep providers informed of any herbal remedies they are taking. What is the nurse's **best** response?

    1. "The client's chart is not complete without every medication the client is taking listed."
    2. "Herbal remedies can interact with traditional medications and can cause significantly harmful results."
    3. "The interactions between herbal remedies and other medications are listed on herbal remedy labels; however, many clients do not take the time to read it."
    4. "Providers are mandated to report interactions between herbal remedies and traditional medications under the Dietary Supplement and Nonprescription Consumer Protection Act."

9. A client states that she took ma huang (ephedra) in 2002 and would like to restart taking the herbal remedy today to help with weight loss. What is the correct response by the nurse?

    1. "Clients with a history of cardiovascular disorders should not take ma huang. We need to do a full cardiac workup before starting the herbal remedy."
    2. "Clients should avoid using caffeine with this herbal remedy."
    3. "This herbal remedy has been banned for sale in the United States following a FDA ruling in 2004 and it's use should be avoided."
    4. "The herbal remedy has been shown to be effective for weight loss and can only be purchased overseas."

10. A client is interested in using herbal remedies asks the nurse how they will know what condition it will treat or cure from looking at the bottle. The nurse explains that due to the Dietary Supplement Health and Education Act of 1994, which statement may be seen on an herbal remedy container?

      1. "Reduces risk of cancer"

      2. "Eliminates pain associated with rheumatoid arthritis"

      3. "Decreases symptoms of menopause"

      4. "Helps support the respiratory system"

REFERENCES

Alcorn, J., Burton, R., & Topping, A. (2015). BCG treatment for bladder cancer, from past to present use. *International Journal of Urological Nursing, 9*(3), 177–186. doi:10.1111/ijun.12064

American Cancer Society. (2018). *Cancer facts and figures 2018.* Retrieved from https://www.cancer.org/content/dam/cancer-org/research/cancer-facts-and-statistics/annual-cancer-facts-and-figures/2018/cancer-facts-and-figures-2018.pdf

ASHP Guidelines on Handling Hazardous Drugs. (2006). *American Journal of Health-System Pharmacy, 63*(12), 1172–1191. doi:10.2146/ajhp050529

Beaver, C., & Magnan, M. (2015). Minimizing staff exposure to antineoplastic agents during intravesical therapy. *Clinical Journal of Oncology Nursing, 19*(4), 393–395. doi:10.1188/15.cjon.393-395

Bhatnagar, S., & Gupta, M. (2016). Integrated pain and palliative medicine model. *Annals of Palliative Medicine, 5*(3), 196–208. doi:10.21037/apm.2016.05.02

Burchum, J. & Rosenthal, L. (2019). *Lehne's pharmacology for nursing care* (10th ed.). St. Louis, MI: Elsevier.

Canning, S., Waterman, M., Orsi, N., Ayres, J., Simpson, N., & Dye, L. (2010). The efficacy of *Hypericum perforatum* (St. John's Wort) for the treatment of premenstrual syndrome: A randomized, double-blind, placebo-controlled trial. *CNS Drugs, 24*(3), 207–225.

CDC. (2004). Preventing occupational exposures to antineoplastic and other hazardous drugs in health care settings. doi:10.26616/nioshpub2004165a

Eilers, J., Harris, D., Henry, K., & Johnson, L. A. (2014). Evidence-based interventions for cancer treatment-related mucositis: Putting evidence into practice. *Clinical Journal of Oncology Nursing, 18*(s6), 80–96. doi:10.1188/14.cjon.s3.80-96

Held-Warmkessel, J. (2015). Looking into hyperthermic intraperitoneal chemotherapy. *Nursing, 45*(1), 65. doi:10.1097/01.nurse.0000458941.58372.1f

Karch, A. M. (2017). *Focus on nursing pharmacology* (7th ed.). Philadelphia, PA: Wolters Kluwer.

Katzung, B. (2018). *Basic and clinical pharmacology* (14th ed.). New York, NY: McGraw-Hill Education.

Mashhadi, N. S., Ghiasvand, R., Askari, G., Hadriri, M., Darvishi, L., & Mofid, M. R. (2013). Anti-oxidative and anti-inflammatory effects of ginger in health and physical activity: Review of current evidence. *International Journal of Preventive Medicine, 4*, S35–S42.

Miguel, R. (2000). Interventional treatment of cancer pain: The fourth step in the World Health Organization analgesic ladder? *Cancer Control, 7*(2), 149–156. doi:10.1177/107327480000700205

National Center for Complementary and Integrative Health. (2018, January). *Dietary and herbal supplements.* Retrieved from https://nccih.nih.gov/health/supplements

Parks, L., & Routt, M. (2015). Hepatic artery infusion pump in the treatment of liver metastases. *Clinical Journal of Oncology Nursing, 19*(3), 316–320. doi:10.1188/15.cjon.316-320

Rahman, K., & Lowe, G. M. (2006). Garlic and cardiovascular disease: A critical review. *Journal of Nutrition, 136*(3), 736S–740S.

Spoelstra, S., & Sansoucie, H. (2015). Putting evidence into practice: Evidence-based interventions for oral agents for cancer. *Clinical Journal of Oncology Nursing, 19*(3), 60–72. doi:10.1188/15.s1.cjon.60-72

Vallerand, A. H. & Snoski, C. A. (2018). *Davis's drug guide for nurses* (16th ed.). Philadelphia, PA: F.A. Davis Company.

World Health Organization. (1986). *Cancer pain relief.* Retrieved from Geneva website: ISBN 92 4 156100 9.

CORRECT ANSWERS AND RATIONALES

CHAPTER 1

1. **D 3.** The ALT level is high, indicating possible liver impairment, which could lead to alterations in drug metabolism. The provider should be notified about the laboratory result and to obtain a possible dosage adjustment, as the dose may need to be reduced for alterations in liver function. An elevated WBC is frequently the reason for antibiotic use; it is not a reason to withhold an antibiotic, as this is frequently a reason for administration of an antimicrobial medication. The serum creatinine is on the low end of normal and does not pose a risk of alterations in excretion. The serum albumin level is within normal range and does not pose a risk of alterations in medication distribution.
   Client Need Category: Physiologic integrity
   Cognitive Level: Analyze

2. **C 3.** Administration of three medications that with high affinities for protein will lead to competition for protein-binding sites. Ultimately, the medication with the strongest affinity to bind with protein will bind to a greater degree, leaving a higher amount of circulating free drug of the other two medications available for use in the bloodstream. This increase of circulating free drug increases the risk of toxicity, and serum drug levels should be assessed with dosing adjustments by the prescriber as needed. The serum albumin level of 6.2 g/dL (62 g/L) is higher than normal, which may lead to more drug–protein binding, which could result in subtherapeutic levels, not toxicity. The client on hemodialysis is at risk of subtherapeutic levels, as medications are commonly dialyzed out of circulation with hemodialysis. While the client prescribed four medications for hypertension is at greater risk of drug–drug interactions, this does not imply risk of toxicity.
   Client Need Category: Physiologic integrity
   Cognitive Level: Analyze

3. **M 4.** A medication with a narrow therapeutic index has an increased risk of causing toxicity. The first action by the nurse should be to assess the client for any signs and symptoms of toxicity caused by the medication, as the greatest priority is the client's safety and well-being. If signs of toxicity are present and found in the nurse's assessment, the nurse would then request an order for a serum drug level to evaluate the exact serum concentration of the medication in the client's system, which may guide the treatment plan ordered by the provider. Although reviewing the most recent liver and renal function should be done for all clients receiving any medications, this is not the priority at this

(continued)

E Easy   **M** Moderate   **D** Difficult   **C** Challenge

time and does not address therapeutic range. Dosing adjustments are necessary if signs of toxicity are present and/or serum drug levels are either below or above the normal range.

Client Need Category: Physiologic integrity

Cognitive Level: Apply

4. **ⓒ 205 mg total daily dose.**

Formula: Converting pounds to kilograms = pounds/2.2

18 lb/2.2 = 8.2 kg

25 mg/kg/day = 25 (8.2 kg) = 205 mg total daily dose

The total daily dose is represented by the total milligrams, not the volume. The preparation of the medication as 125 mg/5 mL will be considered when calculating the volume (mL) to administer based on the calculated dose (mg).

5. **ⓒ 4.** The nurse can suggest and implement nonpharmacologic techniques such as biofeedback, massage, and/or guided imagery in an effort to enhance the effectiveness of pain medication. Increasing the frequency of dosing may occur, but this is not the priority at this time as other nonpharmacologic interventions should be attempted first. The decreased effectiveness of the medication could be the result of tolerance to the medication, not toxicity. Physical dependence may occur when medications are used for prolonged periods of time; however, that would be evident if the client was experiencing a withdrawal syndrome, not tolerance.

Client Need Category: Physiologic integrity

Cognitive Level: Apply

6. **Ⓜ 1.** The medication should be held, and the prescriber should be notified to ascertain the correct dose for the medication. The nurse should not administer the recommended dose of the medication according to the drug manual, as it has not been prescribed and is outside of the nurse's scope of practice to determine dosing. It is not necessary to contact the pharmacist, as the nurse has already researched the dosing parameters for the mediation using an approved resource. Given that the client has a mild allergic reaction, it is not necessary to assess for anaphylaxis unless the client's condition has worsened.

Client Need Category: Physiologic integrity

Cognitive Level: Apply

7. **ⓒ 2.** The amount of protein in the bloodstream will alter drug distribution, not metabolism. Liver function is the primary factor in the metabolism of most drugs. All of the other statements are correct.

Client Need Category: Physiologic integrity

Cognitive Level: Apply

8. **ⓒ 3.** It takes ~4 half-lives of a medication for it to be metabolized and removed, provided metabolism and elimination functions are intact. For a medication with a half-life of 6 hours, 4 half-lives would be ~24 hours. The client should notice the effects of a medication, even with a one-time dose. The effects of the medication may start to decline after one half-life; however, this does not answer the client's question. It would also be important to consider the client's individual characteristics, including renal and hepatic function

Ⓔ Easy   **Ⓜ** Moderate   **Ⓓ** Difficult   **ⓒ** Challenge

as well as any genetic alterations that may alter medication metabolism, if known. There is interclient variability with all medications, so the average of four half-lives may vary from client to client. The nurse should be aware of typical metabolism and half-lives of medications and can answer the client's question without contacting the prescriber.

Client Need Category: Physiologic integrity

Cognitive Level: Apply

9. **Ⓔ 4.** When a medication is taken with food, the presence of food can alter its absorption pattern and decrease its effectiveness. When a medication is directed to be taken on an empty stomach, it should be taken 1 hour before or 2 hours after a meal. The nurse should not advise the client to take an additional dose, as this may lead to toxicity. Side effects may be less when taken with food, since absorption is decreased. The risk of toxicity is low when absorption is delayed by food.

Client Need Category: Physiologic integrity

Cognitive Level: Apply

10. **Ⓔ 2.** The priority of the nurse is to assess the client, including obtaining vital signs. Hemodialysis would be indicated if the poison cannot be removed in less invasive ways (activated charcoal, administration of an antidote, etc.). The nurse may insert a nasogastric tube and/or obtain blood work; however, the priority is to assess the client's baseline status to prepare for the initiation of any emergency interventions that may be required.

Client Need Category: Physiologic integrity

Cognitive Level: Apply

11. **Ⓜ 2.** The nursing process begins with client assessment followed by determining a nursing diagnosis, planning interventions, implementing care, and ending with an evaluation of that care. Evaluating the effectiveness of the medication therapy would be the next nursing responsibility.

Client Need Category: Physiologic integrity

Cognitive Level: Apply

12. **Ⓜ 3.** In most cases, the trade and generic versions of medication are equivalent, and the generic form is less expensive. Medications may have several brand names if marketed by a variety of companies. The chemical name is not used outside of the development phase.

Client Need Category: Physiologic integrity

Cognitive Level: Analyze

13. **Ⓓ 2.** The nurse should obtain baseline information prior to the administration of any medication so that the medication's effectiveness can be properly evaluated. Comparing vital signs, especially temperature, will help determine if the antibiotic is effectively managing the bacterial infection. Nausea and vomiting are possible side effects and will not help in the evaluation of medication effectiveness. Identifying allergies and taking a medication history are both vital but not related to evaluating medication effectiveness.

Client Need Category: Physiologic integrity

Cognitive Level: Apply

Ⓔ Easy   Ⓜ Moderate   Ⓓ Difficult   Ⓒ Challenge

14. Ⓜ **3.** Supratherapeutic signs and symptoms indicate a need to reduce or titrate downward the medication dosage as prescribed. Too high a dose of heparin will result in bleeding such as in the case of bright red blood noted in the stool. Ingesting red foods such as beets can result in red stool, but in this case, possible bleeding would be addressed first. Blood in the stool does not indicate an allergy. Increasing the dose of heparin may result in additional bleeding and is not appropriate in this client situation.

Client Need Category: Physiologic integrity

Cognitive Level: Analyze

15. Ⓜ **2.** Disruption of the blood–brain barrier (BBB) has an important part in cellular damage in neurologic diseases, including acute and chronic cerebral ischemia, brain trauma, multiple sclerosis, brain tumors, and brain infections. This damage and its ultimate effect on the BBB create problems with the distribution by which a medication exits the bloodstream and enters cells to exert its effect(s). Absorption depends on factors such as blood flow, surface area at the site of administration, perfusion and circulation, gastric pH, and the presence or absence of food in the stomach (for oral administration). The metabolism or breakdown of a medication commonly occurs in the liver. Disorders of the liver are primary barriers to effective medication metabolism. Excretion is the mechanism through which medication is removed from the body. Excretion is dependent on renal function and perfusion.

Client Need Category: Physiologic integrity

Cognitive Level: Apply

16. Ⓜ **1.** Topical absorptions via transdermal patches can be altered if lesions, burns, or breakdowns are present at the application site. Atherosclerosis affects the distribution of medications, while the other options would affect absorption of oral medications.

Client Need Category: Physiologic integrity

Cognitive Level: Analyze

17. Ⓒ **1, 2, 4, 5.** The implementation phase allows the nurse to complete the action of medication administration and follow through with the interventions designed during the planning phase. Interventions focus on methods to increase the effectiveness of medications through the use of nonpharmacologic adjuncts in nursing care, proper drug administration using the six rights of medication administration, and providing appropriate client education and consideration of client safety measures. Assessing how the client slept would be a part of the evaluation phase of the process.

Client Need Category: Physiologic integrity

Cognitive Level: Apply

18. Ⓓ **1, 2, 5.** No drug is perfect, and this can lead to medication nonadherence. Factors that contribute to nonadherence include cost, side effects, and ease of administration. While lifelong medication therapies and anger over the need for medication can be problematic, they tend to be issues that clients resolve in time and are not as likely to cause nonadherence.

Client Need Category: Physiologic integrity

Cognitive Level: Analyze

Ⓔ Easy　　Ⓜ Moderate　　Ⓓ Difficult　　Ⓒ Challenge

19. **D 4.** If the nurse is unfamiliar/uncertain about a prescribed medication, the drug reference manual on the unit would be the first resource to utilize to help clarify or enhance understanding of the medication. If the prescription remains unclear, or the nurse is not certain as to why the client is receiving the medication, the nurse should then consult with the prescribing health care provider. The nurse can also utilize the pharmacist, however this would not be the initial resource for the nurse. Asking for clarification from other nurses on the unit will not be the initial or best resource for medication clarification.

    Client Need Category: Physiologic integrity

    Cognitive Level: Apply

20. **D 1.** The liver is not completely developed until close to 3 years of age, slowing metabolism of medications, which can lead to toxic levels. None of the other medical conditions directly affect medication metabolism.

    Client Need Category: Physiologic integrity

    Cognitive Level: Analyze

21. **C 1, 5.** Distribution of medications throughout the body differs in older adults due to the decreased amount of total protein, lower amounts of body water and lean mass, and higher amounts of body fat. With age, liver function and hepatic blood flow decline and drug metabolism is slowed. Renal function also declines with age and is the most common reason for drug toxicity in older adults. Ease of administration and ability to swallow pills may impact adherence to a medication regimen, but it does not relate to adverse effects or toxicity. Ingestion of meat or poultry will not affect medication effects, side, or adverse effects. Height and/or weight is not used to adjust medication dosing in older clients.

    Client Need Category: Physiologic integrity

    Cognitive Level: Apply

22. **C 3.** Ethnic origin should also be considered when prescribing medications, as the genetic makeup varies by ethnicity. For example, Asian clients metabolize medications in the CYP450 2D6 system (e.g., SSRIs) more slowly, necessitating lower dosages to prevent toxicity. None of the other options accurately describe typical reactions of Asians to SSRI therapy.

    Client Need Category: Physiologic integrity

    Cognitive Level: Apply

23. **M 3.** Schedule I represents the medications with the highest potential for abuse that can cause both physical and psychological addiction. The withdrawal symptoms are severe and can even be fatal if left untreated. Treatments for such addictions are available and have been shown to be successful.

    Client Need Category: Psychosocial integrity

    Cognitive Level: Analyze

24. **C 2.** Poisons ingested orally within the past 3 hours or less can be treated with medications or other methods to decrease the gastric absorption. Knowing when the poison was ingested will be vital in determining the most appropriate means of poison removal. Assessing the child's level of consciousness, type of detergent, and allergy history will also be addressed; however, these questions will not direct the treatment strategy for the ingestion.

    Client Need Category: Physiologic integrity

    Cognitive Level: Analyze

E Easy   **M** Moderate   **D** Difficult   **C** Challenge

25. Ⓜ **2.** Activated charcoal should not be administered to clients with gastric perforations, bowel obstructions, or those at risk for gastric perforation since a healthy/functioning GI tract is required for successful treatment. None of the other options present a risk to the GI tract or the administration of activated charcoal.

Client Need Category: Physiologic integrity

Cognitive Level: Apply

CHAPTER 2

1. Ⓔ **4.** Administering potassium replacement in the setting of impaired renal function can lead to hyperkalemia, which can cause several adverse effects. Normal hourly urine output is ≥30 mL/hr. The nurse should notify the prescriber and anticipate an evaluation of the client's renal function prior to the administration of potassium. Potassium chloride should be administered over at least 60 minutes; infusing in 30 minutes may also cause adverse effects and will not address the urinary output. Administering the medication via the oral route may still lead to hyperkalemia in the setting of renal dysfunction. While increasing oral intake of fluids may be necessary if the low urine output is due to dehydration, that is not the priority action at this time.

Client Need Category: Physiologic integrity

Cognitive Level: Apply

2. Ⓓ **1.** Low magnesium and potassium levels can both lead to cardiac dysrhythmias, some of which are fatal. Knowing this, the first action of the nurse should be to assess the cardiac rhythm. The sodium is mildly elevated and does not indicate a need for seizure precautions. The calcium level is mildly decreased; adding foods high in calcium may occur; however, the cardiac rhythm related to the potassium and magnesium levels presents the greatest threat to the client and is the nurse's first priority. The phosphorus level is normal.

Client Need Category: Physiologic integrity

Cognitive Level: Analyze

3. Ⓓ **2.** The laboratory values indicate dehydration, with a high concentration of solutes (sodium) and a low concentration of water, as evidenced by the increased serum osmolality. The priority for this client is an increase in hydration using hypotonic fluids to prevent worsening of electrolyte imbalance and increased fluid volume. Treating the nausea with a medication such as ondansetron will be required once fluid volume status is attempted to be restored to prevent additional fluid losses. Insertion of an NG tube and taking the client for the CT scan will occur once the fluid volume losses are addressed.

Client Need Category: Physiologic integrity

Cognitive Level: Apply

4. Ⓜ **1.** Erythropoietin alfa can lead to the development of thrombi if administered to clients with hemoglobin levels >12 mg/dL (7.45 mmol/L). Knowing this potential adverse effect, the nurse should question the order. The medication should not be administered. A hemoglobin level of 13 mg/dL (8.07 mmol/L) does not warrant a blood transfusion with packed red blood cells or any other blood product. Blood transfusions are usually reserved for a

Ⓔ Easy   Ⓜ Moderate   Ⓓ Difficult   Ⓒ Challenge

hemoglobin level <8 mg/dL (4.96 mmol/L). Allergy history should be determined before any medications are administered; however, this is not the nurse's priority.

Client Need Category: Physiologic integrity

Cognitive Level: Apply

5. **C 2, 5.** A medication list is necessary to determine if there are other medications the client is taking that may impair clotting, such as aspirin or other nonsteroidal anti-inflammatory drugs (NSAIDs). The aPTT level will detect alterations in coagulation for clients with hemophilia, whereas the PT and INR will remain unchanged. Treatment of hemophilia A is with factor VIII, not IX. Preparing for a blood transfusion is not the priority until all laboratory results are obtained unless the client is currently bleeding uncontrollably, which is not the case.

Client Need Category: Physiologic integrity

Cognitive Level: Apply

6. **E 125 mL/hr.**
Formula: volume (mL)/time (hours) = flow rate in mL/hour
250 mL/2 hours = 125 mL/hr

Client Need Category: Physiologic integrity

Cognitive Level: Apply

7. **E 1.** The first action by the nurse should focus on relieving the cause of the client's shortness of breath by stopping the infusion. The nurse should then elevate the head of the bed. Immediately following, administer oxygen, and notify the prescriber.

Client Need Category: Physiologic integrity

Cognitive Level: Apply

8. **C 2, 3, 4, 5.** A serum sodium level of 127 mEq/L (127 mmol/L) places the client at risk for seizures. The nurse should initiate seizure precautions in the event that a seizure occurs. This includes side rail pads, having suction available at the bedside, and obtaining IV access. Lorazepam can be used to not only treat anxiety but also stop seizure activity should it occur. Telemetry is indicated for alterations in potassium and magnesium levels and is not necessary at this time.

Client Need Category: Physiologic integrity

Cognitive Level: Apply

9. **M 3.** Phlebitis is a common side effect of potassium chloride infusions. The best action by the nurse is to stop the infusion and restart at a new intravenous site. Slowing the infusion may decrease the phlebitis; however, it is best practice to avoid continued injury to that vein. Warm compresses may be applied for pain management once the site is discontinued. The infusion may continue at an alternate site without the need for an oral formulation.

Client Need Category: Physiologic integrity

Cognitive Level: Apply

10. **C 2, 3, 4, 6.** Potatoes, strawberries, spinach, and legumes are high in potassium. Carrots are high in vitamin A, and yogurt is high in calcium.

Client Need Category: Physiologic integrity

Cognitive Level: Apply

E Easy **M** Moderate **D** Difficult **C** Challenge

11. **C 2.** A decrease in GFR below 60 mL/min indicates altered renal function, which can lead to hypermagnesemia with possible adverse reactions such as cardiac dysrhythmias. The BUN is decreased, which does not imply renal dysfunction. Potassium and sodium do not affect MOM.

 Client Need Category: Physiologic integrity

 Cognitive Level: Apply

12. **C 1, 3, 4.** Treatment of hyperkalemia may include any or all of the following: insulin, loop diuretics, sodium bicarbonate, and/or sodium polystyrene sulfonate. Magnesium would not decrease potassium levels. Spironolactone is a potassium-sparing diuretic and would increase the potassium level further.

 Client Need Category: Physiologic integrity

 Cognitive Level: Apply

13. **D 3.** Elevated calcium levels in the blood can lead to accumulation of calcium in the form of kidney stones (nephrolithiasis). Symptoms of kidney stones include severe flank pain, hematuria, low-grade fever, and groin pain. Low levels of sodium or potassium and high levels of phosphate will not result in kidney stones.

 Client Need Category: Physiologic integrity

 Cognitive Level: Apply

14. **M 28 gtt/min**

 First, convert volume in liters to milliliters. Knowing 1 L = 1,000 mL, 2 L = 2,000 mL

 Then, calculate volume per hour. Formula: Volume (mL)/time (hours) = 2,000 mL/12 hours = 167 mL/hr

 Next, calculate gtts/min using the formula: volume per hour in mL × drop factor (gtt/mL)/time in minutes

 167 × 10/60 = 1,670/60 = 27.8, which rounds up to 28 gtt/min

 Client Need Category: Physiologic integrity

 Cognitive Level: Apply

15. **C 4.** A low-grade fever may occur during administration of blood products. If the client's temperature is <100.4°F (38°C), the nurse can administer acetaminophen, which is a fever reducer, and continue the infusion while monitoring the client closely. The rate does not need to be slowed for a low-grade fever as it may be with volume overload. Unless the client has shortness of breath or an oxygen saturation below 95%, oxygen is not necessary. The infusion will need to be stopped if the client's temperature continues to increase or the client develops other signs or symptoms of transfusion reactions.

 Client Need Category: Physiologic integrity

 Cognitive Level: Analyze

CHAPTER 3

1. **D 4.** Losartan, an angiotensin receptor blocker, can cause hyperkalemia, which can lead to potentially fatal dysrhythmias. The potential hyperkalemia should be investigated and treated immediately to avoid additional heart complications. Common symptoms

E Easy   **M** Moderate   **D** Difficult   **C** Challenge

of elevated potassium include weakness, nausea, palpitations, and chest pain. Checking the BP will not provide additional information about the client's symptoms or potassium level. Salt substitutes contain high amounts of potassium, which would worsen the existing hyperkalemia. It is not within the nursing scope of practice to advise the client to hold a medication without consulting the prescriber.

Client Need Category: Physiologic integrity

Cognitive Level: Analyze

2. **3.** The client's signs and symptoms indicate worsening of heart failure. For this reason, the furosemide, spironolactone, and lisinopril should be continued, but dose adjustments may be required upon discussion with the prescriber. The nurse should hold the digoxin for client heart rate <60 beats/min. Furosemide should not be held, as this would worsen edema and shortness of breath. Withholding all medications may result in acute exacerbation of symptoms. Administering all medications could result in severe bradycardia caused by the digoxin.

Client Need Category: Physiologic integrity

Cognitive Level: Analyze

3. **4.** Rivaroxaban is an anticoagulant used for the treatment or prevention of DVT. Due to its anticoagulant properties, bleeding is the most common and the most potentially serious side effect. Darkening of the stools may indicate bleeding in the gastrointestinal tract, which would require immediate evaluation. Warfarin, not rivaroxaban, interferes with vitamin K. Foods with higher levels of vitamin K, such as canola and vegetable oils, need to be consistent while taking warfarin. Heparin and warfarin both require regular lab work to check bleeding times, rivaroxaban does not. Treatment and prevention of DVT will continue beyond the time that the extremity is swollen and/or the DVT is resolved.

Client Need Category: Physiologic integrity

Cognitive Level: Apply

4. **2,3.** ST-segment elevation is diagnostic for an ST-segment elevation myocardial infarction (STEMI). During this acute process, the nurse's priority is to administer medications, which will decrease the size of the infarct and improve perfusion, including aspirin, nitroglycerin, beta-blockers, and morphine. Aspirin should be administered immediately for its antiplatelet effects. Serum lab testing for cardiac-specific troponin levels should be assessed immediately as an additional assessment of cardiac muscle damage. Oxygen should only be administered if the oxygen saturation is <93% to avoid oxygen toxicity and free radical production. Diltiazem, a calcium channel blocker, is used during episodes of variant angina or atrial tachydysrhythmias; it is not used in the treatment of STEMI. While nitroglycerin should be administered, it should only be given one tablet at a time every 5 minutes for a maximum of three tablets.

Client Need Category: Physiologic integrity

Cognitive Level: Apply

5. **3.** Colesevelam is a medication used to lower LDL cholesterol levels. In addition, it can also be used as an adjunct treatment for type-2 diabetes mellitus. The client should expect blood sugar levels to decrease, not increase, when colesevelam is taken with metformin. Colesevelam should be taken apart from other medications, as it may interfere with absorption. Constipation is a common side effect; increasing water and fiber would

(continued)

 Easy   Moderate   Difficult   Challenge

be an appropriate intervention to reduce constipation. Metformin dosing may be lowered if blood sugars lower while taking colesevelam.

Client Need Category: Physiologic integrity

Cognitive Level: Apply

6. **C 2.** Lovastatin is used to lower cholesterol and is frequently prescribed following a myocardial infarction. One potential adverse effect of lovastatin is severe muscle breakdown, known as rhabdomyolysis. This is a potentially fatal condition characterized by intense muscle pain, elevated creatine kinase levels, and the release of myoglobin in the urine. Tea-colored urine is the result of the myoglobin being excreted by the kidneys. Ventricular dysrhythmias, such as premature ventricular contractions, are common after STEMI and reperfusion treatment. While the BP is on the low side, it is not the most important finding requiring intervention. Bilateral crackles in the lungs may be a result of the recent STEMI and should be investigated further, but the tea-colored urine is the priority based on the newly prescribed lovastatin.

Client Need Category: Physiologic integrity

Cognitive Level: Analyze

7. **D 3.** The laboratory values indicate thrombocytopenia, supratherapeutic heparin, and low hemoglobin. All of these findings increase the risk of bleeding in a client on a heparin infusion. The first action by the nurse is to stop the infusion to prevent further lowering of the aPTT and platelet counts and notify the prescriber. The nurse will also assess for signs of bleeding, but the infusion should not be continued. Increasing or continuing the dose of heparin may result in worsening of the laboratory values and further increasing the risk of bleeding or hemorrhage.

Client Need Category: Physiologic integrity

Cognitive Level: Analyze

8. **C 3.** Gemfibrozil can increase the effects of warfarin, increasing the client's risk of bleeding. The nurse should consult with the prescriber and discuss this medication interaction prior to administering an increased dose of warfarin. The nurse should review the PT and INR levels, but this is not the priority and would not account for the newly prescribed gemfibrozil and its potential effects on bleeding times. Holding the gemfibrozil is not necessary.

Client Need Category: Physiologic integrity

Cognitive Level: Analyze

9. **C 1.** Verapamil is a calcium channel blocker that results in decreased automaticity, AV-node conduction, and cardiac contractility. The normal range for a PR interval is 0.12 to 0.2 ms. A PR interval of 0.3 ms suggests an AV-node heart block, which would require holding the medication and notifying the prescriber. The medication may be continued; however, since this is a new finding, the nurse should hold the medication until the prescriber is aware of the ECG change. Verapamil will help to reduce heart rate and should be administered for a ventricular rate of 125 beats/min. The atrial-to-ventricular ratio of 4:1 is an expected finding for a client in atrial flutter. Occasional PVCs would not warrant withholding the verapamil.

Client Need Category: Physiologic integrity

Cognitive Level: Analyze

E Easy   **M** Moderate   **D** Difficult   **C** Challenge

10. **C** **1, 2, 4.** The rhythm on the telemetry strip is consistent with supraventricular tachycardia. Based on the client's symptoms, the nurse should administer oxygen for the shortness of breath and tachycardia. Asking the client to bear down/perform the Valsalva maneuver is a noninvasive technique that can help decrease heart rate. Adenosine is the pharmacologic treatment of choice for clients with supraventricular tachycardia. Pacer pads are used for symptomatic bradycardic rhythms, not tachycardic rhythms. Amiodarone is approved for use in ventricular dysrhythmias and also commonly used for atrial fibrillation; it is not used to treat supraventricular tachycardia.

    Client Need Category: Physiologic integrity

    Cognitive Level: Analyze

11. **C** **1, 2.** Decreasing dietary sodium will aid in the reduction of fluid retention, which can relieve symptoms of HF. Furosemide, a loop diuretic, is the most effective medication for reducing excess fluid volume to improve symptoms of HF. It is beyond the nurse's scope of practice to recommend dose adjustments of any medications. Increasing fluid intake will lead to worsening of symptoms through the increased fluid volume. Increasing dietary potassium will not improve cardiac function and may promote hyperkalemia in client's taking medications that increase potassium levels, such as spironolactone and losartan.

    Client Need Category: Physiologic integrity

    Cognitive Level: Apply

12. **C** **2.** Lower extremity edema may be a sign of heart failure, a potential adverse effect of metoprolol. This should be investigated further for additional signs and symptoms (weight gain, jugular vein distention, shortness of breath); and the prescriber should be notified. A heart rate of 62 is within normal limits. Diminished breath sounds in the left lower lobe are abnormal; however, they are unrelated to hypertension or metoprolol. The blood glucose level is high, which may be a side effect of beta$_1$ blockade, but this is not the priority assessment requiring immediate intervention.

    Client Need Category: Physiologic integrity

    Cognitive Level: Analyze

13. **C** **4.** Prazosin, an alpha 1 adrenergic antagonist, can cause first-dose hypotension and possible loss of consciousness. For this reason, the client should be advised not to get out of bed without assistance. The nurse should offer to ambulate with the client to prevent falls secondary to the side effects of the medication. The medication can be administered with or without food and should be given at bedtime. The client should also be placed on fall precautions. Raising all side rails is a form of restraint and should not be done.

    Client Need Category: Physiologic integrity

    Cognitive Level: Apply

14. **C** **1375.2 units/hr.**

    Formula: weight in kg = weight in lbs/2.2

    168/2.2 = 76.4 kg

    Initial dose = 80 units/kg bolus and 18 units/kg/hr infusion

    Bolus = 80 units × 76.4 kg = 6,112 units

    Initial dose of infusion = 18 units × 76.4/hour = 1375.2 units/hr

    Client Need Category: Physiologic integrity

    Cognitive Level: Apply

E Easy   **M** Moderate   **D** Difficult   **C** Challenge

15. **C 27.5 mL**

    25,000 units/500 mL = 50 units/mL

    Solving for x

    $$\frac{50\ \text{units}}{1\ \text{mL}} = \frac{1375.2\ \text{units}}{x\ \text{mL}}$$

    $50x = 1375.2$

    $x = 1375.2/50$

    $x = 27.5$ mL/hr

    Client Need Category: Physiologic integrity
    Cognitive Level: Apply

16. **M 2.** Furosemide is a loop diuretic and blocks sodium and water reabsorption in the ascending loop of Henle, which results in a loss of water and electrolytes. It may lead to dehydration, hypokalemia, hypomagnesemia, hyponatremia, and hypochloremia. Hypoxia may be present if the client has heart failure, and this may be improved with the administration of furosemide.
    Client Need Category: Pharmacological and parenteral therapies
    Cognitive Level: Apply

17. **C 1.** Nifedipine is a calcium channel blocker and blocks calcium channels in the blood vessels, which causes vasodilation and improves perfusion of coronary arteries. Hydralazine is an arterial vasodilator and dilates the arteries. Both agents are used in treatment of hypertension and not congestive heart failure.
    Client Need Category: Pharmacological and parenteral therapies
    Cognitive Level: Remember

18. **C 3.** The nurse should instruct the client that NSAIDs reduce the effectiveness of thiazide diuretics and should be taken infrequently. A nurse should teach the client that hydrochlorothiazide is a diuretic, which blocks sodium and water absorption by the distal convoluted tubule in the kidney. A client taking this medication should be taught to reduce their sodium intake and check their blood pressure frequently. Unless the client also has heart failure and is utilizing the diuretic to reduce circulating fluid volume, it is not necessary to preform frequent weight checks.
    Client Need Category: Pharmacological and parenteral therapies
    Cognitive Level: Apply

19. **M 2.** A client taking spironolactone, a potassium-sparing diuretic, should be taught to avoid foods high in potassium such as bananas, spinach, and yogurt. The client should also be instructed in decreasing their sodium levels.
    Client Need Category: Pharmacological and parenteral therapies
    Cognitive Level: Remember

20. **D 1.** Lisinopril is an angiotensin-converting enzyme inhibitor, which causes vasodilation and a decrease in the blood pressure. If a cough develops, the client can be switched to an angiotensin II receptor blocker (ARBS), which blocks the angiotensin II receptors in the kidney. One of the ARBS is losartan. Hydralazine is an arterial vasodilator. Furosemide is a loop diuretic, and verapamil is a calcium channel blocker.
    Client Need Category: Pharmacological and parenteral therapies
    Cognitive Level: Apply

E Easy   **M** Moderate   **D** Difficult   **C** Challenge

21. **C 5.** Verapamil is safe to administer during pregnancy to manage hypertension. Pregnant clients should not be given any anti-hypertensive medication that affects kidney function such as angiotensin-converting enzyme (ACE) inhibitors such as lisinopril, angiotensin II receptor blockers (ARBs) such as losartan, and diuretics such as furosemide. These medications also have potential teratogenic effects and should be avoided. There are many cautions for use of hydralazine during pregnancy, especially in the third trimester. Since other safer anti-hypertensive medications are available, this medication should be avoided in pregnancy.

    Client Need Category: Health promotion and maintenance

    Cognitive Level: Remember

22. **C 4.** Diltiazem is a calcium channel blocker that blocks calcium channels, which causes vasodilation and improves perfusion of the coronary arteries. The client should be instructed in increasing fluids and fiber to prevent constipation that occurs as the medication relaxes the smooth muscle of the small intestine. The client should be instructed to check BP and heart rate prior to administering the medication and hold for HR < 60 beats/min and/or systolic BP < 90 mm Hg. Diltiazem does not affect the urine output like a diuretic; therefore, weekly weight is not necessary to monitor medication effectiveness. The medication does not produce a cough as a cough is associated with angiotensin-converting enzyme (ACE) inhibitors.

    Client Need Category: Pharmacological and parenteral therapies

    Cognitive Level: Apply

23. **E 3.** Digoxin has a narrow therapeutic range and the level should be checked prior to the administration of the dose. Normal range of digoxin which is a cardiac glycoside is 0.8 to 2 ng/mL (1.02 to 2.56 nmol/L). Normal white blood cell (WBC) count is 4,000 and 11,000 per mcL of blood. A normal range of potassium is between 3.6 and 5.2 millimoles per liter (mmol/L) of blood. The normal range of the BUN level is 7 to 20 mg/dL (2.5 to 7.1 mmol/L). An elevated white blood cell count is not a contraindication to the use of digoxin.

    Client Need Category: Pharmacological and parenteral therapies

    Cognitive Level: Apply

24. **E 4.** A systolic BP > 100 mm Hg is a normal finding; digoxin will not affect BP. Digoxin is a cardiac glycoside that inhibits sodium–potassium ATPase enzyme, which slows the heart rate and strengthens the contractions. The medication has a narrow therapeutic range, and the client should be instructed to check their apical heart rate for 1 full minute prior to administration of the medication. The client should also be instructed that an early symptom of toxicity is nausea and vomiting, and this should be reported immediately to the provider.

    Client Need Category: Pharmacological and parenteral therapies

    Cognitive Level: Apply

25. **C 1, 2, 4.** A client having an acute MI would be treated with a variety of medications. Morphine assists with the pain. Nitroglycerin is administered to decrease oxygen demand and dilation of the veins to reduce chest pressure. Metoprolol is a beta 1 selective adrenergic antagonist to slow the heart rate down to reduce conduction and contractility. Lisinopril is an angiotensin converting enzyme (ACE) inhibitor which decreases blood pressure by way of kidneys. This is usually used for chronic hypertension and not an acute MI. Warfarin is an oral anticoagulant and is used in long term anticoagulation and not the acute phase of an MI.

    Client Need Category: Pharmacological and parenteral therapies

    Cognitive Level: Remember

    E Easy   **M** Moderate   **D** Difficult   **C** Challenge

26. **C 1.** Gemfibrozil is prescribed for clients with an elevated triglyceride or VLDL and the goal is <150 mg/dL (1.69 mmol/L). VLDL contains the highest amount of triglycerides. VLDL is considered a type of bad cholesterol, because it helps cholesterol build up on the walls of arteries. Gemfibrozil can lower the triglyceride level and increase the HDL. An HDL level of 60 milligrams per deciliter (mg/dL) of blood or higher is recommended. HDL that falls within the range of 40 to 59 mg/dL is normal but could be higher. Having HDL under 40 mg/dL increases the risk of developing heart disease. LDL cholesterol levels should be <100 mg/dL. Total cholesterol levels <200 mg/dL are considered desirable for adults. A reading between 200 and 239 mg/dL is considered borderline high, and a reading of 240 mg/dL and above is considered high.

    Client Need Category: Reduction of risk potential

    Cognitive Level: Understand

27. **C 3.** The client should be instructed that the clopidogrel should be taken 12 hours from omeprazole, they should not be taken together or 4 hours apart. Clopidogrel is an anti-platelet and can cause GI upset, which is why the client is now prescribed omeprazole, a protein pump inhibitor. Metoprolol is a beta-blocker, and furosemide is a diuretic. The clopidogrel, metoprolol, and furosemide can be taken at the same time.

    Client Need Category: Pharmacological and parenteral therapies

    Cognitive Level: Apply

28. **E 1.** The nurse should instruct clients receiving any medications for clotting disorders carry a risk of bleeding. Instructions should include avoiding IM injections and unnecessary venipuncture, use of soft bristle toothbrush and electric razor, and avoiding the use of other medications that promote bleeding such as aspirin. The client should also be placed on fall precautions but does not need to only use the bedside commode. Telling the client to prepare for discharge is not a component of patient teaching specific to dabigatran.

    Client Need Category: Pharmacological and parenteral therapies

    Cognitive Level: Apply

29. **D 1.** Lovastatin is a HMG-CoA reductase inhibitor or statin that lowers LDL cholesterol. The medication works best when administered at night. The medication lowers LDL cholesterol and does not affect the BP. In addition, the client does not need to weigh themselves but should be instructed to return for laboratory values in 3 to 4 months. The medication does not affect the client feeling rested.

    Client Need Category: Pharmacological and parenteral therapies

    Cognitive Level: Apply

30. **E 1.** Sodium nitroprusside is a venous and arterial vasodilator, which will bring down the BP of the chronic renal failure client. The medication does not assist with decreasing pain or anxiety. Medications for pain would be morphine or a benzodiazepine to reduce anxiety. Nitroglycerin is used to decrease oxygen demand and coronary spasms for stable and unstable myocardial infarctions.

    Client Need Category: Pharmacological and parenteral therapies

    Cognitive Level: Apply

E Easy   **M** Moderate   **D** Difficult   **C** Challenge

CHAPTER 4

1. **E 1.** A spacer is a device that attaches directly to the MDI and works to increase the amount of medication that is delivered to the lungs. When using a spacer, less of the drug remains on the oropharyngeal mucosa, decreasing the risk of oropharyngeal candidiasis. Hand–mouth coordination is required with use of all MDIs; they cannot work passively as a nebulizer can. However, some spacers may have a one-way valve, decreasing the need for such coordination.

   Client Need Category: Physiologic integrity

   Cognitive Level: Application

2. **C 4.** Oropharyngeal candidiasis (oral thrush) and dysphonia (hoarse voice) are the most common side effects of using inhaled glucocorticoids; however, their risk can be diminished by rinsing and gargling with water after each dose and/or using a spacer. Otherwise, inhaled glucocorticoids may slow the rate of growth, but a client's adult height will not be affected. Calcium and vitamin D supplements should be taken along with participation in weight-bearing exercise to help decrease the risk of bone loss that may occur when inhaled corticosteroids are used over long periods of time. Long-term use of inhaled glucocorticoids may increase the risk of cataracts and glaucoma.

   Client Need Category: Physiologic integrity

   Cognitive Level: Apply

3. **D 1.** It is essential that clients contact their health care provider if they need to use a short-acting beta$_2$-agonist rescue inhaler more than twice weekly. Short-acting beta$_2$ agonists may cause tachydysrhythmias, angina, and seizures when taken in excessive amounts. Oral beta$_2$ agonists are to be used for long-term control only; they cannot act quickly enough to abort an oncoming attack. Long-acting inhaled beta$_2$ agonists are dosed on a fixed schedule, not an as needed basis. To provide quick relief, beta agonists must be administered via inhalation.

   Client Need Category: Physiologic integrity

   Cognitive Level: Analyze

4. **D 2.** The withdrawal of glucocorticoids should be done slowly to allow time for the adrenal glands to fully recover, which may take 6 to 8 weeks. The time taken for the adrenal glands to recover is directly related to the length of time the client has been taking oral glucocorticoids rather than to the dosage taken. Signs and symptoms of glucocorticoid withdrawal syndrome include hypotension, hypoglycemia, myalgia, arthralgia, and fatigue.

   Client Need Category: Physiologic integrity

   Cognitive Level: Analyze

5. **M 3.** The treatment goals of COPD are to reduce the client's symptoms, prevent progression of the disease, and prevent exacerbations of COPD. COPD is complicated by the fact that many clients have comorbidities, and a complete recovery is not possible. Treatment instead focuses on preventing a progression of the disease. All clients with COPD may be treated with long-acting bronchodilators for management of COPD; if the client stops responding to the long-acting bronchodilator, glucocorticoids can be given. Lastly,

   (continued)

 E Easy   **M** Moderate   **D** Difficult   **C** Challenge

systemic glucocorticoids provide a substantial improvement in outcomes when used for COPD exacerbations.

Client Need Category: Physiologic integrity

Cognitive Level: Application

6. **C 1, 2, 5.** Side effects of PED-4 inhibitors include diarrhea, weight loss, nausea, back pain, insomnia, headache, and depression. Hypertension is not a known side effect of this medication. This drug helps reduce cough (and inflammation).

Client Need Category: Physiologic integrity

Cognitive Level: Apply

7. **C 4.** Anticholinergics like ipratropium bromide can cause side effects such as dry mouth, blurred vision, photophobia, constipation, and tachycardia. Urinary retention, not an increase in voiding, may also occur. Gastric upset and postural hypotension are not known side effects of this medication.

Client Need Category: Physiologic integrity

Cognitive Level: Apply

8. **C 3.** Intranasal glucocorticoids (fluticasone) are the most effective medication for the treatment of seasonal and perennial allergies. Oral sympathomimetics (pseudoephedrine) can only relieve nasal congestion; they do not reduce rhinorrhea or sneezing. Oral antihistamines are most effective when taken prophylactically.

Client Need Category: Physiologic integrity

Cognitive Level: Apply

9. **C 2.** Most first-generation antihistamines have significant anticholinergic effects, whereas second-generation antihistamines are largely devoid of anticholinergic side effects. Sedation is a major issue with first-generation antihistamines. Second-generation antihistamines all work equally as well and do not cross the blood–brain barrier as much as do first-generation antihistamines, which is why they produce much less sedation.

Client Need Category: Physiologic integrity

Cognitive Level: Apply

10. **D 3.** Pseudoephedrine can cause vasoconstriction and is therefore contraindicated for anyone with a history of cardiovascular disease. Topical sympathomimetics, not oral ones, have a risk of rebound congestion when they are used for more than a few days. Pseudoephedrine and ephedrine are both associated with abuse by causing CNS stimulation, and individuals have limits on their daily and monthly purchases of the medication.

Client Need Category: Physiologic integrity

Cognitive Level: Analyze

11. **M 2.** Combination over-the-counter cold remedies can be beneficial to a client. However, they frequently include medications the client does not need. Therefore, the client should be educated to choose a product that only contains medications to treat the symptoms he/she currently has. There is no proof of efficacy of over-the-counter cold remedies for pediatric clients; use of these medications should be limited to those over the age of 6 per the American Academy of Pediatrics, the Canadian Paediatric Society, and Health Canada. Antihistamines are frequently added to combination over-the-counter cold

E Easy　　**M** Moderate　　**D** Difficult　　**C** Challenge

remedies to help suppress mucus secretion (and can sometimes worsen the situation by thickening the mucus, not allowing it to drain). In addition, caffeine may be added as well to combat against the sedation caused by the antihistamine. It is important to remember that cold medications are used to treat the symptoms of a cold and cannot cure a cold. The common cold is a self-limiting virus, with no known cure.

Client Need Category: Physiologic integrity

Cognitive Level: Apply

12. **Ⓜ 2.5 mL**

Universal formula is used: $\dfrac{D(\text{desired amount}) \times V(\text{volume})}{H(\text{amount on hand})} = \text{Dose}$

$\dfrac{15 \text{ mg} \times 5 \text{ mL}}{30 \text{ mg}} = 2.5 \text{ mL}$

Client Need Category: Physiologic integrity

Cognitive Level: Analyze

13. **Ⓔ 1.** Rebound congestion occurs when intranasal decongestants such as oxymetazoline are taken for more than a few days. The client should be instructed to stop the medication, although an intranasal glucocorticoid may be added as the oxymetazoline is tapered to decrease discomfort. Discontinuation of the oxymetazoline is the priority action of the nurse.

Client Need Category: Physiologic integrity

Cognitive Level: Analyze

14. **Ⓜ 3.** Albuterol should be used cautiously for clients with a history of coronary artery disease, arrhythmias, hypertension, hyperthyroidism, seizure disorders, diabetes, glaucoma, and hypokalemia. A history of coronary artery disease, arrhythmias, or hypokalemia is most concerning because ventricular ectopy and/or ischemia may occur. There are no known contraindications for clients with a history of chickenpox or gout.

Client Need Category: Physiologic integrity

Cognitive Level: Apply

15. **Ⓔ 2 tablets.**

$\dfrac{\text{Order}}{\text{Supply on hand}} = \dfrac{40 \text{ mg}}{20 \text{ mg}} = 2 \text{ tablets}$

Client Need Category: Physiologic integrity

Cognitive Level: Analyze

CHAPTER 5

1. **Ⓓ 1.** Early signs of systemic toxicity are tinnitus, diplopia, lightheadedness, and a metallic taste in the mouth. If not treated, nystagmus, slurred speech, and tremors may develop followed by seizures, respiratory depression, and coma. The prescriber should be notified, and the nurse should be prepared to initiate further emergency interventions if necessary. Allergic reactions are extremely rare for an amide-type anesthetic such as lidocaine but would include signs or symptoms such as pruritus, urticaria, laryngeal edema, facial

(continued)

 Easy   Moderate   Ⓓ Difficult   Ⓒ Challenge

swelling, nausea, and vomiting. Lastly, lidocaine given topically could still result in systemic toxicity or an allergic reaction; particular caution should be given when the medication is applied to mucous membranes where the absorption rate is extremely high.

Client Need Category: Physiologic integrity

Cognitive Level: Analyze

2. **D** **4.** The use of opiates should be used with caution for clients with a history of respiratory disorders, a head injury, benign prostatic hyperplasia, hypotension, liver disorders, or inflammatory bowel disease. Hypertension, renal disease, or gout would not exclude a client from taking morphine to treat pain postoperatively.

Client Need Category: Physiologic integrity

Cognitive Level: Apply

3. **E** **2.** The use of central nervous system depressants while taking morphine can result in profound sedation and respiratory depression. Use of alcohol while taking an opiate should be avoided. The use of opioids may result in cough suppression. Instruct clients to cough at regular intervals. Additionally, the use of opioids is contraindicated during pregnancy as well as during labor and delivery. When taken during the time of conception, opioids can increase the risk of spina bifida and congenital heart defects. Finally, the combination of opioids and an anticholinergic such as antihistamines can exacerbate the symptoms of constipation and urinary retention that occur with opioid use.

Client Need Category: Physiologic integrity

Cognitive Level: Apply

4. **E** **1.25 mL**

$$\frac{\text{Order dose} \times \text{quantity}}{\text{On hand amount}} = \text{Desired dose} \quad \frac{12.5 \text{ mg} \times 1 \text{ mL}}{10 \text{ mg / mL}} = 1.25 \text{ mL}$$

Client Need Category: Physiologic integrity

Cognitive Level: Analyze

5. **M** **2.** With initial use of opioids, many clients experience nausea and vomiting. An antiemetic can be given to help minimize the symptoms; however, tolerance does quickly develop. Nausea and vomiting are signs of neither an allergic reaction to an opioid nor an opioid overdose.

Client Need Category: Physiologic integrity

Cognitive Level: Analyze

6. **E** **1.** Respiratory depression is limited with the use of pentazocine, making it an ideal choice for the relief of mild-to-moderate pain in clients with a history of respiratory disorders. In addition, it does not cause euphoria and therefore the abuse liability is fairly low. Pentazocine actually increases the workload on the heart and should not be used for pain relief in clients having a myocardial infarction. As pentazocine is an agonist–antagonist opioid, special care must be taken for clients that are physically dependent on morphine or other opioid agonists when transitioning to pentazocine. Clients must be withdrawn from the opioid agonist first to avoid abstinence syndrome from occurring. Both morphine and pentazocine can be given via several different routes of administration, by mouth, intravenously, intramuscularly, and subcutaneously.

Client Need Category: Physiologic integrity

Cognitive Level: Apply

E Easy   **M** Moderate   **D** Difficult   **C** Challenge

7. **C 1, 2, 3, 4, 5.** Naloxone is an opioid antagonist and when given to client experiencing an opioid overdose, all the effects of the opioid are reversed, including sedation, euphoria, respiratory depression, pain relief, and abdominal cramping. Caution should be taken for clients physically dependent on opioids as the administration of naloxone will result in an immediate withdrawal reaction.

Client Need Category: Physiologic integrity

Cognitive Level: Comprehension

8. **E 4.** Tolerance is defined as the requirement of a larger dose of an opioid to produce the same response that could be previously achieved with a small dose of the medication. There is cross tolerance between all opioid agonists; however, cross tolerance does not exist between opioids and agents that depress the central nervous system, including alcohol. Tolerance also develops to respiratory depression; however, it does not for constipation and miosis. The client who has been taking the morphine with good therapeutic effects is not experiencing any signs of opioid tolerance.

Client Need Category: Physiologic integrity

Cognitive Level: Apply

9. **C 1.** Reye syndrome is associated with the use of aspirin in children under the age of 18, particularly following a viral illness such as chickenpox or influenza. Although rare, if left untreated, it has a mortality rate of up to 40%. Signs and symptoms come on quickly and include encephalopathy (confusion, hallucinations, lethargy) and liver damage. If not treated in time, these symptoms can progress to seizure and/or coma. It is a medical emergency, and treatment is aimed at supportive measures—ensuring hydration, electrolyte balance, maintaining cardiorespiratory status, and monitoring liver function. Salicylism symptoms include sweating, dizziness, and ringing in the ears; hypersensitivity reactions are very rare and even more uncommon in children under the age of 18. Symptoms of a hypersensitivity reaction include rhinorrhea, urticaria, bronchospasm, and throat swelling. While the symptoms reported are not typical symptoms of a client with chickenpox, the priority action is to address the administration of aspirin to the child.

Client Need Category: Physiologic integrity

Cognitive Level: Analyze

10. **C 1, 2.** Aspirin is contraindicated for clients with peptic ulcer disease, a history of a hypersensitivity reaction to NSAIDs, and bleeding disorders including hemophilia and vitamin K deficiency. Caution should be taken for clients with an active *Helicobacter pylori* infection, heart failure, hepatic cirrhosis, asthma, nasal polyps, or a history of alcoholism; however, the use of aspirin is not contraindicated. Gout is not an associated risk factor when taking aspirin.

Client Need Category: Physiologic integrity

Cognitive Level: Apply

11. **D 2.** The American College of Gastroenterology recommends that clients with an increased risk for developing ulcers receive prophylaxis with a proton pump inhibitor while taking NSAIDs. Clients at risk include those with a history of peptic ulcer disease,

(continued)

E Easy   **M** Moderate   **D** Difficult   **C** Challenge

currently taking glucocorticoids and older clients. Peptic ulcers are not associated with rheumatoid arthritis, myocardial infarction, or metformin use.

Client Need Category: Physiologic integrity

Cognitive Level: Apply

12. **D 3.** Ibuprofen and other NSAIDs blunt the effect of the vaccination by decreasing the production of antibodies necessary to mount the immune response desired by the vaccination. Ibuprofen can be used in babies as young as 2 months old with positive effects and ibuprofen can be given by mouth and Reye syndrome is associated with aspirin only.

Client Need Category: Physiologic integrity

Cognitive Level: Analyze

13. **C 4.** COX-2 inhibitors increase vasoconstriction within the blood vessels and as a result, increase the risk of myocardial infarction, stroke, and other cardiovascular events. Toxic metabolites are not formed with this medication. The risk of bleeding is not increased in COX-2 inhibitors as they do not inhibit COX-1 and suppress platelet aggregation. Renal impairment may be seen with the use of COX-2 inhibitors, however their use is not associated with liver damage.

Client Need Category: Physiologic integrity

Cognitive Level: Analyze

14. **M 3.** Therapeutic doses of acetaminophen are less than 4,000 mg/day, and acetaminophen overdoses account for almost 50% of all acute liver failure clients in the United States. The early signs of acetaminophen overdose are nausea, vomiting, diarrhea, sweating, and abdominal pain and may progress into liver failure if not treated. Signs of liver damage do not appear for 2 to 3 days after acetaminophen overdose; therefore, early symptoms are often overlooked until too late. Clients must seek immediate treatment for a suspected overdose, and acetylcysteine, the antidote for acetaminophen, is given to treat an overdose along with supportive care. Steven-Johnson syndrome has also been associated with the use of acetaminophen; however, it is characterized by a painful rash and blistering of the skin. It too is a medical emergency and can result in death if left untreated.

Client Need Category: Physiologic integrity

Cognitive Level: Analyze

15. **M 1.** The client is in acute pain and morphine, and an opioid is recommended for acute pain. Aspirin renders platelets inactive and may increase bleeding postoperatively. Ketorolac is anti-inflammatory and used for mild to moderate pain. The client is experiencing severe pain, and an opioid is necessary to assist in the acute pain phase. Pregabalin is indicated for neuropathic pain and not acute pain.

Client Need Category: Physiologic integrity

Cognitive Level: Apply

16. **M 4.** The client is experiencing neuropathic pain. This pain responds to adjuvant analgesics such as anti-inflammatory agent celecoxib. Opioids such as hydromorphone and fentanyl are used as a last resort. Melatonin is used for short-term treatment of troubled sleeping.

Client Need Category: Physiologic integrity

Cognitive Level: Apply

E Easy   **M** Moderate   **D** Difficult   **C** Challenge

CHAPTER 6

1. **E 2.** Combining metronidazole with any amount of alcohol leads to a disulfiram-like reaction, which causes severe nausea and vomiting. Alcohol should be avoided while taking metronidazole. Darker urine, which may be a sign of dehydration, is not a common side or adverse effect of metronidazole. Nausea is a common side effect of the medication that would not require intervention. Dietary changes such as increasing green leafy vegetables will not affect the absorption or effectiveness of metronidazole.
   Client Need Category: Physiologic integrity
   Cognitive Level: Apply

2. **M 2.** Penicillin V potassium includes potassium in its formulation. Tall, peaked T waves on the ECG could be indicative of hyperkalemia, which is a potential adverse effect of penicillin V potassium. Due to the risk of dysrhythmias in the setting of hyperkalemia, the nurse would need to notify the provider of these findings immediately. An elevated WBC count is expected in the presence of a bacterial infection and does not require immediate intervention. Hypoactive bowel sounds, while abnormal, do not occur secondary to this medication and do not require immediate alert of the provider. The absolute neutrophil count is normal.
   Client Need Category: Physiologic integrity
   Cognitive Level: Analyze

3. **E 1.** The symptoms are consistent with "red man" syndrome, a type of hypersensitivity reaction caused by vancomycin. Treatment consists of discontinuing the infusion immediately, followed by administration of antihistamines. The medication may be resumed and infused at a slower rate, at the discretion of the prescriber, after antihistamines are administered. Until the reaction is treated, the priority action of the nurse is to stop the infusion. Epinephrine is not indicated for "red man" syndrome. Diphenhydramine is administered. However, the first action by the nurse is to stop the infusion.
   Client Need Category: Physiologic integrity
   Cognitive Level: Analyze

4. **C 4.** The antibiotic clindamycin carries a high risk of causing *Clostridium difficile* infection, a serious and potentially fatal adverse reaction. If a client reports several episodes of diarrhea, the medication should be stopped immediately, and the client should be tested for *C. difficile*. Although diarrhea can occur with many antibiotics, diarrhea associated with clindamycin must be investigated further, and increasing dietary fiber will not resolve the problem. It is not within the scope of practice of the nurse to alter a medication's dosage, and this will not correct diarrhea caused by *C. difficile*.
   Client Need Category: Physiologic integrity
   Cognitive Level: Apply

5. **D 3.** Oral antifungal medications carry a much greater risk of hepatotoxicity, and fatal hepatic necrosis has occurred. For non–life-threatening superficial fungal infections, such as those within toe or fingernails, topical preparations are preferred to avoid hepatotoxicity. Ketoconazole treats fungal, not viral infections. Discoloration of the nails is a harmless
   (continued)

E Easy   **M** Moderate   **D** Difficult   **C** Challenge

effect of nail fungus, which will resolve over several months as the nail grows out. The nurse should instruct the client about the risks of the oral formulation and advise against it.

Client Need Category: Physiologic integrity

Cognitive Level: Apply

6. **E 2.** The first action by the nurse is to determine if the client took the antibiotic as prescribed, because noncompliance with an antibiotic regimen is a common reason for undertreatment of a bacterial infection. Restarting the antibiotic is not appropriate instruction; the client will need to have the urine tested for the presence of infection prior to treatment. Symptoms do not commonly return after completing an antibiotic regimen, unless the bacteria were not susceptible to the antibiotic or the full course of treatment was not completed. Although another infection is possible, that is not the best response by the nurse at this time. The symptoms may be those of a new infection or an under-treated first infection.

Client Need Category: Physiologic integrity

Cognitive Level: Apply

7. **D 3.** Fluoroquinolones such as ciprofloxacin must be administered separately from calcium and calcium-containing supplements to reduce the risk of decreased absorption. The nurse should contact the prescriber to request a change in the time of administration of the calcium so that the antibiotic may be started to treat the bacterial infection without delay. The nurse should not administer both medications at 0800, because this will decrease the absorption and effectiveness of the antibiotic. Holding the ciprofloxacin dose will alter treatment of the infection and should be avoided. The pharmacist is not responsible for changing the antibiotic for the client. The nurse should contact the pre-scriber to make that change.

Client Need Category: Physiologic integrity

Cognitive Level: Analyze

8. **C 2, 3, 4, 5.** Women who are pregnant, adults with chronic illnesses such as asthma, clients who are immunosuppressed by diseases or medications, and individuals caring for immu-nosuppressed individuals should receive the annual influenza vaccination. Young adults without risk factors do not require annual vaccination, although it should be encouraged.

Client Need Category: Physiologic integrity

Cognitive Level: Apply

9. **E 125 mL/hr.**

Rationale: Constant: 250 mL normal saline × 1 hour = 250 mL/hr

250 mL/2 hours = 125 mL/hr

Client Need Category: Physiologic integrity

Cognitive Level: Apply

10. **D 1.** Acyclovir is safe to take during pregnancy and should be continued, especially during the last 5 weeks of the pregnancy to reduce the risk of transmission of the her-pes virus to the baby during delivery. There is no indication that a topical formulation is required while pregnant. The medication should not be discontinued completely; the

E Easy   **M** Moderate   **D** Difficult   **C** Challenge

risk of transmission to the child during birth would be greatly increased. Acyclovir can be taken to suppress future outbreaks, not only during active outbreaks. It is especially important to reduce the risk of outbreaks while pregnant to decrease the risk of transmission to the child.

Client Need Category: Physiologic integrity

Cognitive Level: Apply

11. **Ⓓ 2, 3.** Red-orange discoloration of sweat, saliva, tears, and urine is a harmless side effect of rifampin. The discoloration of tears may stain contact lenses, and these may need to be replaced. Liver injury is a common adverse effect of rifampin, but it does not present with orange discoloration of tears, and it does not indicate a worsening of the disease process. Decreasing dietary beta carotene will not alter this harmless side effect caused by rifampin.

Client Need Category: Physiologic integrity

Cognitive Level: Apply

12. **Ⓓ 2.** Latent tuberculosis is treated with monotherapy using isoniazid. Monotherapy for latent tuberculosis is not a prescribing error. Active tuberculosis would require a second agent, such as rifapentine. Gram stains for tuberculosis direct treatment; however, this is not the correct response to the client's question based upon the type of tuberculosis the client currently has. Treatment will be with one drug; a second drug would not be added unless the client develops active tuberculosis.

Client Need Category: Physiologic integrity

Cognitive Level: Apply

13. **Ⓓ 4.** Fluoroquinolones such as ciprofloxacin can worsen muscle weakness caused by myasthenia gravis. Clients with myasthenia gravis should not take fluoroquinolones for any reason. The nurse should hold the medication and contact the prescriber to request an alternative antibiotic class. The nurse will document the diagnosis; however, this is not the priority nursing action. A higher dose of ciprofloxacin will increase the risk of muscle weakness. The nurse may monitor renal function prior to administering antibiotics, but the ciprofloxacin should be held based on the medical history of the client.

Client Need Category: Physiologic integrity

Cognitive Level: Analyze

14. **Ⓓ 3, 4, 5.** Other potentially nephrotoxic medications should be avoided while administering amphotericin. Medications that can be toxic to the kidneys include cyclosporine (an immunosuppressant), gentamicin (an aminoglycoside), and ibuprofen (a nonsteroidal anti-inflammatory drug). Acetaminophen and fexofenadine are not known to cause renal toxicity and can be used.

Client Need Category: Physiologic integrity

Cognitive Level: Apply

15. **Ⓒ 2, 3.** Boceprevir and lamivudine are antiviral agents used in the treatment of chronic hepatitis B. Interferon alfacon-1 and ribavirin are used to treat hepatitis C. Acyclovir, while an antiviral medication, is not approved to treat hepatitis.

Client Need Category: Physiologic integrity

Cognitive Level: Apply

Ⓔ Easy   Ⓜ Moderate   Ⓓ Difficult   Ⓒ Challenge

16. **D 1.** A superinfection occurs during antibiotic therapy when the normal protective flora has been destroyed from the antibiotic, causing overgrowth of bacteria or fungi. An esophageal yeast infection is the result of this loss of normal flora. Although yeast infections can also occur due to immune suppression and hyperglycemia, these issues are not implied within this question. While it is a second infection, it is not bacterial and is directly related to the antibiotic therapy.

    Client Need Category: Physiologic integrity

    Cognitive Level: Apply

17. **D 2.** The minimum bactericidal concentration is the lowest amount of an antibiotic required to produce killing of bacterial cells. Following the completion of an antibiotic regimen, increased tactile fremitus would indicate continued consolidation of the lung field, which may signify unresolved pneumonia. Sterile sputum cultures and a white blood cell count of 4,500 units/L (4.5×10^9/L) are normal findings. While a productive cough is not normal, the thin clear sputum is more reassuring that the infection has improved than is the increased tactile fremitus.

    Client Need Category: Physiologic integrity

    Cognitive Level: Analyze

18. **M 3.** Immunocompromised clients with a fever of unknown origin should receive antibiotics due to the risks of infection in an immunosuppressed state. Prior to the administration of antibiotics, cultures should be obtained to determine the causative bacteria. Clients who are not immunosuppressed should be evaluated and the infection should be confirmed prior to administering antibiotics. The priority action is to obtain the cultures, followed by reviewing laboratory results and administering the antibiotic.

    Client Need Category: Physiologic integrity

    Cognitive Level: Analyze

19. **D 3.** Erythromycin can lead to accumulation of warfarin, causing toxicity. The client's dose of warfarin may be reduced to decrease the risk of toxicity and bleeding. Increasing the dose of warfarin will increase the risk of toxicity and bleeding further. Increasing or decreasing the erythromycin dose will not have an effect on the increased activity of warfarin.

    Client Need Category: Physiologic integrity

    Cognitive Level: Apply

20. **C 2.** Fluoroquinolones are associated with a risk of tendon rupture. The risk increases with advanced age, strenuous activity, and corticosteroid use. For older clients who exercise vigorously and/or are taking oral corticosteroids, an alternative antibiotic class should be prescribed to avoid the risk of tendon rupture. Completing an antibiotic for a urinary tract infection does not indicate a need to withhold the medication. Fluoroquinolones do not have a cross-sensitivity with penicillin and are safe to administer to a penicillin-allergic client. Fluoroquinolones are administered daily or twice daily, compared to more frequent dosing of other antibiotics, so compliance may be enhanced.

    Client Need Category: Physiologic integrity

    Cognitive Level: Analyze

21. **C 2.** Headache is frequently the first symptom of ototoxicity caused by gentamicin. The risk of ototoxicity is related to high trough levels of gentamicin. The nurse should first

E Easy   **M** Moderate   **D** Difficult   **C** Challenge

review the trough level prior to notifying the prescriber. Administering acetaminophen may treat the headache; however, it is more important to review potential causes of the headache, because ototoxicity from aminoglycosides such as gentamicin is irreversible. Calcium gluconate is used to treat neuromuscular blockade, not ototoxicity, caused by aminoglycosides.

Client Need Category: Physiologic integrity

Cognitive Level: Analyze

22. **C 2.** Trimethoprim as monotherapy is approved only for the treatment of urinary tract infections. The nurse should contact the prescriber to request an alternate antibiotic to treat a skin infection, because this medication cannot be used. Increasing the dose will not improve its effectiveness for a skin infection, and it should not be administered as prescribed. Taking the medication with a full glass of water is not necessary and will not alter its effectiveness or absorption for use in this instance.

Client Need Category: Physiologic integrity

Cognitive Level: Analyze

23. **C 3.** *Escherichia coli* is usually sensitive to TMP/SMZ. However, loop and thiazide diuretics that have a sulfa component may have a cross-sensitivity allergic reaction with other sulfa-containing medications, such as TMP/SMZ. Thus, sulfa-containing medications should be avoided to reduce the risk of allergic reaction. Renal damage with TMP/SMZ occurs from an accumulation of crystalluria, not calcium-containing stones. Recent childbirth is not a contraindication to using TMP/SMZ; the medication should be avoided during late pregnancy to reduce the risk of kernicterus in the fetus.

Client Need Category: Physiologic integrity

Cognitive Level: Analyze

24. **C 2, 4.** Cefepime is a fourth-generation cephalosporin and can reach the cerebrospinal fluid (CSF) and treat CNS infections. Metronidazole is also approved for treating CNS infections. Although penicillin G can also enter CSF, it cannot be administered orally due to the inactivation of the medication by gastric enzymes. Oral vancomycin is used only for the treatment of intestinal infections such as *Clostridium difficile*. Ciprofloxacin is not approved for use in treating CNS infections.

Client Need Category: Physiologic integrity

Cognitive Level: Apply

25. **C 4.** If a throat culture is negative for bacterial growth and streptococcal pharyngitis is not present, then the antibiotic should be stopped immediately to reduce the formation of drug-resistant microbes. Antibiotics should be continued for the full duration prescribed, even if symptoms have resolved. Using a probiotic will help reduce gastrointestinal upset, such as diarrhea, but will not reduce the risk of drug resistance. The dose and duration of an antibiotic is based on the bacteria and disorder being treated. The lowest dose may increase drug-resistant organism development if the dose is not adequate to kill the offending bacteria.

Client Need Category: Physiologic integrity

Cognitive Level: Apply

E Easy   **M** Moderate   **D** Difficult   **C** Challenge

26. **C 1,200 mg/dose.**

    32 lb = 14.5 kg, which rounds up to 15 kg

    15 kg × 240 mg/kg/day = 3,600 mg/day

    3,600 mg/day ÷ 3 doses = 1,200 mg/dose

    Client Need Category: Physiologic integrity

    Cognitive Level: Apply

27. **C 200 gtt/min.**

    Microtubing always has a drop factor of 60 gtt/mL

    100 mL × 60 (gtt/mL)/30 minutes

    Client Need Category: Physiologic integrity

    Cognitive Level: Apply

28. **C 1, 5.** The most serious adverse effect of ethambutol is optic neuritis, which can lead to permanent visual changes. If the client experiences blurred vision, or changes in visual sense of colors, the medication should be stopped. Elevated uric acid levels, not elevated blood glucose, may occur. Nausea is a common (not adverse) side effect. Jaundice is not a known adverse effect of ethambutol.

    Client Need Category: Physiologic integrity

    Cognitive Level: Apply

29. **D 2.** Intramuscular injections of aminoglycosides such as amikacin peak 30 minutes after administration of the medication. Fifteen minutes will not allow enough time for the medication to be absorbed, resulting in a falsely low peak level. Forty-five or sixty minutes after administration may also result in falsely low peak level, as some of the medication may have been metabolized by this time.

    Client Need Category: Physiologic integrity

    Cognitive Level: Understand

30. **D 2.** Tetracycline may cause hepatotoxicity. Other hepatotoxic agents (alcohol, acetaminophen) should be avoided to reduce the risk of liver injury/damage. Photosensitivity is a possible adverse reaction; however, sunlight exposure to be limited to 30 minutes at most (not 2 hours). Decreased calcium in bones occurs in infants, not adults, so calcium supplementation is not necessary. Tooth discoloration occurs in children under the age of 8 or in fetal development of pregnant women after the 4th month of pregnancy.

    Client Need Category: Physiologic integrity

    Cognitive Level: Apply

CHAPTER 7

1. **E 4.** The hemoglobin A1c is a diagnostic measure of the average 3-month blood sugar level of the client. A level of 6.5% and above is considered abnormal (above 6% for prediabetes), which suggests that the current medication regimen is not adequately controlling

E Easy   **M** Moderate   **D** Difficult   **C** Challenge

the blood sugar levels. Hemoglobin A1c levels are not altered with food or when fasting, as it represents an average of glucose levels over the preceding 3 months.

Client Need Category: Physiologic integrity

Cognitive Level: Apply

2. **C 4.** Metformin decreases glucose production without increasing insulin production, causing no risk of hypoglycemia. The blood sugar value does not need to be checked daily while taking metformin unless it is combined with insulin or another medication that risks hypoglycemia. It may be taken without regard to meals, and doses should not be skipped to allow for maximum effect.

Client Need Category: Physiologic integrity

Cognitive Level: Apply

3. **M 4.** NPH insulin peaks anywhere from 6 to 14 hours after administration. During peak action of the insulin, hypoglycemia is most likely to occur. Symptoms of hypoglycemia include altered mental status, hunger, tremors, and diaphoresis. Prior to intervening, the nurse must confirm that the patient is experiencing hypoglycemia by checking the capillary blood glucose level. The nurse would then administer a simple carbohydrate to increase the blood glucose level. Administering more insulin would worsen the hypoglycemic state and is contraindicated. Checking the oral temperature and urine output are not priority nursing actions during a hypoglycemic episode.

Client Need Category: Physiologic integrity

Cognitive Level: Analyze

4. **M 2.** Canagliflozin is an SGLT-2 inhibitor, which increases glucose excretion via the urine. For this reason, hypoglycemia is a common side effect and the client should be educated on signs and symptoms of hypoglycemia and self-monitoring of blood glucose. The glucosuria increases the risk for urinary tract and vaginal infections; clients should be taught the signs and symptoms of these infections while taking canagliflozin. While urination may increase, clients should be advised to continue all other prescribed medications unless directed otherwise by his/her prescriber. This medication may cause hyperkalemia, so clients may need to decrease their potassium intake.

Client Need Category: Physiologic integrity

Cognitive Level: Apply

5. **D 2.** The combination of NPH and regular insulin is acceptable practice. The nurse must first verify the medication order prior to mixing the insulin for administration. To avoid contamination of the regular insulin with NPH insulin, one must inject air into the NPH vial, then inject air into the regular insulin vial, and then draw up the regular insulin followed by drawing up the NPH insulin (clear then cloudy).

Client Need Category: Physiologic integrity

Cognitive Level: Apply

6. **M 2.** Levothyroxine adverse effects include headache, insomnia, anxiety, tachycardia, heat intolerance, and shortness of breath. This is related to supratherapeutic levels of levothyroxine, placing the client in a hyperthyroid state. Polyuria, cold extremities, and pallor are

(continued)

 Easy   Moderate   Difficult   **C** Challenge

not side or adverse effects of levothyroxine. These findings represent signs and symptoms of hypothyroidism.

Client Need Category: Physiologic integrity

Cognitive Level: Analyze

7. **C 1, 4, 5.** A supratherapeutic dose of levothyroxine would put the client into a hyperthyroid state. Symptoms of hyperthyroidism include elevated heart rate, often >100 beats/min, increased energy and decreased ability to sleep, and increased appetite. This condition leads to more frequent bowel movements and an elevation in blood pressure.

Client Need Category: Physiologic integrity

Cognitive Level: Analyze

8. **D 4.** The platelet count, TSH, and white blood cell counts are all within normal limits and do not signify any reasons to withhold the prescribed methimazole. A free T4 level of 0.2 ng/dL is below the normal range, which would signify a decrease in circulating thyroid hormones below the acceptable range, placing the client at risk for hypothyroidism. For this reason, the provider will likely have the nurse instruct the client to withhold the next dose of the medication. Methimazole works to decrease thyroid hormones in the setting of hyperthyroid states. This level would alert the nurse that the dose may need to be decreased to prevent further lowering of circulating thyroid hormones.

Client Need Category: Physiologic integrity

Cognitive Level: Analyze

9. **D 3.** The data in the question indicate that the client is now presenting in a hypothyroid state as evidenced by high TSH and low free T4. The client will now require exogenous thyroid hormone replacement in the form of the synthetic hormone levothyroxine. Methimazole and radioactive iodine are not indicated at this time as the client is no longer in a hyperthyroid state.

Client Need Category: Physiologic integrity

Cognitive Level: Analyze

10. **C 3.** The above signs and symptoms and recent history of illness combined with hyperthyroidism are indicative of thyrotoxicosis (thyroid storm). Nursing interventions are focused on limiting the synthesis of thyroid hormones via medications while simultaneously providing client care directed at lowering metabolic demands. The priority intervention is the administration of antithyroid medications (PTU) to decrease circulating thyroid hormones, which will directly decrease the metabolic rate, including heart rate, blood pressure, and temperature. Next, the nurse must aggressively work to lower core body temperature and treat any cardiac dysrhythmias that occur.

Client Need Category: Physiologic integrity

Cognitive Level: Analyze

11. **M 48 mcg/day.**
Weight conversion from pounds to kilograms is 7/2.2 = 3.2. Multiply weight by dose of 15 mcg, to equal 48 mcg/day.

Client Need Category: Physiologic integrity

Cognitive Level: Apply

E Easy   **M** Moderate   **D** Difficult   **C** Challenge

12. **C 3.** Desmopressin acetate is a synthetic version of antidiuretic hormone (ADH). DI is characterized by low circulating levels of ADH, which results in elevated serum osmolality, increased diuresis with low urine specific gravity, and elevated electrolyte levels secondary to hemoconcentration. Administering excess amounts of desmopressin acetate may result in water intoxication, which would result in low serum osmolality levels <280 mOsm/kg (280 mmol/kg). The low blood pressure is consistent with hypovolemia, indicative of continued excessive diuresis. An elevated serum osmolality and serum sodium indicate poorly or untreated DI, which would require continued treatment with desmopressin acetate. Urine specific gravity should begin to rise as urine becomes more concentrated via the administration of exogenous ADH.

Client Need Category: Physiologic integrity

Cognitive Level: Analyze

13. **C 2, 5.** Indomethacin is a nonsteroidal anti-inflammatory drug (NSAID) known to increase the kidney's ability to recognize and utilize antidiuretic hormone (ADH) in the setting of nephrogenic DI. Utilizing ADH will result in a decrease in urine output, which will decrease serum osmolality and increase the specific gravity of the urine. While it is also used in inflammatory conditions and to decrease pain and joint inflammation associated with gout, that is not the indication with DI. Blood pressure will increase as more circulating volume is maintained through the use of ADH. Serum sodium will decrease as the serum osmolality decreases and the serum becomes less hemoconcentrated.

Client Need Category: Physiologic integrity

Cognitive Level: Analyze

14. **M 3.** Prednisone therapy can result in weight gain, fluid retention, hypertension, and hyperglycemia. Clients may need to decrease sodium intake to help with fluid retention and subsequent blood pressure elevations. Prolonged use of this medication longer than 7 to 10 days may result in adrenal suppression, necessitating the slow taper of the medication, allowing the adrenal glands to resume normal functioning and production of corticosteroids. Failure to taper the dose may result in adrenal insufficiency and Addisonian crisis, which can progress to severe hypotension and shock.

Client Need Category: Physiologic integrity

Cognitive Level: Apply

15. **E 1, 2, 3.** Clients who take continuous prednisone may develop adrenal suppression if the dose is too low to provide an adequate stress response. Symptoms of adrenal crisis will occur if exogenous prednisone doses are too low. Symptoms of adrenal crisis include hypotension, tachycardia, and hyponatremia. Corticosteroid excess (not insufficiency) with prednisone presents with fluid retention and subsequent hypertension, hyperglycemia, and purplish abdominal striae.

Client Need Category: Physiologic integrity

CHAPTER 8

1. **M 4.** The first response by the nurse should be to ascertain more information from the client about the characteristics of bowel movements to determine if additional diagnostics, such as an abdominal X-ray, are needed. Frequency of bowel movements does not

(continued)

E Easy   **M** Moderate   **D** Difficult   **C** Challenge

imply constipation. If the client also reports hard, small stool that is painful or difficult to pass, that is indicative of constipation. Asking about prior use of laxatives is not the best response by the nurse and does not address this present concern. The nurse should not request a laxative until more information is obtained.

Client Need Category: Physiologic integrity

Cognitive Level: Apply

2. **D 1.** Promethazine has a potential adverse effect of local tissue injury and extravasation. If the client reports burning or pain during infusion, the infusion must be discontinued immediately to prevent further tissue injury. Following discontinuation, the nurse may assess the area and apply a warm compress. The rate should not be slowed, because this will not alter the risk associated with tissue injury from this medication. The area should be assessed for redness or swelling after the infusion is discontinued.

Client Need Category: Physiologic integrity

Cognitive Level: Analyze

3. **C 3.** The rhythm strip demonstrates a prolonged QT interval (>0.4 seconds). Ondansetron may cause prolongation of the QT interval and should not be used when the QT interval is prolonged at baseline due to the potential for fatal dysrhythmias. Dexamethasone, promethazine, and lorazepam do not alter the intervals of electrical activity in the heart and could be used to treat the client's nausea.

Client Need Category: Physiologic integrity

Cognitive Level: Analyze

4. **C 2, 3.** Avoiding known triggers that induce nausea and eating upon waking are two ways to help reduce nausea. Pregnancy-induced nausea is worse on an empty stomach; frequent snacks, small frequent meals, and avoiding prolonged fasting may help to reduce nausea. Dietary fat may increase nausea; carbohydrates have been known to help reduce nausea. Acupuncture, not massage, is another alternative that may help reduce nausea. While staying hydrated is important, drinking 8 to 10 glasses of water per day will not help reduce the symptom of nausea.

Client Need Category: Physiologic integrity

Cognitive Level: Apply

5. **C 4.** Loperamide is an analog of meperidine. However, loperamide does not cross the blood–brain barrier and therefore has no central nervous system effects such as euphoria. For this reason, loperamide has no abuse potential. The nurse should reassure the client that it will not lead to relapse or cause any type of high. Diphenoxylate has a risk of abuse at high doses and should be avoided in clients with a history of opioid abuse.

Client Need Category: Physiologic integrity

Cognitive Level: Apply

6. **C 1, 4, 5.** Excessive diarrhea may lead to dehydration as well as acid–base and electrolyte imbalances. Dehydration leads to hemoconcentration and decreased urinary output, which will be evidenced by low serum osmolality (<275 mOsm/L). Urinary output <30 mL/hr would be expected. Bicarbonate is lost in the stool and contributes to metabolic acidosis; the bicarbonate level would be low (<22 mEq/dL), not high. The loss of magnesium and

E Easy **M** Moderate **D** Difficult **C** Challenge

potassium via stool results in signs and symptoms of hypokalemia and hypomagnesemia, such as flat T waves on the electrocardiogram and muscle cramps.

Client Need Category: Physiologic integrity

Cognitive Level: Apply

7. **C 2, 3.** Prolonged use of proton pump inhibitors (PPIs) such as omeprazole can lead to decreased absorption of certain electrolytes, such as magnesium (hypomagnesemia) and calcium. The client should be made aware of the potential effects of decreased absorption of calcium, such as osteopenia, osteoporosis, and bone fractures. Hyperkalemia, stomach cancer, and renal insufficiency are not long-term effects associated with PPIs.

Client Need Category: Physiologic integrity

Cognitive Level: Apply

8. **C 4.** Misoprostol is pregnancy category X and should never be administered to a female client who is, or may become, pregnant. A human chorionic gonadotropin (hCG) level of 25 mIU/mL (30 IU/L) or greater is considered positive for pregnancy. While the other values are slightly abnormal, they would not require as immediate action by the nurse when compared to the hCG level and the potential adverse effects of misoprostol use in pregnancy.

Client Need Category: Physiologic integrity

Cognitive Level: Analyze

9. **D 2.** Peptic ulcer disease (PUD) caused by *Helicobacter pylori* is treated using antibiotics (not antifungals) and acid-reducing medications, such as proton pump inhibitors. Nonsteroidal medications (NSAIDs) may worsen or exacerbate PUD, but acetaminophen is safe to take. Increasing the acidity of the diet will not result in eradicating the bacteria; antibiotics are required to accomplish this.

Client Need Category: Physiologic integrity

Cognitive Level: Apply

10. **D 3.** Ranitidine is a histamine-2 receptor antagonist that directly reduces the production of gastric acid, thus decreasing symptoms of GERD. Sucralfate is used in peptic ulcer disease to provide a coating over ulcers, allowing them to heal in the acidic environment of the stomach. Sucralfate will not decrease acidity of gastric acid and will not provide any symptom relief from GERD. Strength of medications cannot be compared between ranitidine and sucralfate, as they have different uses and mechanisms of action. Using both medications is not required since sucralfate does not reduce gastric acidity and will not treat GERD. Sucralfate is not systemically absorbed and does not have any systemic side effects.

Client Need Category: Physiologic integrity

Cognitive Level: Analyze

11. **C 2.** Pantoprazole, a proton pump inhibitor, carries a risk of pneumonia related to decreased gastric acidity, which allows more bacteria to grow. If the bacteria move upward through regurgitation, vomiting, and aspiration, the client may develop pneumonia. The priority based on the symptoms of the client would be to assess the lungs. Tactile fremitus would be increased at an area of consolidation, indicating possible pneumonia. Additional assessments will be completed to rule out other sources of infection following a respiratory assessment.

Client Need Category: Physiologic integrity

Cognitive Level: Analyze

E Easy   **M** Moderate   **D** Difficult   **C** Challenge

12. **C 4.** Temporary and reversible hearing loss may occur with clarithromycin. A rash may be a sign of a serious adverse reaction such as Stevens-Johnson syndrome. The provider should be notified immediately if a rash occurs. Diarrhea is a common side effect of antibiotics. One episode is not cause for concern. If the frequency were more than several episodes per day, the client would need to notify the provider to rule out *Clostridium difficile*. Taste alteration is a common side effect of clarithromycin and is not dangerous.

    Client Need Category: Physiologic integrity

    Cognitive Level: Apply

13. **D 3.** Bisacodyl suppository will aid in constipation relief starting within 15 minutes. This laxative option and route will aid in reduction of the client's symptoms most quickly. Docusate will exert constipation relief actions more slowly. While the client does have nausea, treating the constipation may reduce that symptom. Ondansetron would not be the priority medication at this time. Ranitidine, a histamine-2 receptor antagonist, is not indicated for any of the client's symptoms.

    Client Need Category: Physiologic integrity

    Cognitive Level: Apply

14. **C 2, 3, 4.** An elevated absolute neutrophil count is indicative of bacterial infection. TPN is high in dextrose and may increase the risk of bacterial infections. Elevated or decreased blood glucose levels may occur while a client is receiving TPN. If the TPN contains insulin, hypoglycemia may occur. If the TPN does not contain insulin, hyperglycemia is common. If the client develops a bacterial infection that is progressing to sepsis, a decrease in blood pressure and mean arterial pressure will occur, indicating decreased tissue perfusion. Absent bowel sounds are not an adverse effect of TPN, because it is administered parenterally and has no effect on the gastrointestinal system. 2+ peripheral pulses are a normal assessment finding.

    Client Need Category: Physiologic integrity

    Cognitive Level: Analyze

15. **D 6.9 mg/day.**

    First convert, pounds to kilograms: 38/2.2 = 17.3 kg

    Next, calculate the dose: 0.1 × 17.3 = 1.73 mg

    Next, calculate the total daily dose: Every 6 hours = 4 doses in 24 hours: 1.73 mg × 4 doses = 6.9 mg/day

    Client Need Category: Physiologic integrity

    Cognitive Level: Apply

CHAPTER 9

1. **E 4.** There are many risk factors associated with breast cancer including inherited genetic abnormalities, family of breast cancer in a first-degree relative, age >55 years or older, early menarche, nulliparity, first full-term pregnancy after age 30, no history of breastfeeding, late age of menopause, use of hormone replacement therapy or oral contraceptives, high fat diet, obesity, high amount of alcohol use, smoking tobacco, and prior thoracic radiation therapy.

    Client Need Category: Health Promotion and Maintenance

    Cognitive Level: Apply

    E Easy   **M** Moderate   **D** Difficult   **C** Challenge

2. **C** **3.** A systemic treatment for cancer uses drugs to stop the growth of cancer cells, either by killing the cells or by stopping them from reproducing. Drugs that exert their maximal effect during specific phases of the cell cycle are termed cell cycle–specific agents. Chemotherapeutic agents that act independently of the cell cycle phases are termed cell cycle–nonspecific agents. Chemotherapy is administered to stop the growth of cancer cells, regardless of whether surgical intervention is not possible or unavailable.

Client Need Category: Pharmacologic and parenteral therapies

Cognitive Level: Analysis

3. **C** **2.** The greatest adverse effects of chemotherapy are associated with gastrointestinal system. Therefore, teaching should focus primarily on this system. However, chemotherapy-related toxicities involve the hematopoietic, integumentary, neurologic, genitourinary, reproductive, pulmonary, cardiovascular, and endocrine systems. Chemotherapeutic agents also affect electrolyte balance.

Client Need Category: Reduction of risk potential

Cognitive Level: Apply

4. **C** **1.** Chemotherapy agents are rated according of the risk of causing nausea and vomiting. Cisplatin, mechlorethamine, streptozotocin, cyclophosphamide, doxorubicin, ifosfamide, and dacarbazine are in the highest risk category. Docetaxel and methotrexate are in the low risk category. Bleomycin is in the minimal risk category.

Client Need Category: Reduction of risk potential

Cognitive Level: Apply

5. **D** **2.** The client's sodium level should be most troubling to the nurse. The sodium level is elevated as the normal sodium level is 135 to 145 mEq/L. Diagnostic indicators of dehydration related to anorexia and cisplatin, which is associated with a high risk of causing chemotherapy-induced nausea and vomiting, include electrolyte imbalance, elevated hemoglobin/hematocrit, elevated blood urea nitrogen/creatinine, tachycardia, hypotension, decreased urine output and jugular venous pressure, and weight loss. The normal potassium level is 3.5 to 5.5 mEq/L. The normal magnesium level is 1.5–2.5 mEq/L. The normal calcium level is 8.6–10.2 mg/dL.

Client Need Category: Reduction of risk potential

Cognitive Level: Apply

6. **E** **2.** Nurses need to assess changes in oral tissue sensation, burning and pain, decreased tolerance to temperature extremes of food, sore throat, ability to maintain oral fluid and nutritional intake, and speech and swallowing status. All of the assessments are normal except for the soreness with swallowing. This could indicate mucositis, and the prescriber should be contacted as severe oral mucositis may impact swallowing, fluid and nutritional intake, speech, and quality of life.

Client Need Category: Reduction of risk potential

Cognitive Level: Apply

7. **E** **2.** Myelosuppression, a common side effect of many chemotherapy agents, refers to suppression of bone marrow functioning characterized by decreased levels of WBCs, neutrophils (neutropenia), hemoglobin and hematocrit levels (anemia), and platelets (thrombocytopenia). An elevated WBC would indicate an infection. Myelosuppression

(continued)

E Easy   **M** Moderate   **D** Difficult   **C** Challenge

results in decreased, not increased, hemoglobin levels. Electrolyte disturbances such as a low potassium level are associated with chemotherapy-induced nausea and vomiting.

Client Need Category: Physiologic Adaptation

Cognitive Level: Apply

8. **E 3.** Ondansetron is a serotonin 5 HT3 antagonist used to prevent nausea and vomiting effects associated with the etoposide. The medication will not increase the neutrophil or sodium level. Ondansetron will not improve the client's appetite.

Client Need Category: Pharmacologic and parenteral therapies

Cognitive Level: Apply

9. **D 4.** Ondansetron is a serotonin agent used to prevent nausea and vomiting with chemo-therapy. Ondansetron has two common adverse effects: headache and constipation. The nurse should provide clients with education regarding management of constipation, which includes adding fluids and fiber to the diet. The medication does not cause depression.

Client Need Category: Pharmacologic and parenteral therapies

Cognitive Level: Apply

10. **C 1.** The most widely cited algorithm for pharmaceutical pain management is the World Health Organization analgesic ladder that suggests a stepwise approach. Step 1 includes use of nonopioid analgesics (i.e., acetaminophen or nonsteroidal anti-inflammatory drugs) with or without adjuvant medications such as antidepressants or anticonvulsants. Step 2 includes use of low-potency opioids with or without adjuvant medications. Step 3 includes use of high-potency opioids such as morphine or oxycodone with or without adjuvant medications. Step 4 includes integrative therapies and analgesic interventions.

Client Need Category: Reduction of risk potential

Cognitive Level: Apply

11. **E 1.** Physical tolerance develops over time in all patients receiving opioids such that they will require increased doses to maintain the same amount of pain control. Abrupt cessa-tion of opioids will result in withdrawal syndrome. Drug craving is use of a drug without the need for analgesia effect. There is no potential toxicity with a client asking for increas-ing doses as long as the dosing is still within the upper limits of the medication.

Client Need Category: Reduction of risk potential

Cognitive Level: Apply

12. **E 1.** Prednisone is a glucocorticoid agent that decreases the inflammatory response of cells and has weight gain, hyperglycemia, and mood effects as common side effects. Toremifene is a hormonal agent used in breast cancer and can cause endometrial cancer and thromboembolic events. Irinotecan is cell cycle–nonspecific chemotherapy agent that can cause myelosuppression and diarrhea. Cisplatin is a platin alkylating agency that damages DNA resulting in impaired cell functioning and reproduction process and can cause delayed hypersensitivity, nausea, vomiting, and renal, neuro-, and ototoxicity.

Client Need Category: Pharmacologic and parenteral therapies

Cognitive Level: Apply

13. **E 4.** Thrombocytopenia is diagnostic indicator of a low platelet count of <150,000 mcL, and clients with this condition experience frequent nosebleeds and abnormal bruising.

E Easy **M** Moderate **D** Difficult **C** Challenge

Anemia is diagnosed by low values of hemoglobin and hematocrit, and most clients experience fatigue. Neutropenia is diagnosed by a neutrophil count <1,500 mcL, and clients have an increase in the number of infections.

Client Need Category: Pharmacologic and parenteral therapies

Cognitive Level: Apply

14. Ⓜ **2.** Chemotherapy agents are considered hazardous drugs, and special handling is required including personal protective equipment (PPE) and adherence to chemotherapy handling guidelines. Nurses who work with chemotherapy agents must be certified to handle them. Generally, all clients are well cared for in an acute care hospital, and the use of PPE may be appropriate to any and all clients in the hospital. Not all chemotherapy clients who are hospitalized have supportive and engaged families.

Client Need Category: Reduction of risk potential

Cognitive Level: Apply

15. Ⓒ **1, 2, 3, 5.** During discharge instruction, the nurse should teach the client to seek a medical evaluation for the following signs and symptoms: unexplained weight loss, pain, skin changes including those involving warts, moles, or sores that do not heal, changes in bowel or bladder habits, persistent cough, hoarseness or sore throat, unusual bleeding or discharge, a thickening or lump in the breast or other part of the body, continued indigestion or trouble swallowing, and white patches inside the mouth or white spots on the tongue. Dry patches of skin on the heels of the feet do not require a medical evaluation.

Client Need Category: Reduction of risk potential

Cognitive Level: Apply

CHAPTER 10

1. Ⓒ **3.** Systemic muscarinic toxicity can occur with an overdose by direct-acting muscarinic agonists such as bethanechol, as well as by cholinesterase inhibitors. Additionally, some poisonous mushrooms can result in muscarinic toxicity. Symptoms of muscarinic poisoning include excessive salivation, increased tearing, blurred vision, bronchospasm, diarrhea, bradycardia, and hypotension. Treatment includes giving a muscarinic blocking agent such as atropine and providing treatment for symptomatic relief.

Client Need Category: Physiologic integrity

Cognitive Level: Apply

2. Ⓓ **1.** A muscarinic agonist such as bethanechol is used to treat urinary retention in postoperative clients, postpartum clients, and clients diagnosed with an atonic bladder. It should not be used to treat urinary retention secondary to an obstruction due to the increased pressure in the urinary tract. Additionally, bethanechol can cause bronchoconstriction, so it is contraindicated for clients with asthma and can also cause an increase in heart rate and may even result in dysrhythmias for clients with hyperthyroidism. It is therefore contraindicated for use by clients with hyperthyroidism as well.

Client Need Category: Physiologic integrity

Cognitive Level: Analyze

Ⓔ Easy   Ⓜ Moderate   Ⓓ Difficult   Ⓒ Challenge

3. **Ⓔ 3.** Continuous cardiac monitoring is necessary when giving epinephrine intravenously due to the increased risk of hypertension and cardiac arrhythmias. Epinephrine cannot be given orally due to the fact that it would be broken down in the gastrointestinal tract, additionally when given subcutaneously absorption is slowed due to the constriction of the blood vessels around the site of injection. Intramuscular injection is the preferred method of administration. Finally, epinephrine should be used cautiously in clients with diabetes due to the risk of hyperglycemia.

Client Need Category: Physiologic integrity

Cognitive Level: Apply

4. **Ⓒ 4.** Muscarinic antagonists (anticholinergics) including atropine are contraindicated for clients with glaucoma, intestinal atony, urinary tract obstruction, and tachycardia. They can be used for clients with asthma, albeit with caution. Constipation may be a side effect of taking atropine, and clients should be instructed to increase their dietary fiber and fluid intake. Laxatives may be used if constipation is severe.

Client Need Category: Physiologic integrity

Cognitive Level: Analyze

5. **Ⓓ 2.** The activation of beta$_2$ receptors in the skeletal muscles causes an increase in the contraction of muscles, resulting in tremors. Other side effects may include hyperglycemia, and beta$_2$ receptor activation relaxes smooth muscle, causing bronchodilation.

Client Need Category: Physiologic integrity

Cognitive Level: apply

6. **Ⓜ 1.** Propranolol (a beta-blocker) may be a contraindication for clients with a history of asthma due to the fact that propranolol is nonselective and the beta$_2$ blockade results in bronchoconstriction in the lungs. It is important that the provider be notified first and the condition is then accurately documented as a component of the client's medical history.

Client Need Category: Physiologic integrity

Cognitive Level: Analyze

7. **Ⓒ 4.** Ideally, the first dose of this medication should be small and given before going to bed to prevent against the first-dose effect. Approximately 1% of clients faint within an hour after receiving their first dose of prazosin. Prazosin may be taken with or without food, and although the inhibition of ejaculation may occur while taking prazosin, it is reversible and will resolve with the discontinuation of the medication. It is crucial that the client be aware of the risk of first-dose effect. Reflex tachycardia (not bradycardia) is an adverse effect of prazosin. A beta-blocker may be started if needed to help counteract this effect.

Client Need Category: Physiologic integrity

Cognitive Level: Analyze

8. **Ⓓ 1.** Alpha antagonist medications lower blood pressure by the dilation of the arterioles, directly reducing arterial pressure, and venous dilation, decreasing cardiac output and reducing arterial pressure indirectly. The alpha blockade results in the relaxation of smooth muscle, helping to treat condition such as benign prostatic hyperplasia. In addition, nasal congestion is a side effect of the alpha blockade; alpha antagonist medications

Ⓔ Easy   **Ⓜ** Moderate   **Ⓓ** Difficult   **Ⓒ** Challenge

can not treat nasal congestion. Lastly, the alpha blockade may result in an increased heart rate and reflex tachycardia by triggering the baroreceptor reflex.

Client Need Category: Physiologic integrity

Cognitive Level: apply

9. **C 1, 2, 3.** Adverse effects of these medications include bradycardia, the precipitation of heart failure (symptoms including shortness of breath, swelling of the extremities, weight gain related to fluid retention), and rebound cardiac excitation. Bronchoconstriction can occur, placing clients with asthma and/or other obstructive airway disorders at risk, and hypoglycemia is also an adverse effect which of particular importance for clients with diabetes.

Client Need Category: Physiologic integrity

Cognitive Level: Apply

10. **M 2.** Nonselective beta-adrenergic blockers are contraindicated for use due to the client's history of asthma. However, this does not mean the client will never experience beta$_2$ blockade–related side effects. At higher doses of the medication, beta$_1$-selective adrenergic antagonists lose their selectivity and block beta$_2$ in addition. The dosing ranges of the medications are not dependent on beta receptor specificity and there is no known increased risk of developing diabetes while taking a beta$_1$-selective adrenergic antagonist.

Client Need Category: Physiologic integrity

Cognitive Level: Apply

CHAPTER 11

1. **M 1.** Alzheimer disease is a common type of dementia. Treatment is with acetylcholinesterase inhibitors and *N*-methyl-D-aspartate (NMDA) receptor antagonists. Parkinson disease is a chronic neurodegenerative disorder that is characterized by motor and non-motor symptoms, and treatment involves medications that increase the level of dopamine in the brain. Multiple sclerosis, a chronic, neurodegenerative, autoimmune disease of the central nervous system, requires medications that modify the disease course, treat exacerbations, and mange the multiple symptoms of the disease. Epilepsy or seizure disorder, a chronic central nervous system disease that affects individuals with recurrent seizures episodes, involves treatment with antiepileptic drugs that alter chemical activity to stop excitatory processes.

Client Need Category: Pharmacologic and parenteral therapies

Cognitive Level: Apply

2. **C 1, 3.** Parkinson disease has cardinal motor features of resting tremor, bradykinesia, and rigidity. Confusion of person, place, and time are associated with Alzheimer disease. Sexual dysfunction and motor weakness are associated with multiple sclerosis. Altered level of consciousness is associated with complex partial seizures.

Client Need Category: Reduction of risk potential

Cognitive Level: Apply

E Easy   **M** Moderate   **D** Difficult   **C** Challenge

3. **D 1.** Phenytoin is a narrow-spectrum first-generation antiepileptic medication. The medication works on the sodium channels, and the sodium levels should be assessed prior to administration of the medication. The potassium level is not affected by phenytoin. The white blood cell count is imperative for a documented infection. Phenytoin does not affect the hemoglobin or hematocrit levels.

   Client Need Category: Reduction of risk potential

   Cognitive Level: Apply

4. **E 2.** Phenobarbital depresses the central nervous system (CNS) activity by causing CNS and respiratory depression. The respiratory rate of 8 breaths/min is much lower than a normal rate of 12 to 24 breaths/min. The normal heart rate is 60 to 120 beats/min. The normal blood pressure is <130/80 mm Hg. The pain rating of 2 is characterized as mild and does not need immediate action.

   Client Need Category: Physiologic Adaptation

   Cognitive Level: Apply

5. **C 1, 2.** Carbamazepine, oxcarbazepine, and lacosamide are narrow-spectrum first-generation antiepileptic medications that work on the sodium channels. However, only carbamazepine and oxcarbazepine are used for generalized and partial seizures. Lacosamide is used for partial-onset seizures. Valproic acid increases availability of the gamma-aminobutyric acid neurotransmitter and works with generalized, partial, partial complex, and absence seizures. Phenobarbital is a first-generation antiepileptic medication that depresses central nervous system activity and is used with generalized and complex partial seizures as well as status epilepticus.

   Client Need Category: Pharmacologic and parenteral therapies

   Cognitive Level: Analyze

6. **C 2.** Zonisamide is a broad-spectrum, second-generation antiepileptic medication that works on the sodium and calcium channels and is used as either monotherapy or adjunctive therapy in generalized or partial seizures. The medication can cause drowsiness, anorexia, and nausea. The other responses are not related to the mechanism of action of zonisamide.

   Client Need Category: Pharmacologic and parenteral therapies

   Cognitive Level: Apply

7. **C 1, 2, 3, 5.** Clinical manifestations of multiple sclerosis may include diplopia or double vision, sensory changes, motor weakness or impairment, fatigue, imbalance, spasticity, bladder and/or bowel disturbances, depression, and cognitive impairment. Insomnia or difficulty sleeping is not a clinical manifestation associated with multiple sclerosis.

   Client Need Category: Reduction of risk potential

   Cognitive Level: Apply

8. **C 4.** Interferon beta-1b suppresses the immune response through various mechanisms causing flu-like symptoms. The nurse should administer acetaminophen or ibuprofen as prescribed prior to administration of the medication to help combat the symptoms. Depression is a clinical manifestation and should be assessed after the interferon beta-1b injection. Obtaining a full set of vital signs and assessing laboratory values

E Easy   **M** Moderate   **D** Difficult   **C** Challenge

are important nursing interventions but should occur after the administration of the medication.

Client Need Category: Pharmacologic and parenteral therapies

Cognitive Level: Apply

9. **D 4.** Carbidopa–levodopa is a drug administered for PD; it is used for symptomatic management of bradykinesia, rigidity, and tremors. The nurse observes that the client has an increase in the movement disorders associated with PD. The nurse can suggest increasing the frequency of the medication. A larger dose will not assist with symptom management. The client's family and mood do not directly impact the mechanism of action of the carbidopa–levodopa and are therefore not relevant in this context.

Client Need Category: Pharmacologic and parenteral therapies

Cognitive Level: Apply

10. **C 3.** Nurses are responsible for teaching clients and families about expectations of treatment. A nurse caring for a client with Alzheimer disease needs to communicate that the medications used do not slow the progression of the disease. Responding with "Not all drugs work the same on all Alzheimer patients" does not provide an information regarding the disease process. Having a family meeting and writing down the thoughts are therapeutic, but the nurse needs to communicate about Alzheimer disease and its progression.

Client Need Category: Pharmacologic and parenteral therapies

Cognitive Level: Apply

11. **M 4.** All antiepileptic drugs (AEDs) have a Federal Drug Administration warning regarding the possible risk of suicidal ideation while on the medication. The child is more at risk during the initial stages of the diagnosis. Therefore, the nurse should recognize this statement and reteach about the medications. AEDs will make the child more tired and sleepy. So allowing the child to rest throughout the day, allowing extra time for morning care, and helping with meals and doctor appointments are all expected statements of understanding.

Client Need Category: Pharmacologic and parenteral therapies

Cognitive Level: Apply

12. **M 3.** Topiramate is a broad-spectrum antiepileptic drug (AED), which works on the sodium channels and enhances gamma-aminobutyric acid activity. The medication is contraindicated in pregnancy and in women trying to get pregnant. The nurse needs to communicate this to the client. Sulfa allergies are cross-referenced to zonisamide, another AED. The medication can be taken in the morning with a full glass of water but that is not the priority with the medication. The medication does not affect blood pressure.

Client Need Category: Pharmacologic and parenteral therapies

Cognitive Level: Apply

13. **E 1.** EEGs are used to diagnose and identify seizure types. There is no diagnostic test for MS, AD, or PD. These three disorders require a complete health history, physical exam, and ruling out of other reversible causes.

Client Need Category: Reduction of risk potential

Cognitive Level: Apply

E Easy   **M** Moderate   **D** Difficult   **C** Challenge

14. **(M) 2.** PD is a chronic neurologic disorder caused by the degenerative destruction of the dopamine neurotransmitter. The medications for PD increase the level of dopamine in the brain or work as agonists. Serotonin is not overproduced in PD. PD does not involve myelin. Multiple sclerosis is a chronic, neurogenerative, autoimmune disease of the central nervous system, and the medications used stop the autoimmune destruction of myelin.

Client Need Category: Physiologic Adaptation

Cognitive Level: Apply

15. **(C) 1, 3, 4.** Medication used in MS can be grouped into three main categories: agents that modify acute exacerbations, agents that modify the disease, and agents that manage symptoms. Medications used in MS do not assist with diagnosis; there is no conclusive diagnostic test for MS. The medications for MS do not slow the progression of the disease but modify the disease.

Client Need Category: Pharmacologic and parenteral therapies

Cognitive Level: Apply

CHAPTER 12

1. **(E) 3.** First-generation (typical) antipsychotics primarily treat the positive symptoms of psychosis (such as hallucinations and delusions). They are not as effective as second-generation (atypical) antipsychotics at treating the negative symptoms of psychosis, such as lack of motivation, poverty of speech, and social withdrawal.

Client Need Category: Physiologic integrity

Cognitive Level: Analyze

2. **(E) 4.** All responses reflect information that should be included in the teaching of a client starting clozapine therapy. However, clozapine poses a potentially lethal risk of agranulocytosis. Therefore, regular monitoring of WBC levels is the highest priority.

Client Need Category: Physiologic integrity

Cognitive Level: Apply

3. **(M) 4.** Anticholinergic effects include dry mouth, constipation, urinary retention, and dry eyes/blurred vision. These are side effects of typical and atypical antipsychotic agents.

Client Need Category: Physiologic integrity

Cognitive Level: Analyze

4. **(D) 1.** Clients with severe lithium toxicity (>3.5 mEq/L/mmol/L) may experience impaired consciousness, nystagmus, seizures, coma, oliguria/anuria, and myocardial infarction. Clients with moderate lithium toxicity (2.0 to 3.5 mEq/L/mmol/L) may experience excessive urine output, tremors, confusion, irritability, and psychomotor retardation. Clients with mild lithium toxicity (1.5 to 2.0 mEq/L/mmol/L) may experience blurred vision, tinnitus, gastrointestinal upset (nausea, vomiting, diarrhea), and ataxia.

Client Need Category: Physiologic integrity

Cognitive Level: Analyze

(E) Easy   **(M)** Moderate   **(D)** Difficult   **(C)** Challenge

5. **D 3.** Benzodiazepines (including diazepam) are intended for short-term use; buspirone is intended for long-term, daily use. Frequently, they are prescribed together at initiation of therapy for rapid symptom relief. Diazepam is tapered/discontinued after the full clinical effect of buspirone has been achieved (3 to 6 weeks). Buspirone has no sedative effect and does not lead to tolerance or dependence.

   Client Need Category: Physiologic integrity

   Cognitive Level: Analyze

6. **C 1, 3, 5.** Benzodiazepines can potentially cause CNS depression, including drowsiness and lightheadedness. They are also known to cause decreased respiratory rate; clients' respiratory function should be regularly assessed while taking benzodiazepines. Anterograde amnesia may also occur. They may cause hypotension and dizziness (not hypertension) and tinnitus (not hearing loss).

   Client Need Category: Physiologic integrity

   Cognitive Level: Analyze

7. **M 2.** Benzodiazepines are indicated for short-term use. They are indicated for short-term management of anxiety disorders (including panic disorder), acute alcohol withdrawal, trauma disorders, insomnia, and for preoperative sedation. They are not indicated for psoriasis or tachycardia. They may be used for short-term management of manic symptoms of bipolar disorder.

   Client Need Category: Physiologic integrity

   Cognitive Level: Apply

8. **C 2.** All the responses should be included in client teaching for phenelzine, but the highest priority is to teach clients to avoid the many foods and medications that interact with phenelzine. Most of phenelzine's food and medication interactions can cause hypertensive crisis, which is life threatening. It is therefore the highest teaching priority.

   Client Need Category: Physiologic integrity

   Cognitive Level: Apply

9. **D 1.** These are all symptoms of serotonin syndrome (in addition to muscle twitching, diarrhea, headache, and dilated pupils). Mania, akathisia, panic attacks, cardiac rhythm changes can occur when abruptly discontinuing tricyclic antidepressants. Nausea, lethargy, orthostasis, headache can occur when abruptly discontinuing selective serotonin reuptake inhibitors (SSRIs) antidepressants. Blurred vision, urinary retention, orthostasis, constipation are anticholinergic symptoms that can occur while taking tricyclic antidepressants.

   Client Need Category: Physiologic integrity

   Cognitive Level: Analyze

10. **C 1, 3, 5.** The full effect of fluoxetine may take 6 to 8 weeks to occur. Risk of suicide may increase with the initiation of treatment with antidepressants, and clients should be closely observed for any changes in their behavior or reports of suicidal ideation. If abruptly discontinued, SSRIs can result in a withdrawal syndrome, including dizziness, headache, nausea, tremors, and anxiety, and can persist for 1 to 3 weeks after the medication has stopped. The medication does not cause sedation, seizures, or tachycardia and should be taken regularly; it is not prescribed on an as needed basis.

    Client Need Category: Physiologic integrity

    Cognitive Level: Analyze

E Easy   **M** Moderate   **D** Difficult   **C** Challenge

CHAPTER 13

1. **C 2, 4, 5.** The drug of choice for the treatment of trichomoniasis is metronidazole. This medication can cause side effects such as vomiting if used with alcohol and can cause a metallic taste in the mouth. Alcohol should be avoided for 24 hours after the medication regimen is completed. Disulfiram should not be used for 2 weeks following the completion of the metronidazole regimen, as the combination of the two medications can cause confusion or acute psychosis. Trichomoniasis is a sexually transmitted infection; therefore, all partners need to be treated and all the medicine must be taken for effective treatment. Gastrointestinal symptoms such as nausea, vomiting, and/or epigastric pain are very common with the use of metronidazole.
   Client Need Category: Physiologic integrity
   Cognitive Level: Analyze

2. **C 3.** Hormone therapy is the most effective treatment for vasomotor symptoms. Any woman with a uterus must not take unopposed estrogen, such as estradiol. A progesterone agent like norethindrone must accompany the estrogen to prevent endometrial hyperplasia and carcinoma. Metronidazole is an antibiotic used in the treatment of bacterial vaginal infections and will not improve symptoms of menopause. Fluconazole is an antifungal medication used to treat fungal infections, such as candida (yeast).
   Client Need Category: Physiologic integrity
   Cognitive Level: Apply

3. **C 3.** Steroid treatment reduces the risk of lung problems for babies who are born early, particularly for those born between 29 and 34 weeks of pregnancy. Pregnant women cannot receive this medication with current low serum platelet levels. The uric acid level is within normal limits and is not a contraindication to receiving betamethasone acetate. While the urinary protein level is elevated, it is also not a contraindication to betamethasone acetate. The serum potassium level is slightly elevated; however, betamethasone acetate may result in hypokalemia (not hyperkalemia) and would thus not require the nurse to hold the medication.
   Client Need Category: Physiologic integrity
   Cognitive Level: Analyze

4. **D 1.** Rho (D) immune globulin is used to prevent an immune response to Rh-positive blood in people with an Rh-negative blood type. The mixing of blood can lead to medical problems such as anemia, kidney failure, and shock. Rh-positive clients (A+ for example) do not need Rho (D) immune globulin injections. Proteinuria, elevated blood pressure, and a B- blood type are not contraindications to the administration of Rho (D) immune globulin.
   Client Need Category: Physiologic integrity
   Cognitive Level: Analyze

5. **C 2, 4, 5.** Cigarette smoking increases serious cardiovascular side effects from estrogen-containing oral contraceptives, especially over 35. The risk is further increased with a greater number of cigarettes smoked per day. Due to the increased risk of thromboembolic events, clients over 35 that smoke cannot use any products that contain estrogens, such as norelgestro-

E Easy   **M** Moderate   **D** Difficult   **C** Challenge

min/ethinyl estradiol. Norethindrone alone or etonogestrel subdermal would be acceptable options, as progesterone can be used without an estrogen component. Condoms are always a safe preventative measure, although they are not as effective as an oral contraceptive.

Client Need Category: Physiologic integrity

Cognitive Level: Analyze

6. **D 3.** Dicloxacillin is safe to use during lactation, supplementation with formula is not necessary. A member of the penicillin class, it should not be used if any there is any prior hypersensitivity. A new infection, called a superinfection, can develop while the original infection is being treated. When penicillin-type medications are used, one possible super-infection is *C. difficile*.

Client Need Category: Physiologic integrity

Cognitive Level: Apply

7. **C 1.** The most common treatment for endometriosis is combination hormonal contracep-tives. Factor V Leiden is a clotting disorder, and thromboembolic disorders are a contrain-dication for combination therapy. Migraines without visual disturbance, such as an aura, are not a contraindication of estrogen and progesterone therapy. Benign breast disorders are often improved with contraceptive therapy, and there is no risk associated with diabe-tes or a history of diabetic ketoacidosis.

Client Need Category: Physiologic integrity

Cognitive Level: Analyze

8. **E 1.** Oxytocin stimulates uterine contractions. In some clients, the placenta cannot tolerate the constant squeezing and in turn will cause a drop in the fetal heartbeat. This hypoxic situation can lead to sequela such as brain damage. Oxytocin needs to be discon-tinued if late decelerations occur multiple times. Even though the blood pressure reading of 162/98 requires intervention, this is not a direct result of oxytocin use. A maternal tem-perature of 101.4°F (38.6°C) would need to be evaluated and watched but is unrelated to oxytocin. Group beta strep bacteria will need to be treated with antibiotics but is caused by flora found in the body, not from oxytocin use.

Client Need Category: Physiologic integrity

Cognitive Level: Analyze

9. **M 3.** The human papillomavirus-9-valent vaccine will protect individuals ages 9 to 45 from 9 of the most common HPV strains (6, 11, 16, 18, 31, 33, 45, 52, 58). It will not cure any of these strains a client may have already contracted during sexual contact. One of the most common side effects is syncope.

Client Need Category: Physiologic integrity

Cognitive Level: Analyze

10. **D 2.** A dangerous side effect of misoprostol is uterine rupture. If that occurs, the fetal heart rate will be undetectable. The priority nursing intervention would be to contact the provider and locate the ultrasound machine to retrieve a visual image of what is occur-ring. The other interventions would not be successful if the uterus has opened, as the fetus would no longer be perfused and is at risk for death.

Client Need Category: Physiologic integrity

Cognitive Level: Analyze

E Easy   **M** Moderate   **D** Difficult   **C** Challenge

11. **E** **3.** Magnesium sulfate causes respiratory depression. If the respirations are <12 per minute, the first action should be to stop the infusion. Next, the provider will be notified, but the medication must be stopped first to prevent harm to the client. If the client is experiencing hypermagnesemia, calcium gluconate may be administered. Oxygen may be administered if the client is experiencing respiratory distress or a decrease in oxygen saturation; however, neither of those conditions are evident in this scenario, and stopping the infusion as the first action may help to prevent these conditions from occurring.

Client Need Category: Physiologic integrity

Cognitive Level: Analyze

12. **D** **4.** Methylergonovine is an oxytocic medication that is administered to promote uterine contractions. This medication is indicated for treatment of postpartum hemorrhage caused by uterine atony or subinvolution, and the desired effect is an increase in uterine tone and decreased or stopped lochia. An increase in blood pressure is an adverse effect of the medication, not a sign of medication effectiveness. This medication is not used in the treatment of breast pain.

Client Need Category: Physiologic integrity

Cognitive Level: Apply

13. **M** **1.** Some antibiotic therapy can decrease the effectiveness of oral contraceptives. The client needs to be instructed to use a backup method, like a condom, for the entire duration of the antibiotic therapy. At no point should the client stop taking her pills, double up, or require any type of blood testing related to the antibiotic regimen.

Client Need Category: Physiologic integrity

Cognitive Level: Analyze

14. **D** **1.** This medication is safe to use while breast-feeding, so the client does not need to wean off the medication. However, it should be used with caution in pregnancy. As with any type of depression, asking about self-harm is a vital component of the assessment of the client's safety. Pyridoxine should be taken daily to help reduce depressive symptoms.

Client Need Category: Physiologic integrity

Cognitive Level: Analyze

15. **M** **1.** There is a risk of thromboembolic effects associated with estrogen therapy. Signs and symptoms of a deep vein thrombosis include calf redness and swelling. The client should be instructed to stop the medication and be seen by the provider immediately. An ultrasound would be indicated. A client should never be told to monitor, ignore, or self-treat these symptoms as the presence of a deep vein thrombosis places the client at risk for pulmonary embolism, which can be fatal.

Client Need Category: Physiologic integrity

Cognitive Level: Analyze

16. **D** **1.** Several oral contraceptive formulations have been Food and Drug Administration approved to treat acne. Combination norethindrone/ethinyl estradiol has an acne indication, as the estrogen helps to decrease acne. Medroxyprogesterone acetate, norethindrone alone, or levonorgestrel (the active ingredient in the intrauterine device) are progesterone-only preparations, with a potential side effect of acne.

Client Need Category: Physiologic integrity

Cognitive Level: Apply

E Easy   **M** Moderate   **D** Difficult   **C** Challenge

17. **C** **2, 3, 4, 5, 6.** Nonsteroidal anti-inflammatory drugs such as ibuprofen are not safe to use in pregnancy due to fetal harm. Acetaminophen-based products are considered safe as well as guaifenesin. Nonpharmacologic therapies would include increasing oral fluid intake and humidifying room air to decrease congestion.

    Client Need Category: Physiologic integrity

    Cognitive Level: Analyze

18. **D** **2.** Contraception must begin with the confirmation that no pregnancy exists. Therefore, beginning a contraceptive without a menses or withdrawal bleed would not be indicated. Secondary amenorrhea is often related to pregnancy or hormone imbalance. Laboratory testing would be indicated at this time. If results are normal, the client may begin medroxyprogesterone, which will stimulate a withdrawal bleed once the medication is complete. After the withdrawal bleed, the client may begin contraception. A laparoscopy is not indicated for secondary amenorrhea.

    Client Need Category: Physiologic integrity

    Cognitive Level: Analyze

19. **C** **2.** The medication needs to be repeated if vomiting happens within 3 hours of taking the medication. There is no blood test that would reveal its effectiveness. If the client does not get a period when she expects one, she should have a human chorionic gonadotropin drawn at that time to rule out pregnancy. There is no age restriction on this medication and is available over the counter.

    Client Need Category: Physiologic integrity

    Cognitive Level: Analyze

20. **E** **2.** Ultrasound and endometrial biopsy would be indicated to rule out abnormalities of the uterine lining. Postmenopausal bleeding at any age or any duration can be indicative of endometrial cancer. Oral contraceptives would not be used in a postmenopausal client, as this increases the risk for estrogen-dependent cancers. A client may need progesterone therapy to stop the bleeding; however, a diagnosis must be made prior.

    Client Need Category: Physiologic integrity

    Cognitive Level: Analyze

21. **D** **2.** Testosterone replacement therapy requires laboratory testing as it can increase the erythropoietic effects of the hematocrit. However, the medication does not affect blood pressure. Taking the medication as prescribed is correct, and the client should use protection to prevent sexually transmitted infections.

    Client Need Category: Physiologic integrity

    Cognitive Level: Apply

22. **M** **3.** Sildenafil is a PDE5 inhibitor, which increases and preserves cGMP levels in the penis making an erection harder and long lasting. The medication can cause a small reduction in blood pressure, but this is not the indication for the medication. The medication does not slow the heart rate nor augment the development of testosterone.

    Client Need Category: Physiologic integrity

    Cognitive Level: Apply

E Easy   **M** Moderate   **D** Difficult   **C** Challenge

23. **Ⓜ 1.** Nitroglycerin is a nitrate and is contraindicated with PDE5 inhibitors, as the combination may cause severe hypotension. Lisinopril is an angiotensin-converting enzyme inhibitor and would be used with caution with sildenafil. Clonidine is a centrally acting vasodilator and would be used with caution with sildenafil. Metoprolol is a beta-1–specific adrenergic antagonist and would be used with caution with sildenafil.

    Client Need Category: Physiologic integrity

    Cognitive Level: Apply

24. **Ⓓ 1.** Finasteride decreases the size of the prostate, which also decreases the PSA level. Alfuzosin is an alpha-1 adrenergic blocker, which relaxes the smooth muscle of the bladder neck and prostate and increases the urine flow but does not decrease the PSA level. Tadalafil is a PDE5 inhibitor used for erectile dysfunction in client with BPH with no effect on the PSA level. Labetalol is a nonselective beta-blocker that lowers heart rate and blood pressure and does not decrease the PSA level in BPH.

    Client Need Category: Physiologic integrity

    Cognitive Level: Analyze

25. **Ⓒ 1, 3.** The client is experiencing prostatitis, an inflammation of the prostate. An anti-inflammatory such as ibuprofen and an antibiotic such as ciprofloxacin are warranted. Acetaminophen has properties to address pain and fever, but not inflammation. Lisinopril is an angiotensin-converting enzyme inhibitor used for hypertension. Morphine is an opioid and not warranted for the prostatitis. Sildenafil is a PDE5 inhibitor used for erectile dysfunction.

    Client Need Category: Physiologic integrity

    Cognitive Level: Apply

CHAPTER 14

1. **Ⓜ 1.** Placing pressure on the tear ducts (inner corner of the eye) for up to 1 minute after administration of the eye drops will limit systemic absorption. Vigorously rubbing the eyes is not recommended, and dry mouth and decreased urination are not known side effects of beta-blockers. Finally, clients do not need to avoid food or drink after administering the medication.

    Client Need Category: Physiologic integrity

    Cognitive Level: Apply

2. **Ⓒ 2.** Allergic reactions, including conjunctivitis or eyelid swelling, occur in ~10% of clients who take dorzolamide. If this occurs, the client should contact their provider and discontinue the use of the medication. The side effects listed for latanoprost, timolol, and brimonidine are all expected and harmless side effects.

    Client Need Category: Physiologic integrity

    Cognitive Level: Apply

3. **Ⓜ 1.** Benefits of the medication may take several days to develop and weeks for it to have its maximal effect. The medication can be given topically, usually prescribed as cromolyn 4% concentration, 1 to 2 drops per eye every 4 to 6 hours. The use of contact lenses should

be suspended during treatment with cromolyn, and eye irritation and tearing may occur as side effects while using the medication.

Client Need Category: Physiologic integrity

Cognitive Level: Analyze

4. **C 1, 3, 2, 4, 5.** The client should be taught to avoid touching the dropper tip against eye or any other part of the body as well as the correct procedure for administration. The correct procedure is to tilt the head back, pull down lower lid of the eye, and administer one eye drop while looking up. Keep the eye closed for up to 5 minutes to increase absorption and avoid blinking or squeezing eyes shut. In addition, compress the lacrimal sac for up to a minute to avoid systemic absorption. If more than one drop is prescribed, repeat the process, waiting at least 5 minutes between drops.

Client Need Category: Physiologic integrity

Cognitive Level: Analyze

5. **D 1.** Glucocorticoids are contraindicated for clients with a systemic fungal infection. A history of migraines, gout, or a concurrent diagnosis of otitis externa would not prevent the client from taking dexamethasone to treat uveitis.

Client Need Category: Physiologic integrity

Cognitive Level: Analyze

6. **C 3.** The American Academy of Pediatrics released a set of guidelines for treating acute otitis media in children in 2013. Per these guidelines, observation became a treatment option and is defined as the management via symptomatic relief for 2 to 3 days allowing of the acute otitis media to resolve on its own. If the symptoms not clear up or get worse, then antibiotic therapy is recommended, amoxicillin 40 mg/kg PO twice daily for 10 days, or if resistant strain with severe symptoms, ceftriaxone 50 mg/kg IM for 3 days. Other antibiotic options exist as well.

Client Need Category: Physiologic integrity

Cognitive Level: Apply

7. **D 190.5 mg.**

   Rationale

   $$1 \text{ kg} = 2.2 \text{ lbs} \quad \frac{1 \text{ kg} \times 56 \text{ lbs}}{2.2 \text{ lbs}} = 25.4 \text{ kg}$$

   $$\text{Dosage} \times \text{weight} = \text{Dose} \quad 7.5 \frac{\text{mg}}{\text{kg}} \times 25.4 \text{ kg} = 190.5 \text{ mg}$$

   Client Need Category: Physiologic integrity

   Cognitive Level: Analyze

8. **M 2.** Pain management is also recommended in the treatment plan for otitis media. Medications such as acetaminophen or ibuprofen are most commonly used; however, stronger pain medications can be prescribed if necessary. The American Academy of Pediatrics also recommends the use of topical anesthetic ear drops for pain relief in children over the age of 5 with an intact tympanic membrane. Many otitis media infections are viral in nature and will clear up on their own; antibiotics are not necessary for a cure in this case.

Client Need Category: Physiologic integrity

Cognitive Level: Apply

 E Easy   **M** Moderate   **D** Difficult   **C** Challenge

9. **E** **3.** Although the fluoroquinolone/glucocorticoid combination medication is expensive, the glucocorticoid reduces the swelling caused by the inflammation and decreases pain, while the fluoroquinolone treats the infection. Additionally, the glucocorticoid may increase the likelihood of antibiotic resistance developing to the fluoroquinolone. The glucocorticoid does not decrease the adverse effects of the fluoroquinolone, and the two medications can be prescribed together.

Client Need Category: Physiologic integrity

Cognitive Level: Analyze

10. **C** **4.** Since the client has diabetes mellitus, a contraindication to topical therapy, and multiple sclerosis, which may make it difficult to administer a topical medication properly, a fluoroquinolone given orally is the best option. The American Academy of Otolaryngology recommends topical treatment for uncomplicated otitis externa, as they are more effective and less antibiotic resistance is seen. Additionally, systemic side effects are avoided. However, there are contraindications to topical therapy, including clients with diabetes, immunodeficiencies, and individuals who would have difficulty administering topical medications properly. Systemic medications, such as oral fluoroquinolones, are recommended in these cases. Hydrocortisone/neomycin/polymyxin B combination solution is administered topically.

Client Need Category: Physiologic integrity

Cognitive Level: Apply

CHAPTER 15

1. **D** **2.** Allopurinol has the potential to result in a potentially fatal hypersensitivity reaction. Signs and symptoms include fever and rash. The medication should be stopped immediately, and the provider should be notified. While a temperature may also be indicative of infection, obtaining a CBC is not the priority if the client develops a fever while taking allopurinol. Administering acetaminophen may be a nursing action to treat the fever after holding the medication and notifying the provider. Reassessing the client in 30 minutes without intervention may lead to severe client harm or death if the client is having a hypersensitivity reaction to allopurinol.

Client Need Category: Physiologic integrity

Cognitive Level: Analyze

2. **C** **4.** Alendronate, a bisphosphonate medication, has the potential to cause esophagitis, which may present as indigestion, trouble swallowing, or reflux. Without identification and intervention, this may lead to esophageal ulceration or rupture. Although aspirin and prednisone also have side effects that include gastric distress and ulceration, the risk of esophagitis from alendronate would be the nurse's greatest concern. Allopurinol is not associated with indigestion.

Client Need Category: Physiologic integrity

Cognitive Level: Apply

3. **E** **1, 3.** A positive tuberculin skin test may indicate tuberculosis. Etanercept administered to a client with tuberculosis may result in disseminated disease, which may be fatal.

E Easy   **M** Moderate   **D** Difficult   **C** Challenge

Bilateral crackles may be indicative of heart failure, which may worsen while taking etanercept. If a client screens positive for tuberculosis, etanercept should not be administered. The risks and benefits should be considered, and the medication should be used with caution. Etanercept increases the risk of bleeding, not clot formation or unilateral edema. Etanercept does not cause changes in gastric motility. Etanercept can cause increase or decrease in white blood cell count, but platelet counts are not affected by this medication.

Client Need Category: Physiologic integrity

Cognitive Level: Analyze

4. **C** **3.** During acute illness, clients on chronic glucocorticoids should increase their dose. Chronic glucocorticoid use depresses adrenal activity, which results in an inability of the adrenal glands to exert a stress response during illness. Increasing the dose of prednisone will counteract the adrenal suppression caused by chronic glucocorticoid use. Stopping or decreasing the dose or leaving the dose of prednisone unchanged will impair the client's ability to build an appropriate stress response and may result in severe hypotension that is potentially fatal.

Client Need Category: Physiologic integrity

Cognitive Level: Analyze

5. **C** **1, 3, 5.** Methotrexate may result in liver and kidney injury. Baseline and periodic evaluations of kidney function via creatinine and aspartate aminotransferase are required. Methotrexate is pregnancy category X; a negative pregnancy test is required prior to starting treatment due to the risk of fetal harm and death. Methotrexate is not used to treat gout and has no impact on uric acid levels. Electrolyte levels are not affected by methotrexate.

Client Need Category: Physiologic integrity

Cognitive Level: Apply

6. **D** **3.** Raloxifene increases the risk of clotting; the risk of deep vein thrombosis, pulmonary embolism, and stroke are increased. Easy bruising may indicate decreased clotting that is not associated with raloxifene. Unlike estrogen, which increases the risk of breast cancer, raloxifene decreases the risk of certain breast cancers. Blood-tinged sputum may be indicative of a possible pulmonary embolus, which requires immediate intervention. Paresthesias and pain of the lower extremities require intervention; however, this is not the priority and is not associated with raloxifene.

Client Need Category: Physiologic integrity

Cognitive Level: Analyze

7. **C** **3, 4, 5.** Prednisone is a glucocorticoid that decreases inflammation during an acute gout flare. Naproxen and indomethacin are both nonsteroidal anti-inflammatory drugs that decrease pain and inflammation during an acute gout flare. Allopurinol is approved for the prevention of gout flares; it will not treat an existing flare. Acetaminophen is not approved for the treatment of gout. Although it is a pain reliever, it does not have any anti-inflammatory properties and would not be effective in treating the inflammation associated with a gout flare.

Client Need Category: Physiologic integrity

Cognitive Level: Apply

E Easy   **M** Moderate   **D** Difficult   **C** Challenge

8. **E** **1.2 mL.**
   Use the formula: D/H × Q (where D = desired dose, H = amount on hand, and Q = quantity) = 30/200 × 8 = 1.2 mL
   Client Need Category: Physiologic integrity
   Cognitive Level: Apply

9. **C** **2, 4, 5.** Toxicity occurring secondary to calcium citrate and vitamin D is due to hyper-calcemia. Signs of hypercalcemia include constipation (not diarrhea), hypertension (not hypotension), flank pain due to calcium deposits in the kidney, anxiety, depression, memory loss, and bone pain.
   Client Need Category: Physiologic integrity
   Cognitive Level: Apply

10. **D** **3.** Misoprostol is a prostaglandin analog that aids in the protection of gastrointes-tinal mucosa in clients at risk of nonsteroidal anti-inflammatory drug–induced ulcers. Misoprostol does not enhance effectiveness of aspirin and has no role in treating joint stiffness. The use of the two medications together is for gastric protection from chronic aspirin use and is not a prescribing error.
    Client Need Category: Physiologic integrity
    Cognitive Level: Analyze

CHAPTER 16

1. **C** **2.** With opioid use, constipation is expected. A bowel regimen should be started pro-phylactically along with opioid use. The other answers are correct.
   Client Need Category: Physiologic integrity
   Cognitive Level: Apply

2. **M** **3.** The pain that this client is describing is classic neuropathic pain. The fact that the client has spinal metastasis is more evidence of this. Opioids and ibuprofen do not fully address neuropathic pain.
   Client Need Category: Physiologic integrity
   Cognitive Level: Apply

3. **E** **4.** Gastric distress and bleeding are side effects of NSAIDs. The darker stools indicate that this client is having gastrointestinal bleeding, which needs to be addressed right away as a circulation issue. Headache is a normal side effect and still feeling some degree of pain is also normal. Eating more than usual is not necessarily a negative finding and not a typical symptom of NSAIDs.
   Client Need Category: Pharmacologic and parenteral therapies
   Cognitive Level: Analyze

4. **C** **1, 2, 4.** The client needs to be placed upright in order to be able to breathe more effectively. Anxiety is a common symptom with dyspnea and can exacerbate dyspnea, so should be treated. Opioids decrease the sensation of breathlessness. When giving anx-

E Easy   **M** Moderate   **D** Difficult   **C** Challenge

iolytics and opioids, care should be taken to give the anxiolytic, wait and reassess effect. If the dyspnea is worse, then the ordered opioid can be given. High flow oxygen may decrease respiratory drive in COPD clients and is not suggested. Reverse Trendelenburg would not be effective in helping the client breathe.

Client Need Category: Physiologic Adaptation

Cognitive Level: Apply

5. **E 1.** The client with diffuse wheezing, accessory muscle use, and high respiratory rate appears to be in respiratory distress. The client with bilateral crackles has heart failure, but the symptoms do not suggest respiratory distress. The client with the increased respiratory rate appears to be hyperventilating with anxiety. The client with emphysema has a higher rate of breathing, which is an expected finding with this medical condition.

Client Need Category: Management of Care

Cognitive Level: Analyze

6. **C 2, 4.** This client is in heart failure with pulmonary edema. Morphine will decrease dyspnea and lower respiratory rate, and furosemide, a diuretic, will address the fluid overload. Prednisone and bronchodilators would be used for a chronic obstructive pulmonary disease (COPD) exacerbation. Scopolamine is used for upper airway congestion.

Client Need Category: Pharmacologic and parenteral therapies

Cognitive Level: Apply

7. **C 3.** Before treating delirium with neuroleptics, the reversible causes need to be assessed first. Pain is not the only cause of delirium. Because the condition came on suddenly, it would not be dementia, which is progressive.

Client Need Category: Reduction of risk potential

Cognitive Level: Analyze

8. **E 1.** Tardive dyskinesia is a potentially irreversible side effect of haloperidol that presents with lip smacking and grimacing. These findings do not indicate a worsening of the hospice client's condition. Grimacing may indicate discomfort or pain, however, in the setting of lip smacking that is not the most likely cause of this finding. While the health care provider can be contacted to discuss questions the client's family may have, the nurse can answer this question regarding the side effects of medication administration. Increasing the dose of the haloperidol will not alleviate the side effect and may result in toxicity of the medication.

Client Need Category: Pharmacologic and parenteral therapies

Cognitive Level: Apply

9. **C 1.** Stevens-Johnson syndrome causes a red, blistering skin rash that is a medical emergency. While the other assessment findings are abnormal, they may represent common side effects of the medication. Decreased blood pressure, increased heart rate, and anticholinergic effects, such as urinary retention, are potential side effects of quetiapine. The nurse would need to assess for additional symptoms associated with each assessment finding to determine if they require additional assessment; however, the red blistering rash that may indicate Stevens-Johnson syndrome is the priority.

Client Need Category: Pharmacologic and parenteral therapies

Cognitive Level: Analyze

E Easy   **M** Moderate   **D** Difficult   **C** Challenge

10. **C 2.** The assessment suggests that the client has nausea and vomiting due to delayed gastric emptying time, or partial bowel obstruction, which only metoclopramide addresses.

    Client Need Category: Pharmacologic and parenteral therapies

    Cognitive Level: Apply

11. **E 2.** Appetite stimulants are short-term medications to improve appetite. They do not necessarily get the client back to baseline weight and should be stopped if there is no effect within 4 to 6 weeks. Addiction is not a reason to avoid these medications in pallia-tive care.

    Client Need Category: Pharmacologic and parenteral therapies

    Cognitive Level: Apply

12. **C 3.** The client has not had a bowel movement for 4 days. Increasing fiber and fluid and administering sennosides and docusate sodium will not help at this point. The priority is to check for fecal impaction, especially since the client reports a small amount of liquid stool, often found with impaction. If the client is not impacted, an enema would be the next step.

    Client Need Category: Basic Care and Comfort

    Cognitive Level: Analyze

13. **D 2, 3, 4.** With opioids, constipation is very likely, so a prophylactic bowel regimen should be started. Fluids can help with constipation. Immobility is also a cause of constipation, especially with clients who are bedbound or have limited mobility. Taking suppositories every day builds up a dependency. Bulk-forming agents are not suggested for palliative care clients, as they can worsen constipation and cause dehydration.

    Client Need Category: Pharmacologic and parenteral therapies

    Cognitive Level: Apply

14. **E 1.** The client is displaying the hallmark signs of anxiety, such as restlessness, lack of attention, hyperventilation, and pacing. This is supported by the fact that the client's terminal diagnosis is new. Psychosis does not typically come on suddenly, and the client does not have signs of delirium or nausea. Terminal agitation occurs late in the disease process and presents as altered mental status, rapid shallow breathing, pain, and the inability to eat or drink and is a precursor of near-death.

    Client Need Category: Psychosocial integrity

    Cognitive Level: Apply

15. **C 2.** Anxiety can produce symptoms of nausea and vomiting. As the client history sug-gests, holidays and isolation seem to be the driving factors for the emergency department visits, suggesting that the cause of the nausea/vomiting is anxiety based. None of the other choices address the underlying anxiety.

    Client Need Category: Pharmacologic and parenteral therapies

    Cognitive Level: Apply

E Easy   **M** Moderate   **D** Difficult   **C** Challenge

CHAPTER 17

1. **E** **2.** It is critical that the client see his/her provider to rule out other possible causes of increased urinary frequency. In addition, it is essential that the provider be aware of any medications the client is taking, including herbal remedies beside saw palmetto. Saw palmetto has not been banned by the FDA; it is tolerated well by most users and only causes mild side effects, like GI distress or headache. Research to date does not show that the use of saw palmetto affects PSA levels at all. Finally, saw palmetto may cause a decreased sexual drive in male clients; however, the best response is that it is crucial that the client see his provider to rule out any other possible causes of increased urinary frequency.
    Client Need Category: Physiologic integrity
    Cognitive Level: Apply

2. **E** **3.** The use of SSRI antidepressants and St. John's wort is contraindicated due to an increased risk of serotonin-related side effects, which can be very serious. There are many medications that need to be used with caution while taking St. John's wort as the herbal remedy can weaken the effects of the medication, including birth control pills, cyclosporine, digoxin, warfarin, and some HIV drugs. However, there is currently no known interaction with methylphenidate. Neither older adult clients nor clients of childbearing age are excluded from using St. John's wort, although clients should ensure that their provider is aware that they are taking St. John's wort as birth control pills are contraindicated. Caution should be used with clients with an increased risk for falls, because dizziness and fatigue are known side effects.
    Client Need Category: Physiologic integrity
    Cognitive Level: Apply

3. **D** **4.** The US Food and Drug Administration released a statement in 2002 with a warning of a risk of liver damage associated with the use of kava. Providers should be alert for signs and symptoms associated with liver damage including yellowing of the skin and sclera of the eyes, abdominal pain, pruritus, dark urine color, and loss of appetite. Use of kava has also been associated with dry, scaly skin, heart problems, eye irritation, and hypertension. Although a headache may be an early symptom associated with hypertension, the risk of liver damage is a more immediate concern. Skin rash and a loss of peripheral vision are not directly associated with kava use.
    Client Need Category: Physiologic integrity
    Cognitive Level: Apply

4. **C** **2.** The use of milk thistle may result in an allergic reaction, an effect more common in those individuals with an allergy to plants such as ragweed, chrysanthemum, marigold, and/or daisy. A history of gout, anemia, or gallstones does not contraindicate the use of milk thistle. In fact, milk thistle may help those being treated for Cooley anemia and gallstones.
    Client Need Category: Physiologic integrity
    Cognitive Level: Apply

 Easy    Moderate   Difficult   **C** Challenge

5. **E 3 capsules.**

Total dose at 0800 = 300 mg

Capsule size = 100 mg

$$\frac{300}{100} = 3 \text{ capsules}$$

Client Need Category: Physiologic integrity

Cognitive Level: Apply

6. **M 1.** Some individuals experience mouth sores and irritation when chewing fresh leaves. In addition, skin irritation may occur with handling of the plant. Clients should be instructed to use gloves when handling and not ingest the raw leaves if they experience such adverse reactions. Raw leaves do not need to be boiled before use, and the leaves, flowers, and stems, but not the roots, are all active parts of the plant. Feverfew does not need to be grown in a lab environment, planting in one's garden can be beneficial as well.

Client Need Category: Physiologic integrity

Cognitive Level: Analyze

7. **C 2.** In 1994, the Dietary Supplement Health and Education Act (DSHEA) was created and defined herbal remedies as dietary supplements. Herbal remedies are not treated in the same way as other medications and are not subjected to the same rigorous testing for safety and efficacy. Manufacturers do not have to seek FDA approval before selling dietary supplements. However, use of herbal remedies can be done both with provider input and following the FDA guidelines. The FDA has put several measures into place to help improve the quality and safety of herbal remedies including DSHEA, which gave the FDA the authority to take any product that poses a significant risk to the public off the market, helping in some part to ensure client safety. In 2006, the Dietary Supplement and Nonprescription Drug Consumer Protection Act was passed mandating the reporting of serious adverse reactions for dietary supplements and nonprescription drugs, and in 2007, the FDA ruled that standardized manufacturing and labeling of dietary supplements must occur, along with quality control procedures clearly outlined.

Client Need Category: Physiologic integrity

Cognitive Level: Apply

8. **E 2.** Herbal remedies can interact with traditional medications and can cause significantly harmful results. An accurate and complete client chart is important; however, it is not the priority, or best response. Herbal remedy bottle labels do not have to list interactions with traditional medications, in many cases because reliable information is not yet known or studied. The Dietary Supplement and Nonprescription Consumer Protection Act only mandates the reporting of a serious adverse event that occurs while a client is taking a nonprescription drug or herbal remedy, not all interactions. It is important for a provider to report a serious adverse event if one occurs, which is why it is essential to keep a provider informed of any herbal remedies being taken.

Client Need Category: Physiologic integrity

Cognitive Level: Apply

E Easy   **M** Moderate   **D** Difficult   **C** Challenge

9. **D 3.** Ma huang, or ephedra, was banned by FDA for sale in all US markets in 2004 due to elevated risk for cardiovascular complications and stroke. The use of this herbal remedy should be avoided for all individuals. The herbal remedy was taken to help with weight loss and the herbal remedy should not be taken. Clients who used this herbal remedy in the past were told to avoid caffeine, use should be avoided since ban in 2004. Ma huang can still be purchased overseas; however, this is not the best answer as the nurse should ensure that the client is aware that it has been banned for sale in the United States since 2004 and not recommend its use.

Client Need Category: Physiologic integrity

Cognitive Level: Apply

10. **M 4.** The restriction posed on the labeling of herbal remedies states that the products must be labeled as dietary supplements and cannot make any claim stating that the remedy can treat, diagnose, cure, or prevent any disease. However, a label CAN state that the remedy is able to influence a body's structure or function, such as supporting the respiratory system. Therefore, claims such as "reduces risk of cancer," "eliminates pain associated with rheumatoid arthritis," and "decreases symptoms of menopause" cannot be used.

Client Need Category: Physiologic integrity

Cognitive Level: Apply

 Easy  Moderate   Difficult **C** Challenge

INDEX

Note: Page number followed by f and t indicates figure and table respectively.